Spirituality and psychiatry

Spirituality and psychiatry

Edited by Chris Cook,
Andrew Powell and Andrew Sims

RCPsych Publications

RCPsych Publications is an imprint of the Royal College of Psychiatrists,
17 Belgrave Square, London SW1X 8PG
http://www.rcpsych.ac.uk

British Library Cataloguing-in-Publication Data.
A catalogue record for this book is available from the British Library.
ISBN 978 1 904671 71 8

Distributed in North America by Publishers Storage and Shipping Company.

Printed by Bell & Bain Limited, Glasgow, UK.

Contents

Contributors

Imran Ali Consultant in General Adult Psychiatry, Greater Manchester West Mental Health NHS Foundation Trust, Salford Directorate, UK

Cherrie Coghlan Consultant in General Adult Psychiatry, in private practice at Cygnet Hospital Harrow, UK

Christopher C. H. Cook Professorial Research Fellow, Department of Theology and Religion, Durham University, Tutor in Pastoral Studies, Cranmer Hall, St John's College, Durham, and Consultant in Substance Misuse, Tees, Esk and Wear Valleys NHS Foundation Trust, UK

Nicki Crowley Consultant Psychiatrist for Adults of Working Age, Oxfordshire and Buckinghamshire Mental Health NHS Foundation Trust, UK

Larry Culliford Former Consultant Psychiatrist, Brighton and Sussex University Hospitals NHS Trust, Chair of the Thomas Merton Society of Great Britain and Ireland, UK

Sarah Eagger Honorary Clinical Senior Lecturer, Department of Psychological Medicine, Imperial College London, and Consultant Psychiatrist for Older Adults, Central and North West London NHS Foundation Trust, UK

Peter Fenwick Emeritus Consultant in Neuropsychiatry, South London and Maudsley NHS Foundation Trust, Honorary Senior Lecturer in Neuropsychiatry, Institute of Psychiatry, King's College London, and Southampton University, and Consultant Clinical Neurophysiologist, Broadmoor Special Hospital, North London NHS Trust, UK

John Foskett Emeritus Chaplain, South London and Maudsley NHS Foundation Trust, Adviser in Religion and Spirituality, Somerset Partnership NHS Foundation Trust, President of the Association for Pastoral and Spiritual Care and Counselling, and President of the British and Irish Association for Practical Theology, UK

Peter Gilbert Professor of Social Work and Spirituality, Staffordshire University, NIMHE Project Lead on Spirituality and Mental Health, Chair of the National Development Team, and Visiting Professor, Birmingham and Solihull Mental Health Foundation Trust and the University of Worcester, UK

Julia H. Head Specialist Chaplain, Bishop John Robinson Fellow in Pastoral Theology and Mental Health, Joint Team Leader, South London and Maudsley NHS Foundation Trust, and Visiting Lecturer, Heythrop College, University of London, UK

Sheila Hollins Past-President of the Royal College of Psychiatrists, Professor of Psychiatry of Learning Disability at St George's, University of London, UK

Gillie Jenkinson Accredited psychotherapist with UK Council for Psychotherapy and Director of Hope Valley Counselling, UK

Robert M. Lawrence Consultant in Old Age Psychiatry, Honorary Senior Lecturer, South West London and St George's Mental Health NHS Trust and St George's University of London, UK

Christopher MacKenna Anglican priest and a Senior Member of the Jungian Analytic Section of the British Association of Psychotherapists, Director of the St Marylebone Healing and Counselling Centre, London, and Chaplain, Guild of Health, UK

Susan Mitchell former Consultant Psychiatrist in Rehabilitation, and Medical Director at The Retreat, York, UK

Andrew Powell Founding Chair, Spirituality and Psychiatry Special Interest Group, Royal College of Psychiatrists, former Consultant Psychotherapist and Senior Lecturer, St George's Hospital and Medical School London, and the Warneford Hospital and University of Oxford, UK

Oyepeju Raji Consultant Psychiatrist in Learning Disabilities, South West London and St George's Mental Health NHS Trust, London, UK

Tim Read Consultant Psychiatrist, and Honorary Senior Lecturer, Royal London Hospital, UK

Peter Richmond Area Lead Chaplain, Kent and Medway NHS and Social Care Partnership Trust, UK

Glenn Roberts Consultant Psychiatrist in Rehabilitation and Recovery, Devon Partnership NHS Trust, and Lead on Recovery for the Royal College of Psychiatrists, UK

Mohamed Omar Salem Assistant Professor, Department of Psychiatry, Faculty of Medicine and Health Sciences, United Arab Emirates University, UAE

Mike Shooter Past-President of the Royal College of Psychiatrists, Chair of YoungMinds, the Mental Health Foundation, and Children-in-Wales, and Vice-President of the British Association of Counselling and Psychotherapy, UK

Andrew Sims Emeritus Professor of Psychiatry, University of Leeds, and Past-President of the Royal College of Psychiatrists, UK

Tables, boxes and figures

Foreword

During my presidency I became more and more convinced of the importance of promoting mental health and well-being, alongside the treatment of mental illness. But I see mental health as the responsibility of everyone, not just health and mental health professionals. The social care, criminal justice and education sectors and faith-based organisations should all be involved in asserting the centrality of mental health in society, in contributing to the prevention of mental illness and in supporting individuals with mental disorders.

The World Health Organization report in 2004 estimated that 40–50% of mental illness could be prevented through primary intervention. Meanwhile, the World Bank has recognised the contribution of social capital (the extent to which people help each other) to the wealth and well-being of a country (Dasgupta & Serageldin, 2005). The contribution of mutual trust, wilful reciprocity of help and participation in civic society are described as three particular markers of social capital. When social capital is high, individual coping capacity increases, but when it is low, crime rates, divorce and family violence increase.

As psychiatrists we work with people with serious mental disorders, many of whom may have lost meaning and purpose in their lives. Each person's journey of recovery will seek to find new meaning and purpose, hopefully supported by friends and family who have shared values (Care Services Improvement Partnership et al, 2007). Spirituality, defined in this book in part as being 'concerned with matters of meaning and purpose in life, truth and values' is clearly relevant. This sharing of values and belief systems with other members of one's community and achieving a personal equilibrium seem intuitively likely to improve one's coping capacity.

I welcome this book that brings together so many excellent explorations of the difficult to measure construct of spirituality, which is yet rated by service users as a fundamental marker of a good mental health service.

I believe that acquiring the understanding and skills needed to allow our patients to express and explore their own spirituality in relation to their well-being is fundamental. However, many students and practitioners will have had little or no training in how to enquire about an individual's spirituality or religious faith. The absence of spirituality in the curriculum must be addressed by educators.

You, the reader, will be the judge of whether the editors have achieved their aim to write a textbook of psychiatry that approaches the field from a new perspective – that of integrating spirituality into traditional theoretical and service models of mental health and mental illness.

References

Care Services Improvement Partnership, Royal College of Psychiatrists & Social Care Institute for Excellence (2007) *A Common Purpose: Recovery in Future Mental Health Services, Joint Position Paper*. Social Care Institute for Excellence.

Dasgupta, P. & Serageldin, I. (2005) *Social Capital: a Multifaceted Approach*. vol. 1. Oxford University Press.

World Health Organization (2004) *Prevention of Mental Disorders: Effective Interventions and Policy Options. Summary Report*. World Health Organization.

Sheila Hollins
Past-President, Royal College of Psychiatrists

Preface

What kind of book is this and what is it about? Spirituality is not easily defined. Although many perceive it as very important, its controversial nature has led to it being defined in diverse ways. The definition that we have taken, with a view to inclusiveness, is concerned with human experience of relationship, meaning and purpose. This includes a transcendent, or transpersonal, dimension of experience that has traditionally been regarded as being more the domain of religion and theology than psychiatry. But it also encompasses experiences that are very familiar to psychiatry – life within family and society that have usually been viewed in a secular and non-spiritual sense. Such experiences have generally been taken as reflecting personal or interpersonal dynamics, emotions, cognitions and beliefs, which obey the 'laws' of sciences such as psychology, sociology and neurobiology. Immediately, then, this book raises the question of why anything more than science should be necessary. Cannot 'spirituality', whatever it is, be reduced to scientific discourse, a matter of objective consideration without any transcendent or transpersonal dimension?

As will become apparent, the contributors to this book have various implicit or explicit responses to this question. First, that there is a growing body of research supporting the importance of spirituality as an independent and dependent variable of some significance, arguably not reducible to a purely bio-psychosocial level. For some issues approached in this book, such as those on substance misuse, neuroscience and old age psychiatry, the body of research of this kind is already quite considerable. For others, however, such as child psychiatry, learning disability psychiatry and the transpersonal perspective, research is still in its infancy.

Second, there are the voices of service users who assert that spirituality is a dimension of their experience that they wish to be able to discuss without it being labelled in pathological terms. The book contains many examples of this kind drawn from clinical practice. In chapter 3, for instance, we find the story of Julie (case study 3.5), whose therapist apparently failed to understand that thoughts as well as actions can be understood as culpable. Such a notion is familiar to philosophers, theologians and priests, but is easily misunderstood phenomenologically by psychiatrists as magical thinking or delusion. Further, in chapter 5, we encounter Liam, whose physical illness led him to a profoundly spiritual reflection upon his life; a story that does not have a happy ending. This could have all too easily been misunderstood by his family or by professionals seeking to help him as evidence of affective disorder, but the spiritual perspective reminds us that 'negotiating terms' with pain and suffering is a universal and primarily spiritual task for human beings, which offers evidence of spiritual health, not psychopathology.

A third answer to our question arises from the experiences of the authors and other members of the Royal College of Psychiatrists' Spirituality and Psychiatry Special Interest Group, who have found that their reflections upon clinical practice are not complete within the bio-psychosocial mode of thought. In chapter 2, Larry Culliford and Sarah Eagger, quoting David Hay, argue that spirituality has supraordinate and integrating significance in the proper assessment of patients. In chapter 3, Susan Mitchell and Glenn Roberts remind us that working with patients who have psychosis can be deeply challenging for professionals, whose own spirituality offers a potentially sustaining resource – hope. Again, in chapter 6, Andrew Powell and Chris MacKenna remind us that spirituality – that of the therapist as well as that of the patient – is an aspect of the therapeutic alliance that is easily neglected, yet holds great power for good.

This book is, then, at least in part a response to the questions posed by researchers, service users and clinicians, concerning the importance of spirituality as a 'fourth dimension' of mental healthcare. But if it is a book that argues for the importance of this fourth dimension and warns of the pitfalls of neglecting spirituality in both research and clinical practice, what kind of book is it? Is it primarily a textbook offering guidance for evidence-based practice, an academic book pushing at the frontiers of research or a handbook for clinicians seeking to describe new territories?

As originally conceived within the Spirituality and Psychiatry Special Interest Group Executive Committee, the book was intended to be a clinical textbook. We share a concern to positively influence clinical practice. Authors have therefore been encouraged to keep in mind the needs of the trainee preparing for postgraduate examinations in psychiatry and the clinical realities of psychiatric practice. Although they were urged to pay attention to the evidence base insofar as it offers support for their beliefs, they were not asked primarily to address methodological issues or chart current research controversies. We hope you will agree that they have endeavoured to address their remit. However, it also became clear to us when reviewing the authors' contributions that in fact this could not possibly be a textbook in the usual sense. Along with the contributors, we share the conviction of the importance of spirituality in mental healthcare, but we also have diverse perspectives about what exactly that means. Nor would it be reasonable to expect that a textbook on spirituality and psychiatry could be written in the same way as one on, say, psychopathology or substance misuse, or any other area of psychiatry.

This book offers perspectives from various subspecialties of psychiatry, as well as considering the generic task of assessment (chapter 2), the generic perspectives of neuroscience, the transpersonal paradigm, religion (chapters 9, 11 and 12 respectively), and issues of integrating spiritual care in service delivery (chapter 10). It also includes an important reminder (in chapter 13) that there is a 'dark side' to spirituality. However, the book does not attempt to cover systematically all psychiatric diagnoses in the way that a postgraduate textbook of psychiatry would be expected to do. Thus, there are important areas of omission. Notably, affective disorders, eating disorders and those disorders traditionally referred to as 'neuroses' have not received the attention that they might otherwise have had. Furthermore, within some subspecialties of psychiatry it was felt that too little work has been done to date to warrant devoting specific chapters to them; thus, forensic psychiatry and rehabilitation psychiatry are not represented here. We have felt these omissions keenly and hope that future publications will be able to remedy them.

There is, perhaps, another more important reason why this book is not a comprehensive textbook. The field of spirituality and psychiatry is currently at such a stage of development that this book must, of necessity, chart areas of research and promise for the future as much as it can say anything about what is agreed in relation to good clinical practice for the present. It will therefore pose more questions than offer answers and, in places, it will be provocative. For example, we do not expect all readers to find that they agree with Mike Shooter in his analysis of the case of Liam in chapter 5. Neither do we expect all readers to share the transpersonal perspective offered by Tim Read and Nicki Crowley in chapter 11, any more than we expect all readers to identify with one of the religious traditions described in chapter 12. However, we do share a concern that psychiatrists and other mental healthcare professionals should at least be familiar with the questions that are posed and the traditions and other explanatory frameworks that are described here. It is the joint task of exploring and reflecting upon such questions with patients and colleagues, valuing those traditions and frameworks of belief and seeking to integrate them with respect and sensitivity into a person's mental healthcare that is properly the spiritual concern of the good psychiatrist.

Christopher C. H. Cook
Andrew Powell
Andrew Sims

The Spirituality and Psychiatry
Special Interest Group
of the Royal College of Psychiatrists

This short account of the Spirituality and Psychiatry Special Interest Group (SIG) must start with sincere thanks to my fellow psychiatrists who have made the activities of the Group an inspiring contribution to the work of the Royal College of Psychiatrists. In particular, the members of our SIG Executive Committee continue to give unstintingly of their time and energy over and above the heavy demands of clinical work.

Further, our thanks must go to the College itself, which has generously assisted throughout, providing administrative support, website facilities and, not least, in commissioning the publication of this book.

We hope the book will attract the attention of a wide readership of mental health professionals, service users, carers, and spiritual advisors, indeed all who seek to understand the suffering that characterises mental disorder. The publication comes in the decennial of the inauguration of the Spirituality and Psychiatry SIG and it gives me the opportunity briefly to record how we began, the work we have undertaken so far, and some of the future developments we are keen to see taking place.

The idea of starting a spirituality interest group came to me as the culmination of many years of puzzling over the divide between spirituality and psychiatry. Historically, spiritual matters have tended to be viewed as being either outside the remit of mental healthcare or else coming to the attention of the clinician as a symptom of illness, religious delusions being just one such example. However, spirituality has not been seen as important to explore in relation to a person's core values and beliefs, although expressing a fundamental aspect of selfhood and personal identity.

Not so many years ago, it was felt intrusive to ask directly whether patients had suffered sexual abuse. Yet we now know that this area of enquiry, when handled with respect and sensitivity, is not only welcomed by our patients, but leads to a better understanding of problems that have arisen and of how to help the person concerned. This example might seem a far cry from asking our patients about their spiritual and religious beliefs and practices, yet psychiatrists have similarly hesitated to enquire about how such personal beliefs affect how our patients view themselves and their lives, what impact this might have on falling ill, be it contributory or protective, and how it may influence the kind of help a person needs.

Our psychiatric training is knowledge-based and primarily equips us to diagnose and treat. In addition, all trainees now learn psychotherapeutic skills, which might be thought to be sufficient to cover the subject of spirituality; however, we do not find it to be so. There is almost no teaching on spirituality and mental health in UK medical schools or at post-graduate level in the training of psychiatrists. It is hardly surprising, therefore, that many psychiatrists are apprehensive about discussing spiritual matters with their patients. We feel unskilled and unprepared for such a dialogue and worse still, we might even get asked whether we believe in God.

At the same time, disregarding spiritual concerns loses us a valuable opportunity to connect with our patients that has both empathic and diagnostic implications. We know from user surveys that up to a half of patients turn to their religious and spiritual beliefs to help get them through a crisis but that they do not feel comfortable talking about such things with the psychiatrist (Faulkner, 1997). The area of spirituality is certainly prone to communication failure – one patient, who happened to be an interfaith minister, told me how she had tried to talk with the admitting psychiatrist about the Holy Ghost, only to be asked in the ward round the next day if she was seeing ghosts!

It seemed, therefore, that a spirituality group for psychiatrists could encourage us to venture beyond the narrow limits of 'scientific realism' and to explore, without risk of censure, such things as: how to address this covert but serious communication gap that can arise between patient and psychiatrist; how better to distinguish mental illness from spiritual crisis, especially when archetypal spiritual/religious themes predominate; why it is that spirituality is largely ignored by mainstream psychotherapy; what parapsychology might bring to our understanding of the bereaved who experience the presence of deceased loved ones; and how to raise awareness of current research correlating spirituality and positive mental health, to name but a few.

In forming the Spirituality and Psychiatry SIG, one which would align psychiatry with its intended meaning of 'psyche' (soul) and 'iatros' (doctor), I was magnificently supported by a working group consisting of Drs Julian Candy, Larry Culliford, Peter Fenwick and Chris Holman, and Professor Andrew Sims. The proposal that we put forward to the College outlined the need for a special interest group that would provide a discussion forum (having no religious bias and respectful of differences) to explore, among other things: (1) fundamental concerns intrinsic to good mental healthcare such as the purpose and meaning of life, including the problem of good and evil; (2) the need for an integrative approach (mind/body/spirit); (3) specific experiences invested with spiritual meaning, including birth, death and near-death, mystical and trance states, 'paranormal' phenomena and the 'spiritual emergency'; (4) how to distinguish between normal and pathological religious/spiritual experiences in relation to mental health;

(5) how best to develop and provide educational input to the College for the training of psychiatrists, including a professional competencies curriculum based on knowledge, attitudes and skills; (6) the relationship between illness, health and spirituality, and the growing evidence base associating spirituality with positive mental health (the protective effect against depression and outcome research in the treatment of alcohol and substance misuse, to name just two).

We were delighted to find that the College supported the proposal, the required 120 signatures in support of the group were soon raised and the inaugural meeting of the Spirituality and Psychiatry SIG followed in September 1999. Since then, the membership of the group has grown to more than 2000 psychiatrists, around one in seven of College members.

The Spirituality and Psychiatry SIG website www.rcpsych.ac.uk/spirit is fully in the public domain, with regular publications of the newsletter giving details of programmes and talks. The wide range of programmes held at the College to date includes:

- 'What do we mean by spirituality and its relation to psychiatry?'
- 'Fear and faith – the quandary of the psyche under threat'
- 'Avenues to peace of mind'
- 'Forgiveness and reconciliation'
- 'Engaging the spiritual mind'
- 'The healing power of love'
- 'Good and evil – the challenge for psychiatry'
- 'Integrating mind and body: psycho-spiritual therapeutics'
- 'Pathways to peace – East meets West'
- 'Invited or not, God is here: spiritual aspects of the therapeutic encounter'
- 'Minds within minds: the case for spirit release therapy'
- 'Spiritual issues in child psychiatry'
- 'Prayer in the service of mental health'
- 'A fatal wound? Who and what does suicide destroy?'
- 'What inspires the psychiatrist? Personal beliefs, attitudes and values'
- 'Special needs, special gifts – learning disability and spirituality'
- 'Spirituality and religion in later life'
- 'Psychosis, psychedelics and the transpersonal Journey'
- 'Sanity, sex and the sacred: exploring intersecting realms'
- 'Suffering – what is the point of it all?'
- 'Body and spirit'
- 'Spirituality and psychopathology'
- 'Researching spirituality: paradigms and empirical findings'
- 'Mindfulness, meditation and mental health'
- 'Consciousness and the extended mind'

Public conferences have included 'The place of spirituality in psychiatry', 'Beyond death: does consciousness survive?' and 'Healing from within and beyond – the therapeutic power of altered states'.

Texts of papers given at all these programmes can be downloaded from the website publications archive. Additionally, we have links with other bodies such as the National Institute for Mental Health in England, the Scientific and Medical Network, the Dutch Foundation for Psychiatry and Religion, and the Psychiatry and Religion Section of the World Psychiatric Association. A milestone publication has been the leaflet 'Spirituality and Mental Health', approved by the College and available for download from the topic menu on the College website (RCPsych, 2006).

The Spirituality and Psychiatry SIG has consistently advocated a holistic approach – not 'either/or' but 'both/and'. Physical treatments, appropriately and thoughtfully given, especially for severe mental illness, can be life-saving, while psychological understanding is always essential. Yet, if mental illness is to hold the potential for growth through adversity, the wisdom of the soul can bring enormous benefit if only we clinicians are open to the spiritual concerns of our patients.

For psychiatry to serve humanity well, the golden rule 'Do to others as you would have them do to you' is hard to beat. Doctor and patient are in complementary roles – both need the other. Indeed, at heart we are far more alike than we are different, and as we meet on the path of life, there is one medicine constantly at our disposal that even comes free. This is the power of love, lending hope, giving comfort and helping bring peace to the troubled mind.

References

Faulkner, A. (1997) *Knowing Our Own Minds*. Mental Health Foundation.
Royal College of Psychiatrists (2006) *Spirituality and Mental Health*. http://www.rcpsych.ac.uk/mentalhealthinformation/therapies/spiritualityandmentalhealth.aspx

Andrew Powell

CHAPTER 1

Spirituality in psychiatry

Andrew Sims and Christopher C. H. Cook

Within British psychiatry, the notion of linking spirituality with psychiatry developed largely in the 21st century. What follows is the first attempt of the Spirituality and Psychiatry Special Interest Group of the Royal College of Psychiatrists to put their heads together, metaphorically and constructively, and produce a book representing both their diverse views and shared vision for better psychiatric practice. Is the result a manifesto or a shopfront, a confession of our differences or a statement of our common beliefs? We will leave those questions with the reader.

Our first intended readership is the mental health community, including service users and carers, voluntary helpers and mental health professionals of all disciplines in the UK and overseas. Our secondary readership, we would hope, would be all those others who are interested in and concerned with mental illness. We share a belief that an aspiration towards the common good of improved mental health and treatment of mental illness in our communities is a worthy one, and that it is worth striving to turn this into a reality.

Spirituality, including its psychological aspects, is relevant for all psychiatrists, not as an add-on to our already overcrowded curriculum but as an idea 'at the back of one's mind', sometimes coming further forward. It is not to be forgotten, permeating every part of psychiatry and forming the underlying worldview from which one practises. If the psychiatrist remembers to incorporate spiritual values into his or her clinical practice, he or she will need to ask the patient a few pertinent questions, thus taking a spiritual history that assesses needs in this area.

How has spirituality entered psychiatry?

Historically, much psychiatric care has been provided within a spiritual or religious context. In medieval Europe, the shrines of St Mathurin and St Acairius in France or St Dymphna in Flanders held a particular reputation for miraculous cures of people with mental illness. In 1247 the priory of St Mary of Bethlehem was founded in Kent, England, for the care of the insane.

Bethlehem Hospital, later known as Bedlam and now as Bethlem Royal Hospital, is the oldest hospital in the UK for people with mental illness. In the Middle Ages, what little care there was for physical diseases like leprosy was provided by religious houses. Thus, the scene was set for the treatment of mental illness also to develop in cooperation with the Church. The Spanish Renaissance philosopher, Juan Luis Vives, contemporary with Erasmus and Thomas More, gave considerable attention to the humane treatment of people with mental illness, recognising them as suffering from illness and treating them with respect, as human beings. However, Vives, like other Renaissance thinkers and later also Galileo, despite being a devout Christian, came into conflict with the monolithic and inflexible ecclesiastical establishment. This conflict between those regarding madness as illness and Church orthodoxy worsened with the era of witch hunts in the 15th, 16th and 17th centuries.

Sadly, Bethlehem Hospital later became the notorious Bedlam, but in response to the inhumanities that arose there and elsewhere, the so-called 'moral approach' to the care of the insane was to bring about a revolution in care for the mentally ill. In late 18th-century England, this movement was led by William Tuke, a Quaker, who established the Retreat at York for the humane care of people with mental disorders.

Psychiatry as a distinct discipline starts at the beginning of the 19th century. Philippe Pinel wrote in 1801:

> As one takes up mental alienation as a separate object of investigation, it would be making a bad choice indeed to start a vague discussion of the seat of reason and on the nature of its diverse aberrations; nothing is more obscure and impenetrable. But if one wisely confines one's self to the study of the distinctive characteristics which manifest themselves by outward signs and if one adopts as a principle only a consideration of the results of enlightened experience, only then does one enter a path which is generally followed by natural history [Pinel, reprinted 1941: pp. 187–188].

There were remarkable developments in brain localisation and neurohistology during the 19th century in Germany. Wilhelm Griesinger regarded 'mental illnesses' as 'illnesses of the nerves and brain' (1867). The contribution of German psychiatrists to psychiatry, neuropathology and especially to classification, was immense and many of these 19th-century German pioneers remain household names within medicine. However, at the interface of religion and psychiatry, these discoveries had encouraged an attitude of reductionism.

Meanwhile, French psychiatry had reached reductionism by a different route – complex behaviour was thought to occur as a result of unconscious mechanisms, ultimately influenced by the state of the brain. Jean-Martin Charcot's pupil, Pierre Janet, psychologist and neurologist, had established the beginnings of psychotherapy by the end of the 19th century. Religion and faith were not seen as necessary in the equation for explaining human activity.

In Britain, following Charles Darwin's *Origin of the Species* (published in 1859), the concepts of 'natural selection' and 'survival of the fittest' had profound consequences for the care of the mentally ill. In part this was due to the subsequent interest in 'somatology', which discounted everything about man, including his history and personality, that could not be shown to be clearly organic. Another negative influence on treatment arose from the hypothesis of 'degeneration': all psychiatric illness was considered to be inherited and to become more severe in later generations. This ushered in several decades of therapeutic nihilism in psychiatry in Britain and elsewhere, which inhibited the search for new, effective methods of treatment.

By the middle of the 20th century, with science dedicated to material realism and with the arrival of modernism in philosophy, reductionism had come to dominate medicine. Man was 'nothing but' an excessively cerebral erect ape; human behaviour was 'nothing but' Pavlovian conditional or Skinnerian operant conditioned responses. Sigmund Freud had asserted that belief in a single God was delusional and that all religion is a mass neurosis. Psychoanalysis was in conflict with traditional religious attitudes and many churches identified Freud, psychoanalysis and by association the whole of psychiatry, with atheism, antagonism to religion and a challenge to conventional morality.

By the 1960s, there was no sense that the patient's religious beliefs contributed significantly to the psychiatric history, formulation or planning of treatment, and spiritual aspects of the patient's mental health problem were usually ignored. In the standard British textbook of the time (*Clinical Psychiatry*, Mayer-Gross *et al*, first edition 1954, later editions in 1960 and 1969) there are only two references to religion in the index, and it is assumed to be for 'the hesitant, the guilt-ridden, the excessively timid, those lacking clear convictions with which to face life'. During the 1970s more practising Christians began to come into the specialty in the UK and there was also a considerable influx into psychiatry of those from other faiths, most of whom had qualified in medicine overseas. The Scientific and Medical Network was set up in 1974, encouraging the exploration of the interface between spirituality, consciousness and mind.

During the 1980s, like-minded people got together and discussed non-material, religious and spiritual issues. Psychiatrists with spiritual interests gained confidence in expressing their faith and working out the consequences for their professional practice. Religious belief was still not regarded as respectable by the rest of the profession but there was less animosity. The quiet progress of the 1970s and 1980s became more public in the 1990s – in 1991, the Patron of the Royal College of Psychiatrists, His Royal Highness the Prince of Wales, urged an approach to mental healthcare that encompassed body, mind and spirit. Successive presidents of the College (Professor Andrew Sims and Professor John Cox) took up the subject in their addresses at College meetings in 1993 and 2002; a series of conferences on religion and psychiatry was held at the Institute of Psychiatry in London. In 1994, the newly published revision of the *Diagnostic and Statistical Manual* of the American Psychiatric Association (DSM–IV) included for the first time a category of 'religious or spiritual problem'. In 1997, the Archbishop of Canterbury addressed a joint annual meeting of the Royal College of Psychiatrists and the Association of European Psychiatrists.

Attitudes of psychiatrists changed significantly and psychiatry, as a profession, has become more accepting of the spiritual and religious concerns of patients and more interested in the relationship between psychiatry and religion. Research in the area of mental illness and religious belief developed during the 1990s from almost none to an accepted area of enquiry with research funding. Correspondingly, publications on spirituality in the psychological and healthcare literature increased exponentially (Cook, 2004a). The setting up of the Spirituality and Psychiatry Special Interest Group within the Royal College of Psychiatrists at the beginning of the new millennium was the culmination of a half-century of hard-won progress.

What is spirituality?

Spirituality and religion have overlapping but distinctively different meanings that have changed in recent decades, particularly in the case of spirituality. There are many possible definitions of spirituality, but for this book and its specific relevance for psychiatry, we have provided the authors with the following working definition of spirituality as a starting point:

> Spirituality is a distinctive, potentially creative and universal dimension of human experience arising both within the inner subjective awareness of individuals and within communities, social groups and traditions. It may be experienced as relationship with that which is intimately 'inner', immanent and personal, within the self and others, and/or as relationship with that which is wholly 'other', transcendent and beyond the self. It is experienced as being of fundamental or ultimate importance and is thus concerned with matters of meaning and purpose in life, truth and values [Cook, 2004a: pp. 548–549].

This definition was developed from a study of the way in which the concept of spirituality is used in the literature on addiction and spirituality but it arguably applies equally well to other areas of psychiatry. It emphasises the universality of spirituality as a subjective dimension of the experience of being human, at the same time attempting to recognise that this is still, nonetheless, a socially situated phenomenon.

Religion is also susceptible to widely varying definitions – some emphasise the personal and others the social, some emphasise belief and others behaviour, some emphasise tradition and others function, and so on (Bowker, 1997: p. xv). The word religion has the same root as ligament, ligature and oblige. It is that grounding of faith and basis of life to which one regards oneself as being bound for one's survival, a rope that ties one to God[1] and to other believers. For our purpose, it might be helpful to emphasise that religion is concerned with socially and traditionally shared beliefs and experience, but in placing this emphasis we must not lose sight of its personal and subjective dimension.

The word religion does not feature in the indices of most psychiatric textbooks. When referred to at all in hospital, it usually alludes to which denomination, if any, is favoured by the patient, like one's preferred supermarket. In everyday conversation, spirituality might be perceived as more inclusive of the large number of people in our society who profess no traditional religious affiliation. However, unlike religion, spirituality *per se* does not confer the support of a like-minded faith community that can offer social help and encouragement during life crises. The position, at least in the UK, is that when discussing such issues within the medical profession, the word spiritual may be preferable; the word religious carries too much historical baggage. Moreover, religion, despite the majority of believers of all creeds living peacefully, has recently yet again become associated with fanaticism and violence.

For research purposes, it has not proved possible to separate distinct factors of spirituality from religion in patient populations and so most studies are concerned with religious groups and their particular characteristics.

Before returning to our theme of the relationship between spirituality and psychiatry, it is important to give attention to one further concept of relevance to spirituality, religion and psychiatry – mysticism. Mysticism and mystical experience are touched upon in several chapters of this book, and such experiences can be easily misdiagnosed as psychiatric disorders (Cook, 2004b). Mysticism might be considered as a particular, perhaps extreme, manifestation of spirituality. However, it is also frequently (although not always) understood within a religious context. Like spirituality, it is receptive of diverse definitions.

In his *Gifford Lectures* (1901–1902), William James proposed four 'marks' of mystical experience: ineffability, noetic quality, transiency and passivity (James, 1902, reprinted 1985). In common with others, he understood mystical experience as being concerned with relationship with a transcendent, or 'ultimate', reality. This relationship has sometimes been understood in a very individualistic way, emphasising the personal and subjective nature of the experience, but in fact mysticism is concerned with experiences of the relationship of an individual with both a transcendent reality and a community (often, but not always, a community of faith). Stace (1973) has further suggested that mystical states may be 'introvertive' (looking inwards, into the mind) or 'extrovertive' (looking outwards), but he concludes that both types of mystical states are expressions of a fundamental experience of the unity of all things.

---

1   We are mindful, however, that Buddhism traditionally does not assert the existence of God and that religion therefore does not necessarily entail belief in God.

A coalition of like-minded psychiatrists

The Spirituality and Psychiatry Special Interest Group was inaugurated on the cusp of the millennium. Why was it worth instituting and what has it set out to achieve? The Group answers:

> The Special Interest Group was founded in 1999 to provide a forum for psychiatrists to explore the influence of the major religions, which shape the cultural values and aspirations of psychiatrist and patient alike. The spiritual aspirations of persons not identifying with any one particular faith are held to be of no less importance, as well as the viewpoint of those who hold that spirituality is independent of religion. The meetings are designed to enable colleagues to investigate and share without fear of censure the relevance of spirituality to clinical practice. The Special Interest Group aims to contribute a framework of ideas of general interest to the College, stimulating discussion and promoting an integrative approach to mental healthcare. For patients, there is the need to help the service user feel supported in being able to bring spiritual concerns to the fore (www.rcpsych.ac.uk/college/specialinterestgroups/spirituality.aspx).

From its inception, the Spirituality and Psychiatry Special Interest Group has been a coalition of like-minded people, coming from different religious, spiritual and cultural backgrounds but with a shared aspiration. We hold in common a conviction that 'spirituality', whatever it may precisely mean, is immensely important and requires due consideration for patients and ourselves; it should permeate almost every area of psychiatric practice. It has been important to accept, respect and learn from our differences and never to devalue each other. Admittedly, 'Religion can be a source of discord. It can also be a form of conflict resolution ... we need to search – each faith in its own way – for a way of living with, and acknowledging the integrity of, those who are not of our faith' (Sacks, 2002).

This diversity of interest and background is shown in the very wide range of topics discussed at the first 20 Spirituality and Psychiatry Special Interest Group one-day programmes (see p. xvii).

Spirituality of patients

As over two-thirds of the UK population have a stated religion, the notion that UK society is secular is clearly incorrect; the UK is, indeed, a multi-faith society but for 93% of those with a stated religion this is Christianity (Table 1.1).

In contrast with the general population, only a minority of psychiatrists in Britain hold religious beliefs: 73% of psychiatrists reported no religious affiliation as compared with 38% of their patients, and 78% attended religious services less than once a month (Neeleman & King, 1993). Only 39% of female and 19% of male psychiatrists believed in God. However, 92% of psychiatrists in Britain believed that religion and mental illness were connected and that religious issues should be addressed in treatment; 42%

Table 1.1 Religious affiliation of the UK population (Office for National Statistics, 2001)

Denomination	Followers, n (thousands)	%
Christian	42079	71.6
Muslim	1591	2.7
Hindu	559	1.0
Sikh	336	0.6
Jewish	267	0.5
Buddhist	152	0.3
Other religions	179	0.3
All religions	45163	76.8
No religion	9104	15.5
Not stated	4289	7.3
No religion/not stated	13626	23.2
Total	58789	100

considered that religiousness could lead to mental illness, but 58% never made referrals to clergy. There is, therefore, a marked disparity between patients and their psychiatrists in terms of their religious belief and its implications for daily life.

It is unlikely that a psychiatrist will share his or her culture and religion completely with any individual patient. This can be beneficial to the patient, as the relationship will be less influenced by unconscious pressures. This is true not only where the patient comes from a minority ethnic and religious group and is treated by a White, British born and trained psychiatrist. The majority Christian religious group is not a single community but comprises many subgroups with quite extreme differences, especially in religious expression. Take, for example, the difference between a suburban London Pentecostal church and its members and a rural, village community clustered around its parish church. It follows that the psychiatrist who aspires to be sensitive about spirituality and religion also needs to be aware of culture differences.

Psychiatrists also need to be sensitive about genre, defined as the way language is organised to achieve social processes.

> Just as the genre of a mystery story has components of introduction of characters, inciting event, search for clues and the villain, discovery of villain, denouement, etc., so the genre that accomplishes a social process (e.g. a casual conversation that continues and solidifies a friendship) may have elements such as *greeting, approach to neutral topics like weather, approach to a substantive topic (why we are having this meeting), leave taking* [emphasis ours]. Such elements establish a schematic structure that speakers are expected to be familiar with [Fine, 2006: p. 307].

7

The importance of genre, in addition to culture, in any exchange between patient and doctor concerning belief, faith and spirituality cannot be overemphasised.

Religion is a protective factor from and in mental illness. The work demonstrating this is drawn together in the *Handbook of Religion and Health* (Koenig *et al*, 2001). This cites 1200 original research studies and 400 reviews, with chapters on both physical and mental health. In most of these studies, 'religious practice or belief' was added as incidental to the main study. This is, methodologically, a strength in that it shows that research was carried out without positive or negative religious bias. Looking at various factors relevant for mental health, religious involvement was found to be significantly correlated with:

- well-being, happiness and life satisfaction
- hope and optimism
- purpose and meaning in life
- higher self-esteem
- bereavement adaptation
- greater social support and less loneliness
- lower rates of depression and faster recovery from depression
- lower rates of suicide and fewer positive attitudes towards suicide
- less anxiety
- less psychosis and fewer psychotic tendencies
- lower rates of alcohol and drug use and abuse
- less delinquency and criminal activity
- greater marital stability.

Religion can also have negative effects on mental health; in their handbook, Koenig *et al* identify three groups of these (pp. 227–228):

1   Adverse effects on number and type of stressful experiences, due usually to excessive devotion to religious practices and consequent neglect of other responsibilities, or rigid interpretations of scripture which lead to abusive behaviour of others.

2   Adverse effects on attitudes and cognitive thought processes, including rigid and legalistic thinking, excessive guilt, stigmatisation of those whose religious beliefs differ, judgementalism, and justification or concealing of pathological or otherwise maladaptive thoughts, attitudes and behaviours.

3   Impaired coping behaviour, including, notably, failure to seek appropriate medical help owing to inappropriate reliance on religious rituals or counsel.

However, in general, the beneficial effects considerably outweigh the adverse ones. Koenig *et al* explain this in terms of the bio-psychosocial model of psychiatric illness (2001: pp. 222–228).

The conventional wisdom of psychiatry in the past was that people with mental illness were timid, easily influenced and dependent upon others. This has been challenged by work on religious belief and locus of control (Jackson & Coursey, 1988). Many patients consider that they are incapable of independent action and controlled by outside circumstances; these are said to have an external locus of control. In the research on this topic, a sense of personal control (or a degree of perceived choice) is a strong predictor of a subjective feeling of happiness. Although believing that God is 'in control' might appear to suggest an external locus of control, research studies have shown a significant, positive relationship between religious belief and internal locus of control. Critics of religion claim that the person believes him- or herself to be controlled from outside by God or another force, but this is not the case. Those with a religious faith are arguably more independent as individuals and more able to make life decisions, knowing that God is 'with them'.

Spirituality of psychiatrists

The psychiatrists need to have clear aims and aspirations for the treatment of each individual patient. In order to benefit the patient, the psychiatrist is required to listen empathically; and inevitably, he or she has values and standards that are applied, often unconsciously, in clinical practice. There has been much work on values in psychiatry over recent years, much of it pioneered by the Royal College of Psychiatrists Philosophy Special Interest Group and its founding chairman (Fulford *et al*, 2006: part IV).

There has been concern in medicine generally, and psychiatry specifically, about burnout in doctors. Following the inception of the National Health Service (NHS), psychiatrists were able to retire earlier than other consultants through entitlement to Mental Health Officer status. Many took this option and retired from the NHS early, from the age 55 onwards (this employment option has recently been withdrawn). Many have felt exhausted, jaded, worn out and undervalued, no longer had the zest for their work or were not able professionally to continue any longer. For some, renewing their interest in spirituality and/or religious belief in relation to psychiatry at this time has been valuable in approaching their work with fresh vigour.

We now have more information on professional burnout and the health of doctors. Psychiatrists, when compared with other doctors, are more likely to suffer from burnout (Kumar *et al*, 2005), have higher reported rates for depression (Deary *et al*, 1996) and show higher suicide rates (Hawton *et al*, 2001). Methods of dealing with this have concentrated on career counselling, selection for the specialty, training and continuing professional development, recruitment, and having effective systems in place for recognising when things go wrong (Firth-Cozens, 2007). All psychiatrists should be trained to help colleagues with mental health problems, both within psychiatry and in other medical disciplines.

Some psychiatrists, especially as they become more senior in their work, gradually develop existential or spiritual difficulties concerning their professional practice. If they cannot resolve these concerns and deal with their internal doubts, they become more prone to burnout and despondency. An involvement in religious belief and practice or in some type of spirituality is valuable for preventing such existential despair.

Being able to acknowledge one's spiritual being gives a sense of fulfilment which facilitates coping with the stresses of professional life. Since its inception, the Spirituality and Psychiatry Group has clearly met a previously unrecognised need of psychiatrists, as the membership figures show (by 2007, out of a College membership of 13000 members and fellows, the Group had attracted more than 1500 members, nearly 12% of the College membership). At an early meeting of the Spirituality and Psychiatry Group, an elderly psychiatrist said, with considerable emotion, 'All my working life I have wanted something like this, where I could discuss these issues with my colleagues'. Many of us had felt constrained by the rigid template imposed by the psychiatric establishment, which had excluded from consideration spiritual aspects of either the patient or the psychiatrist. Previously, such matters had not been discussed either with patients or in any professional forum.

Spirituality in psychiatric treatment

Spirituality is increasingly being included as a component of psychiatric treatment and also as an independent and dependent variable in treatment research. Furthermore, a variety of faith-based organisations are providing care for people with mental health problems (Koenig, 2005). Koenig proposed ten ways in which religion can improve mental health (2005: pp. 133–139). He includes within his analysis reference to spiritual as well as religious beliefs and we would extend the analysis here to explicitly refer to both throughout. Thus spirituality and religion:

1   Promote a positive worldview.
2   Help to make sense of difficult situations.
3   Give purpose and meaning.
4   Discourage maladaptive coping.
5   Enhance social support.
6   Promote 'other-directedness'.
7   Help to release the need for control.
8   Provide and encourage forgiveness.
9   Encourage thankfulness.
10   Provide hope.

Like Koenig, we recognise that spirituality and religion can also be deleterious to treatment and such pathological forms of spirituality are discussed later in this book (chapter 13). However, psychotherapy and counselling based upon religious frameworks of belief or else offered within the context of a faith community, can bring great benefit when undertaken within proper professional and ethical boundaries and appropriately offered. It is also possible to explore spirituality in the secular treatment setting and organisations like Alcoholics Anonymous explicitly adopt a 'secular spirituality', which is open to people of all faith traditions or none (this will be considered further chapter 8).

Furthering spirituality in mental healthcare in the UK

Historically, people with widely different and strongly held beliefs have not always proved to be natural allies. The strength of the Spirituality and Psychiatry Special Interest Group is that it is a coalition built on mutual respect for each person's beliefs and traditions. The problem with coalitions, whether political or ideological, is that those with strong convictions find it hard to collaborate with others coming from a different ideology. To overcome this barrier to progress, we have had to respect the beliefs of those from different faiths, as well as those not aligned with a faith tradition, recognising that we can make headway together in a way that would not be possible as individuals. It is essential that all those for whom religious and spiritual aspects of psychiatry are important feel able to join and contribute towards the work of the Group. Tolerance and valuing different perspectives has been crucial, an ethos that so far the Group has been able to maintain well.

The Royal College of Psychiatrists needs to produce expert and well-balanced material and opinion from its component parts. In this, the Spirituality and Psychiatry Group has a continuing role and does make comment where appropriate. This book aims to be such a contribution. To fulfil what is expected of us, we need to be aware of the existing spiritual and religious dialogue on each issue of concern, ascribing sources where relevant, taking into account scientific evidence, giving rational argument for our statements and, above all, representing a high standard of psychiatric knowledge and practice. We should also avoid evanescent sensationalism. Only if all these criteria are achieved have we any right to expect others to listen to us and act upon our recommendations; only then can our contribution to professional discourse become an acceptable and valid position, even if not universally agreed.

The Spirituality and Psychiatry Group will have to develop intellectual muscle for its continuing existence and influence. It will need to convince psychiatrists that they, as well as their patients, have emotions. It will need to demonstrate the volitional nature of humankind and remind us that we are not wholly determined in our thought and behaviour by biochemistry and circumstances.

Mental health statutory and voluntary organisations have become much more aware in recent years of the spiritual aspirations of patients and professional staff. The Spirituality and Psychiatry Group will continue to make a contribution to this debate in various different ways; it is increasingly seen as a source for expertise and advice at the interface between spirituality and psychiatric practice. Members of the Group have formed useful links with religious organisations such as churches, mosques and synagogues, and with clergy, especially hospital chaplains or equivalent designations (e.g. spiritual advisors). In the past, relationships were often strained between the two institutions of psychiatry and the Church, but easier communication in recent years has been immensely beneficial to psychiatric patients and their relatives. By drawing on the insights of both institutions, we have aimed to help our patients, to improve training and continuing professional development and to expand the vision of religious ministers and mental health professionals alike. It is important that this is not just the cosy situation of a psychiatrist of one religious persuasion conferring with a like-minded religious leader. Our diversity is a positive contribution we can make and it is necessary for our patients to have confidence in us.

The Spirituality and Psychiatry Special Interest Group has therefore a useful role in giving helpful direction and advice to the College and through the College to other mental health individuals and organisations of users, carers, volunteers and professionals. A specific example of this is planning the training of psychiatrists and other doctors in psychiatry, and also the continuing professional development of trained doctors. The Group has already contributed to this and intends to continue to do so through proposals for the curriculum for professional postgraduate examinations and training, commenting on the required characteristics of trainees and trainers and the interaction between them, and on the accreditation of psychiatric training schemes.

Training in spirituality and psychiatry

In order to introduce spiritual aspects into the training of psychiatrists, we need to help trainees to overcome common prejudices such as 'religion is usually harmful for patients' and 'religion is for the weak, vacillating and dependent'. Training concerning spirituality and psychiatry should consider what is relevant in terms of knowledge, skills and attitudes. In addition, it is important to consider clinical judgement, which is itself a neglected matter associated with the spiritual value of discernment.

We need to look at each level of training for psychiatry: medical undergraduate, postgraduate psychiatrist in training and continuing professional development for the fully trained psychiatrist. Taking a religious or spiritual history should be emphasised; the following example is drawn from the American College of Physicians (Lo *et al*, 1999):

1   Is faith (religion, spirituality) important to you in this illness?
2   Has faith (religion, spirituality) been important to you at other times in your life?
3   Do you have someone to talk to about religious/spiritual matters?
4   Would you like to explore religious/spiritual matters with someone?

Such questions need take very little time, perhaps only a couple of minutes (Koenig, 2004). In more expanded form they might lead on to discussions about whether religious/spiritual beliefs are supportive, anxiety provoking or punitive; whether the patient is a member of any spiritual/religious community; what the patient's relationship with clergy is like; whether there are any spiritual/religious issues the patient would like to discuss in therapy; whether the patient's spiritual/religious beliefs influence the type of therapy he or she would be most at ease with; and how his or her beliefs influence their attitude to medication.

Other concerns to be addressed in the curriculum might include:

- psychiatrist's awareness of and responsiveness to:
    - the need to find a sense of meaning and purpose in life
    - the personal search for answers to deeper questions concerning birth, life and death
    - the difference between spirituality and religion, and their inter-relatedness
    - the relationship of spirituality to the development and expression of individual human values
    - how spirituality informs concepts of good and evil
    - the way in which good medical practice is founded on values that include discernment, compassion, generosity, tolerance, patience, honesty, humility and wisdom
    - the psychiatrist's own value systems and the way that these may influence others
    - the value systems of others and the psychiatrist's own response to these;
- knowledge of:
    - spiritual development as part of personal growth
    - spiritual crises, meditation, prayer and altered states of consciousness, including the near-death experience
    - the spiritual significance of anxiety, doubt, guilt and shame
    - the spiritual importance of love, altruism and forgiveness and their relation to mental health
    - the influence of materialistic goals on personal identity and self-esteem
    - the reciprocal relationship between culture and spiritual/religious beliefs and practices and their consequences for psychiatric practice
    - how the presence or absence of spiritual/religious beliefs and practices in mental healthcare workers may influence clinical decision-making
    - the role in clinical management of spiritual/religious support networks, including chaplaincy and pastoral care departments as well as those in the community
    - quantitative and qualitative research on spirituality and mental health;
- skills in:
    - taking a spiritual history

- being able to stay mentally focused in the present, remaining alert and attentive with equanimity
- developing the capacity to witness and endure distress while sustaining an attitude of hope
- the recognition of his ot her own emotional responses to spiritual disclosures
- honest self-appraisal, in the interest of continuing personal development
- maintaining personal well-being in the interest of patient care.

Conclusion

Psychiatrists and other mental health professionals need to be bilingual, 'fluent in … the language of psychiatry and psychology … and the language of spirituality that focuses on issues of meaning, hope, value, connectedness and transcendence' (Swinton, 2001: p. 174). It is probably fair to say that we have, for too long, neglected one of these languages to our own detriment and the detriment of our patients. That there is now renewed interest in learning the language of spirituality is very encouraging, but like all languages this one needs practice. Just as the language of psychiatry needs to be employed at every stage of assessment, diagnosis and treatment, as well as in all good research and training in mental healthcare, so the language of spirituality needs to permeate our relationships with our patients, colleagues and our whole understanding of the field of psychiatry.

References

American Psychiatric Association (1994) *Diagnostic and Statistical Manual of Mental Disorders (4th edn) (DSM–IV)*. APA.

Bowker, J. (1997) *Oxford Dictionary of World Religions*. Oxford University Press.

Cook, C. C. H. (2004a) Addiction and spirituality. *Addiction*, **99**, 539–551.

Cook, C. C. H. (2004b) Psychiatry and mysticism. *Mental Health, Religion and Culture*, **7**, 149–163

Deary, I. J., Agius, R. M. & Sadler, A. (1996) Personality and stress in consultant psychiatrists. *International Journal of Social Psychiatry*, **42**, 112–123.

Fine, J. (2006) *Language in Psychiatry: a Handbook of Clinical Practice*. Equinox.

Firth-Cozens, J. (2007) Improving the health of psychiatrists. *Advances in Psychiatric Treatment*, **13**, 161–168.

Fulford, K. W. M., Thornton, T. & Graham, G. (2006) *Oxford Textbook of Philosophy and Psychiatry*. Oxford University Press.

Griesinger, W. (1867) Preface to first issue of *Archive for Psychiatry and Nervous Diseases*. In *A History of Psychiatry* (trans. E. Shorter) (1997), p. 76. John Wiley & Sons.

Hawton, K., Clements, A., Sakarovitch, C., *et al* (2001) Suicide in doctors: a study of risk according to gender, seniority and specialty in medical practitioners in England and Wales, 1979–1995. *Journal of Epidemiology and Community Health*, **55**, 296–301.

Jackson, L. E. & Coursey, R. D. (1988) The relationship of God control and internal locus of control to intrinsic religious motivation, coping and purpose in life. *Journal for the Scientific Study of Religion*, **27**, 399–410.

James, W. (1985) *The Varieties of Religious Experience*. Penguin.

Koenig, H. G. (2004) Taking a spiritual history. *Journal of the American Medical Association*, **291**, 2881.

Koenig, H. G. (2005) *Faith and Mental Health*. Templeton.

Koenig, H. G., McCullough, M. E. & Larson, D. B. (2001) *Handbook of Religion and Health*. Oxford University Press.

Kumar, S., Hatcher, S. & Huggard, P. (2005) Burnout in psychiatrists: an etiological model. *International Journal of Psychiatry in Medicine*, **35**, 405–416.

Lo, B., Quill, T. & Tulsky, J. (1999) Discussing palliative care with patients. *Annals of Internal Medicine*, **130**, 744–749.

Mayer-Gross, W., Slater, E. & Roth, M. (1969) *Clinical Psychiatry* (3rd edn). Baillière, Tindall & Cassell.

Neeleman, J. & King, M. B. (1993) Psychiatrists' religious attitudes in relation to their clinical practice: a survey of 231 psychiatrists. *Acta Psychiatrica Scandinavica*, **88**, 420–424.

Office for National Statistics (2001) UK Census. Office *for National Statistics*.

Pinel, P. (1801) *Traité Médicophilosophique* (1st edn, trans. G. Zilboorg (1941) 'A History of Medical Psychology'), pp. 187–188. WW Norton & Company.

Sacks, J. (2002) *The Dignity of Difference*. p. 4. Continuum.

Stace, W. T. (1973) *Mysticism and Philosophy*. Macmillan.

Swinton, J. (2001) *Spirituality and Mental Health Care*. Jessica Kingsley.

CHAPTER 2

Assessing spiritual needs

Larry Culliford and Sarah Eagger

The most important objective in psychiatry is to get alongside the patient
[Poole & Higgo, 2006: p. 2]

There is no better way to 'get alongside' the patient than to enquire sympathetically about what gives his or her life most meaning and what helps most in adversity. These questions necessarily point towards spirituality and in the direction of a person's strengths rather than deficits.

Poole & Higgo (2006), two experienced and committed psychiatrists, encourage a narrative approach to understanding patients and emphasise that as well as any weaknesses operating in their lives, assessment has to include patients' strengths. However, both they and the authors writing on assessment in another recent book (Meaden & Farmer, 2006), emphasise diagnosis and problem-listing. 'Cultural and spiritual issues' are virtually ignored, being mentioned only once in the two texts (in Meaden & Farmer, section on 'Lifestyle assessments', p. 70).

We therefore seek to fill a vital gap in the literature on psychiatric assessment. This chapter expands on an earlier paper (Culliford, 2007a) and is influenced by the profession's growing acceptance of the strengths perspective, 'which posits clients' personal and environmental strengths as central to the helping process' (Hodge, 2001a). As well as asking 'Why' the spiritual needs of psychiatric patients should be addressed, we also ask questions about 'how', 'who' and 'when' (Koenig, 2002). We discuss quantitative v. qualitative approaches, and also narrative v. interpretative frameworks for understanding spirituality as necessarily intrinsic to optimal care-planning in mental healthcare.

Why assess a person's spirituality?

The reasons for assessing spiritual aspects of psychiatric patients' lives, including their spiritual needs, are complex (Culliford, 2002b). In addition to discovering personal and environmental strengths on which to draw, the more obvious include:

1   The very nature of spirituality as a source of vitality, motivation and a healthy sense of belonging and being valued.
2   The long historical relationship between religion, medicine and mental healthcare.
3   The patients' wishes as well as those of carers.
4   The epidemiology of spirituality/religion and mental health.
5   The influence of spirituality/religion on the attitudes and decisions of psychiatric staff.

The nature of spirituality

Spirituality is universal, yet unique to every person. It is essentially unifying and applies to everyone, including those who do not believe in God or a 'higher being'. Ellison has suggested that spirituality:

> enables and motivates us to search for meaning and purpose in life. It is the spirit which synthesizes the total personality and provides some sense of energizing direction and order. The spiritual dimension does not exist in isolation from the psyche and the soma. It affects and is affected by our physical state, feelings, thoughts and relationships [Ellison, 1983].

Spirituality is therefore supraordinate to, and an integrating force for, the other hierarchically ordered dimensions of human life: physical, biological, psychological and social (Culliford, 2002a,b). Nevertheless, it is a dimension that has, until recently, been neglected in both physical and mental healthcare (Swinton, 2001). This neglect can largely be ascribed to the secularisation of the culture in which psychiatry has developed as a mainly science-based discipline. As a consequence, reason has often been given primacy over other major mental faculties: actions, sense perceptions, emotions and, particularly, intuition.

The resulting imbalance among these seamlessly and dynamically interrelated faculties has become entrenched, partly in response to the perceived conflict between religion and science, for example with regard to evolutionary theory. In medicine and psychiatry, dualistic 'either/or' thinking continues to prevail over the more holistic 'both/and' type (Culliford, 2007b). Renewed balance is called for.

Spirituality is a strong factor in people's lives (Hay & Hunt, 2000). The relevance of this for healthcare professionals – and especially for psychiatric staff – is that at times of emotional stress, physical and mental illness, loss, bereavement and death, people necessarily confront what Buckley has called 'the great issues of life' that lie 'far beneath the formal separation of the sciences, and of the sciences from the humanities' (1987: p. 360).

How to talk about spiritual matters with patients?

In dealing with these weighty matters, mental health professionals can help themselves, their colleagues in other disciplines and their patients by using ordinary language rather than religious terminology. What Nolan

& Crawford (1997) call 'the rhetoric of spirituality' does not have to be complex or mysterious.

The most common and possibly most useful method of assessing spiritual needs, 'taking a spiritual history', involves engaging with people (who happen, for the time being, to be patients) as equals in enquiry and discussion, using their own words about what – at the deepest level – makes sense to them and what puzzles them, what motivates them and what holds them back. This is the most direct way to get quickly to the heart of whatever is troubling the patient. It coincides with the essence of good medical practice: two people, doctor and patient, engaged in genuine and meaningful communication about what matters most in terms of physical, mental and spiritual health. It seems worth adding that both may gain from the encounter.

It is not surprising that where spirituality is concerned, patients' needs and wishes coincide (Faulkner, 1997). As Greasley *et al* (2001) note, spirituality is a vital concern for most service users. In a study of spiritual care in mental health practice, Nathan (1997) asked psychiatric patients to describe the most important elements of 'spiritual care' and the potential benefits such care may bring. Their responses are summarised in Boxes 2.1 and 2.2.

Box 2.1   Elements of spiritual care (adapted from Nathan, 1997)

- an environment fostering hope, joy and creativity
- being valued and trusted, treated with respect and dignity
- sympathetic and confidential listening
- help to make sense of, and derive meaning from, illness experiences
- receiving permission, encouragement (and sometimes guidance) to develop spiritually.

Box 2.2   Benefits of spiritual care (adapted from Nathan, 1997)

- healthy grieving of losses enabled (letting go)
- improved self-esteem and confidence
- maximisation of personal potential
- relationships improved (with self, others and with the Absolute/God)
- renewed sense of meaning and purpose
- enhanced feeling of belonging
- improved capacity for solving problems
- insoluble problems, continuing distress and disability more easily endured
- hope renewed.

The effect of spirituality on (mental) health and the case for spiritual assessment

There is now extensive research evidence to suggest a positive relationship between religion, spirituality and health (Koenig *et al*, 2001). However, there are occasions on which spirituality can exert a deleterious effect (see chapter 13). Effects in apparently opposite directions both highlight the need for careful spiritual assessment.

Taking a spiritual history is most clearly necessary when spiritual or religious issues are part of the presenting problem, for example in religious delusions, feelings of rejection (by God or a faith group) and excessive guilt or shame. Although it is acknowledged that religion can have negative effects, confidence is growing in the benefits of spiritual beliefs and practices to both physical and mental health (Plante & Thoresen, 2007); this confidence is based on substantial epidemiological research of improving quality (Koenig *et al*, 2001; Levin, 2001). The authors quoted here suggest that while fewer than 10% of studies report negative effects, 80% identify spiritual/religious beliefs and practices as beneficial, not so much part of the problem as part of the remedy (Box 2.3). In Hodge (2001*a*), for example, spirituality is a significant variable for coping ability and self-esteem, also for recovery from divorce, homelessness, sexual assault and substance abuse. For Ellison & Levin (1998), it is a key factor in personal well-being.

Where spiritual and religious issues are not explicitly to the fore, spiritual assessment might easily be misunderstood in many cases as good, compassionate care and practice by another name. It is more than this, however. Spirituality concerns itself with who a person really is, their essence or soul, thus with such matters as a person's beliefs, values,

---

Box 2.3   Examples of spiritual and religious factors positively affecting mental health

Religion can positively affect mental health:

- through enabling inner resources:
  - greater self-esteem, life satisfaction and happiness
  - improved sense of meaning and purpose (motivation)
  - increased hope;
- through connecting or re-connecting with external resources (e.g. within the person's faith community):
  - increased social support (practical and emotional);
- with specific problems:
  - increased adaptation to bereavement
  - improved recovery from addictions (e.g. Alcoholics Anonymous and similar groups using the 12-step method)
  - decreased levels of anxiety, loneliness and suicide.

motivations, attachments, ideas and ideals (see chapter 1) and these are (or should be) important to all clinicians and patients. Yet, they are frequently overlooked. The need to take a 'spiritual' history reminds us that they are important and that we should look deeply into patients' personal and environmental strengths on a routine and regular basis.

The evidence for a positive relationship between spirituality and health is not that strong in some cases. For example, it is apparently less important (or at least less well demonstrated) for major mental illnesses such as schizophrenia. Nevertheless, spiritual or religious contents of thoughts, delusions and/or hallucinations also require careful assessment, particularly when a diagnosis of 'spiritual emergence' (chapter 11, pp. 227–230) rather than psychosis is a possibility. The need to pay attention to the spiritual history is therefore established in every psychiatric case.

Spiritual elements in staff decision-making

The influence of spirituality and religion on the attitudes and decisions of psychiatric staff is complex. Although curricula exist (Puchalski & Larson, 1998), in the UK the topic has seldom been taught as part of professional competency training as it should be: in terms of knowledge, skills and attitudes. When individual views on the subject have been canvassed, it is not surprising that mental healthcare professionals' attitudes towards spirituality have tended to be negative (Neelman & King, 1993).

At one extreme, clinicians may automatically deem any expression of religiosity or spiritual awareness to be psychopathological. Routinely taking patients' spiritual histories, and becoming more skilful at doing so, will provide staff with both information and material for reflection. The experience and knowledge gained will help correct any previously held attitudinal bias.

At the other extreme, caring efficiently and compassionately for disadvantaged others can legitimately be experienced as vocational. Many mental health workers consider themselves to a degree spiritually guided, somehow involved in a sacred and undeniable calling. For them, assessing patients' spiritual needs is an expression of spiritual care, and therefore fulfilling in itself, as well as a necessary preparation for providing what is required in the circumstances.

What is a psychiatric assessment?

A psychiatric assessment is not primarily formulaic. It involves a dynamic process between a professional and a patient (Poole & Higgo, 2006). Gathering information or data is not sufficient – the knowledge gained must be interpreted, organised, integrated with theory and made meaningful (Rauch, 1993). This is the process of 'formulation'. To quote Hodge (2001a), writing for social workers:

Assessment is critical to the incorporation of strengths into the therapeutic milieu. Without a reliable means for finding consumers' strengths, workers tend to revert to practice models that are based on the identification of problems and deficits [p. 204].

Assessment is therefore defined as: 'the process of gathering, analysing and synthesising data into a useful form, so that it provides a basis for action' (Hodge, 2001a). Assessment methods encourage a systematic approach and provide guidance on the areas that need exploring. The aim is to ensure that only relevant information is gathered, and people's right to privacy is protected.

A person's spiritual dimension is not easy to measure. It has been argued (Reed, 1992) that as a subjective, interior reality, it is difficult to quantify in any manner. Furthermore, attempts at quantification are made more difficult by considerable variation in this reality among different religious and non-religious traditions. Nevertheless, there are several reasons for wanting to quantify spirituality in the healthcare context. These include setting standards of care and reducing risks, thereby contributing towards accountable practice. Quantification can also form the basis for practitioner and patient decision-making and goal setting, and may be important in validating problems in this potentially intangible domain.

An assessment is aimed primarily at seeking to understand a patient's spirituality and what impact it has on their illness. It is not simply to screen for spiritual needs, but to assist staff in appreciating how spirituality functions in the life of each patient. Assessment can be a factor in helping understand how a person copes with illness and also how illness may challenge their personal integrity and belief system. As well as aiding good communication, the assessment process helps identify spiritual variables as important mediators of change and enables healthcare staff to recognise and respond to a patient's spiritual distress. It often calls for a direct, immediate and empathic (compassionate) response. Staff training therefore needs to address this. Teaching third-year medical students shows that this can be highly rewarding (Culliford, 2009).

Assessing spiritual needs: how?

Quantitative methods

Several clinically tested instruments are available for spiritual assessment, including the Royal Free Interview for Religious and Spiritual Beliefs (King et al, 1995), the Spiritual Involvement and Beliefs Scale (Hatch et al, 1998), the multi-dimensional instrument developed by the Fetzer Institute (1999) and Hill & Hood's Measures of Religiosity (1999).

However, using quantitative methods for spiritual assessment, including questionnaires, has been criticised because they fail to capture the subjective nature of human existence (Hodge, 2001a). Vital information can be overlooked, as patients are obliged to tailor descriptions of their experiences to fit the limited choices of a specific scale and its predetermined understanding of how things are.

This type of assessment can, moreover, feel unnecessarily intrusive or dismissive, and the patient may not feel sufficiently valued as an individual. Results obtained from such patients would then be suspect. Empathic staff, picking up someone's reluctant attitude to this approach, may equally lack enthusiasm for engaging with patients in this way, aware that it is harder to foster a collaborative atmosphere using any kind of predetermined and structured pro forma to investigate what is often an intensely private and sensitive area. For these reasons, and because such methods are usually too detailed, they are more suitable for research and audit projects than for clinical use.

Qualitative methods

In the clinical setting, where richness and the emotional tone of information can be of special importance, qualitative methods of enquiry into spirituality work better. These get closer to patients' experience of reality by being person-centred, open-ended and process (rather than structure) orientated.

Taking a spiritual history

The principal qualitative method of spiritual needs assessment in clinical practice involves taking a spiritual history. This is best thought of as a clinical skill to acquire and hone, rather than an activity to be performed by recipe or rote. It is a skill that requires empathic engagement with the patient, and which therefore sanctions the judicious use of both intuition and initiative by the assessor. It may lead, for example, to sensitive exploration of what the patient only hints at or seems to be avoiding; this is to honour and uphold the spiritual values of courage and honesty, whose enemy is concealment, whether conscious or otherwise. It is therefore important to be reasonably systematic and thorough. This type of interview works best in a comfortable, quiet and confidential setting and a gentle, unhurried approach is recommended. More than one conversation may be necessary.

Initial (brief) assessment

Despite the need for thoroughness, it is sometimes necessary to make rapid assessments of psychiatric patients. At such times, two types of questions are useful:

1   What helps you most when things are difficult, when times are hard (such as when you are facing big problems, major losses or other important challenges)?

Reflections on experience and life meaning are usually best considered before specific questions about religion are asked, as in, for example: 'What is really important in your life?' This is a good opening strategy, being inclusive and appealing to those whose life's meaning is not defined in religious terms. The patient's replies usually point to the principal values held and lived by, indicating their major spiritual concerns and practices (Box 2.4).

When taking a spiritual history the aim is to offer a sense of acceptance and validation of the patient's account. It is best therefore to avoid interruption as the story unfolds. However, gentle prompts (such as 'Would you like to say more about that?') may be helpful in encouraging the patient to expand his or her story.

It is also best to build rapport by repeating and paraphrasing salient points, using especially terminology congruent with the patient's spiritual tradition, borrowing words from the patient's own narrative. For example, his or her place of worship and spiritual communion may be a church, synagogue, mosque, temple or gurdwara, or equally a garden, an allotment, the bath, the beach, the riverbank, a lakeside or a hilltop.

2   Do you think of yourself as being either religious or spiritual?

This second question may be amplified by asking about whether the person identifies with being one of the following: atheist, agnostic, unsure, religious, or spiritual (Box 2.5). Note that a person may choose to be identified as both religious and spiritual.

Box 2.4   Spiritual practices

1   Mainly religious:
   - belonging to a faith tradition, participating in associated community-based activities
   - ritual and symbolic practices and other forms of worship
   - pilgrimage and retreats
   - meditation and prayer
   - reading scripture
   - sacred music (listening to, singing and playing), including songs, hymns, psalms and devotional chants.

2   Mainly secular:
   - acts of compassion (including work, especially teamwork)
   - deep reflection (contemplation)
   - yoga, tai chi and similar disciplined practices
   - engaging with and enjoying nature
   - contemplative reading (literature, poetry, philosophy etc.)
   - appreciation of the arts and engaging in creative activities, including artistic pursuits, cookery, gardening etc.
   - maintaining stable family relationships and friendships (especially those involving high levels of trust and intimacy).

Box 2.5   Suggested definitions for spiritual identities

- Atheist: to be atheist is to deny emphatically the existence (even the possibility) of a sacred being, supreme reality, God or other deity.
- Agnostic: to be agnostic is to assert that we cannot truly know about the existence or otherwise of a sacred being, supreme reality, God or other deity.
- Unsure: to be unsure means the person does not know what he or she believes about a sacred being, supreme reality, God or other deity.
- Religious: to be religious is to believe and have faith in a sacred being, supreme reality, God or other gods, and/or to belong to and practise within an organised religion.
- Spiritual: to be spiritual is to experience awareness of relationship with a sacred reality, whether or not also belonging to or practising within an organised religion

Spiritual practices

An appropriate next step, following naturally from a brief appraisal, is to ask in more detail about spiritual practices. Regularly engaging in such activities identifies a person as spiritually engaged as much as holding and expressing spiritual or religious beliefs does. Listing one or more 'mainly secular' spiritual practices may give cause to people who describe themselves as atheist, agnostic or unsure to reconsider their self-assessment, and – whatever beliefs they have – to begin to accept themselves as open to spirituality.

A more detailed spiritual history: six comparable approaches

A brief assessment will often indicate that a more detailed history is required to establish relevant aspects of the patient's background, specific problems related to spirituality or religion, available spiritual support and additional spiritual needs.

Various authorities have independently offered guidance on assessing the religious and spiritual aspects of people's lives. However, they are fairly uniform regarding the topics covered. This allows practitioners to pick the style with which they feel most comfortable. Guides tend to take the form of aides-memoires rather than exact prescriptions.

1   The first approach, outlined in the guide published by the Spiritual Competency and Resource Centre (http://www.spiritualcompetency.com/assess_spirit/ASrshx.asp), focuses on religious background and beliefs as well as spiritual meaning and values (including spiritual practices (Box 2.4), spiritual experiences (Box 2.6) and prayer experiences).

2   In a guide to the assessment of spiritual concerns in mental healthcare, Eagger (2006) lists some simple, non-intrusive questions that can inform the care team's approach. These look, for example, at the place of spirituality or religion in the patient's past or present, the nature of

---

Box 2.6   Some types of spiritual experiences

- Mystical experiences (broadly defined) including personal epiphanies and 'callings'
- Ritualistic experiences – tribal and cult phenomena, often derived from oral traditions
- Formalised experiences – highly structured, relating to a specific doctrine
- Informal, everyday insights (such as becoming aware that 'god is with me' or a spontaneous feeling of love and fellowship with others and/or with nature)
- Spiritual living – spirituality as a deliberate choice, a constant, day-to-day lived experience
- Near-death experiences
- Meaningful dreams
- Psychedelic (drug-induced) experiences

---

its influence (positive or negative, supportive or excluding) and whether it affects the patient's acceptance of and engagement in treatment.

3   The leaflet *Spirituality and Mental Health* (Royal College of Psychiatrists, 2006) suggests five broad areas of questioning: setting the scene, the past, the present, the future, and remedies. These gather a picture of how patients see themselves, their place and purpose in life and their future, and ask whether spirituality or religion might be part of the problem or could be the solution.

4   In an article aimed at healthcare professionals, Puchalski & Romer's (2000) guide to taking a spiritual history uses the mnemonic FICA:
   - Faith and belief (what gives the patient's life meaning)
   - Importance (how important is this to their situation)
   - Community (their place in any social or religious group)
   - Address in care (how they would like their personal spirituality addressed in healthcare).

5   A fifth tool for spiritual assessment involves the HOPE questions (Anandarajah & Hight, 2001). The mnemonic HOPE directs the assessor's attention to four areas of the patient's life:
   - sources of Hope, meaning, comfort, strength, peace, love and connection
   - Organised religion
   - Personal spirituality and Practices
   - Effects on medical (psychiatric) care and End-of-life issues.

6   Finally, another useful mnemonic is SPIRIT (Maugans, 1996):
   - Spiritual belief system
   - Personal spirituality
   - Integration/Involvement in a spiritual or religious community
   - Ritualised practices and Restrictions
   - Implications for medical care
   - Terminal events planning.

This scheme, designed for general practice, is physician-orientated and open to wider dimensions of spirituality. Useful for those who express no formalised religious orientation, including atheists, secular humanists and agnostics, it can be adapted for mental health. It also includes a section on planning for death, which may be particularly helpful in the context of old age psychiatry.

More complex models of spiritual assessment

These six guides do not all emphasise the importance of distinguishing between public events (such as baptism, confirmation, bar mitzvah and other rites of passage) and private experiences (such as conversion, spiritual awakening or transcendent communication/communion with God, a higher consciousness or a 'higher being'). The significance of each, both in the mind of the patient and through the lens of the family faith tradition, is worth clarifying, particularly when the former deviates from, and may be in conflict with, the latter.

More complex models of assessment may be helpful in understanding some patients. Hodge (2001a), for example, recommends an 'initial narrative framework' consisting of three sets of questions, to be followed by an 'interpretative anthropological framework' consisting of six sets. Some of these questions focus on ideas suggested by Nee (1968, quoted by Hodge, 2001a), namely that the human spirit is 'an integrative unity' consisting of 'communion', 'conscience' and 'intuition'. Communion refers here to a person's capacity to relate to and identify with the Ultimate. Conscience is a subjective, ethical guidance system beyond cognitively held beliefs – a person's most deeply adhered to values system. Intuition involves insights entering consciousness directly, bypassing normal information channels and drawing on a kind of reservoir of wisdom or 'sacred knowledge' (Culliford 2007b). Intuition is also closely connected to creativity. These several faculties are seamlessly interlinked in life. Hodge's framework is designed to include all of them in the assessment.

Hodge has developed other methods for engaging with and assessing spirituality. These include 'spiritual lifemaps' (Hodge, 2005), which are 'client-constructed pictorial narratives of a spiritual journey'. This egalitarian method acknowledges patients as the experts in their own situations, thus empowering them and facilitating the construction of therapeutic interventions in partnership with mental health staff. Hodge lists 'spiritual reframing', 'cognitive reframing', 'solution-focused rituals', 'leveraging church-based social support', and 'brevity of life reflection' among such useful interventions, making the strong point that 'being asked to create, to visually depict a spiritual lifemap, may promote self-esteem and enhance self-image', offering the message that the patient 'is capable, important, and has a significant role to play' (Hodge, 2005). This type of message underpins all attempts to communicate with patients about their spiritual lives.

Other tools that may be useful in spiritual assessment are 'spiritual ecomaps' (Hodge, 2000) and 'spiritual genograms' (Hodge, 2001b). The former are diagrammatic tools for assessing marital and family spirituality, depicting the patient's present existential relationships. The latter chart the flow of spirituality over the course of three or more generations of the patient's family. Both are more useful in a family therapy, but can also yield valuable information and insight in individual casework.

Spiritual lifemaps are related to the 'stage models' approach to assessment, in which a series of spiritual developmental stages through which people pass as they mature throughout life is delineated. The originator of this approach, psychology researcher James Fowler, drew on the earlier developmental models of Jean Piaget, Erik Erikson and Lawrence Kohlberg to describe six sequential 'stages of faith' (Fowler, 1981; see also Culliford, 2007a).[1] The patient's stage can be assessed using, for example, the Spiritual Assessment Inventory (Hall & Edwards, 1996), but similar problems apply here as with other quantitative methods of assessment. The stage models approach may seem judgemental, and there is a greater risk of staff reverting to a deficit mindset (looking at weaknesses, rather than strengths) with such highly structured models than with those at the open-ended, narrative end of the continuum.

Another way to discern the patient's degree of spiritual maturity is by way of a 'spiritual autobiography' and stage-specific questions, but caution is required. 'Expert clinicians' are needed to safely and successfully undertake and interpret such an assessment, but the question 'Who can reliably decide who else is more (or less) mature in terms of spiritual growth?' remains self-evidently problematic.

Somewhere in between open-ended and closed structure is Fitchett's model (1993), aimed at systematically producing a complete assessment encompassing all bio-psychosocial–spiritual factors relevant to well-being. Fitchett offers seven holistic dimensions of existence: medical, psychological, psychosocial, family systems, ethnic and cultural, societal issues, and spiritual. Under 'spiritual' he lists seven subcategories: belief and meaning, vocation and consequences, experiences and emotion, courage and growth, ritual and practice, community, and authority and guidance. These labels are worth keeping in mind when taking a spiritual history, as a prompt to enquire about whatever may seem to have been left out.

Assessing spiritual needs: who?

McSherry (2001) argues that no single professional group can be considered to have sole responsibility for the provision of spiritual care. For many health-care staff, NHS trust chaplains are the obvious people to undertake spiritual assessments. However, this solution is too simple, not least because most chaplaincy services are too small to engage with every patient as required.

---

1   Fowler's stages of faith are described in full in chapter 5.

Suitably trained and experienced personnel are needed in every clinical team, and this means staff from all the different professional disciplines.

The Royal College of Psychiatrists (2006) advises that 'Making a spiritual assessment is as important as all other aspects of medical history taking and examination. When making a diagnosis, a psychiatrist should be competent in distinguishing between spiritual crisis and mental illness and able to explore areas of overlap and difference between the two'. The competency of psychiatrists depends largely upon training, which in turn depends largely on curriculum (see chapter 1).

The Chief Nursing Officer's review of mental health nursing (Department of Health, 2006) similarly recommends that all mental health nurses recognise and respond to the spiritual and religious needs of service users. This is to be achieved by mental health service providers ensuring that all nurses have access to sources of information and advice regarding religious and spiritual issues. The report continues that nurses should perform assessments to discover the user's religious and spiritual needs and beliefs. Ross (1998), for instance, argues that the conceptual framework of the nursing process already provides a mechanism for delivering systematic, individualised spiritual care. According to this framework, assessment is to be followed by planning, intervention and evaluation. The nursing literature on spirituality and mental healthcare is extensive, including valuable contributions from Govier (2000) and White (2006).

Govier (2000) developed a nursing model using the 'five dimensions of spiritual care'. He provides prompts in the dimensions of reason, reflection, religion, relationships and restorations. This process is similar to Ross's (1998), but it also invites the nurse to enquire into intimate details of the patient's world and is aimed at grasping the essence of an individual's spiritual experience.

White (2006), in turn, sees spirituality as a process of reflection. She describes a narrative and continuous style of assessment where spirituality is seen and experienced as part of the healthcare process, and is therefore embedded in the quality of the conversations with and about patients. Staff members require grounding in reflective learning and in order to engage in the dialogue of dynamic therapeutic relationships team members need knowledge, skills and confidence. The core of the process White describes involves creating opportunities that allow deeper concerns about meaning and purpose to surface. It involves looking for connections, without being locked into a rigid, formalised assessment process. Using a combination of prompts and questions, a shared multiprofessional assessment tool may be completed by any member of the team, and can be returned to at different stages.

Similarly, Narayanasamy (2001) has a hierarchy of questions regarding religious and spiritual practices that start as general and become more specific. The categories include: meaning and purpose, sources of hope and strength, love and relatedness, self-esteem, fear and anxiety, anger, relation between spiritual beliefs and health, concept of God or deity, and spiritual practices.

Because spiritual healthcare practice involves multidisciplinary teamwork, it is also relevant to note that Egan & DeLaat (1997) write of 'the implicit spirituality of occupational therapy practice'; and Hodge (2004), in turn, recommends that social workers develop 'spiritual competency'. Psychologists, having for many years advocated 'healthy scepticism' about the relevance of spirituality to healthcare (Thoresen, 1999), are also now espousing changing attitudes in its favour (Fontana, 2003; Plante & Thoresen, 2007). Spirituality therefore affects everyone, and it is no longer appropriate to deny its relevance to clinical care.

Spiritual assessment is, therefore, a concern for all clinical disciplines. At the simplest level, all clinicians should be competent to conduct the kind of screening assessments described in this chapter. In more complex cases, a more specialist assessment – by a chaplain or clinician with a special interest – might be required.

Potential drawbacks to spiritual assessment

Timing

Patients are often disorientated and very preoccupied when admitted to hospital. An initial brief assessment is necessary to ensure that correct diets are provided and any immediate religious needs are met, but a deeper and more extensive discussion will need to take place over time to allow people to share their stories and express needs in their own words in the process of developing a trusting relationship. Thus the assessment process depends on trust, rapport and continuity. Relying on the application mechanistically or by rote of assessment methods, such as those discussed earlier, poses a danger of failing to respond to fluctuations in patients' mental states. Communication skills are vital in spiritual assessment. Each clinician must use his or her sensitivity to judge the extent, appropriateness and timing of more extensive exploration; each must know him- or herself to be ready for what may become an intimate and possibly extended conversation at the heart of the patient's concerns.

Is it practical?

Cobb (1998) helpfully reflects on several aspects of spiritual assessment, asking first whether or not it is practical. Professionals may show some apprehension that the task is too difficult or that it might take up too much time to fit into ordinary clinical practice. However, a conversation lasting an hour or more, leaving a patient feeling appreciated as a person and therefore more cooperative with co-planning and receiving healthcare interventions, could save many hours of distress and difficulty, and can contribute to a better outcome. Many authorities would, therefore, consider this time well-invested.

Cobb also raises a concern that the language of spirituality and the concepts used may not be appropriate for all patients. Few will have spent much time on spiritual reflection and many may not have a vocabulary to enable deep or extensive discussions on this topic. He also suggests that spirituality may be particularly important for people with a relatively low level of education.

Finally, Cobb raises the issue of whether the healthcare professional is capable of dealing with consequences of discussing spiritual matters with a patient. As mentioned earlier, this may require an immediate, truthful and genuinely compassionate response. It may also raise emotional tension within the healthcare worker, who may be discomforted, if his or her personal religious and spiritual beliefs (or disbeliefs) are challenged.

There is some ambiguity, and many misconceptions, concerning the issue of 'spirituality', so it is not surprising that the subject can be controversial. Some clinicians remain sceptical, suggesting that it is only appropriate to discuss it with people who are openly religious. Spirituality is deeply subjective, very personal and perhaps beyond scientific enquiry, and some practitioners naturally fear that they will not 'get it right' or ever achieve sufficient competence in assessing it. They may feel unsure about what data are required or how to handle the information, especially if they have not received adequate training and do not have appropriate encouragement and support within the working environment. There are issues, too, around role boundaries (Post *et al*, 2000), and ethical concerns about the possibility of inappropriate proselytising, imposition of religious beliefs or activities (such as prayer) and bias against various spiritual perspectives (Dagi, 1995) on the part of the physician or other healthcare professional.

Attitudes are changing rapidly in the multicultural, multi-faith UK society, although the healthcare perspective can appear to be lagging behind, remaining mainly Judeo-Christian in focus. There is also some risk of fragmentation of care when one healthcare professional is responsible for the assessment and another spiritual care specialist (e.g. a chaplain) is seen as mainly providing the spiritual care; but this simply calls for teamwork. Both are assessors and providers, ideally in collaboration with each other and with the patient. McSherry (2000) advocates greater multidisciplinary and interdisciplinary collaboration and better communication between professions on the topic of spirituality. Carey (1997) has also called for more collaboration between mental health professionals and spiritual advisers from outside the health service.

There are serious concerns about, and drawbacks to, spiritual assessment, owing mainly to a lack of appropriate training, encouragement and support for clinical staff. On the positive side, this deficiency is in the area of spiritual competency, and can therefore be remedied, both as part of initial professional training and later CPD.

Assessing spiritual needs: when?

Healthcare influenced by spiritual skills and values (Culliford, 2002*b*; Royal College of Psychiatrists, 2006) should be offered at first contact between the patient and psychiatric service personnel, whose concern will be 'to get alongside the patient' quickly. If adequately trained and 'spiritually competent', staff members will swiftly be ready to make a brief initial spiritual assessment. A spiritual component, one of caring and compassion, can be conveyed in the very first questions, 'How are you?' or 'What seems to be the problem?' The added message that may or may not be stated is0 'I am here to try and help you'. In order to establish the best possible rapport, it is usually worth making this clear.

An initial brief assessment should be undertaken as soon as conditions of calm and confidentiality allow it, no matter whether the setting is in the community, in day care or on an in-patient ward.

Once contact has been made with the patient and an initial assessment of spiritual needs has been undertaken, the assessment process continues. In some cases, several staff members may, at different times, engage the patient in discussion about spiritual matters. Care programme approach demands that the in-patient primary nurse and the community care coordinator should both be updated with relevant information. Depending on the setting, one or the other should be responsible for keeping a record. Ideally, a shared computerised record will be available to facilitate this.

It may be necessary to use some kind of pro forma with free text entry to record and share information obtained during the spiritual assessment. For example, a few mental health trusts, including the South London and Maudsley NHS Trust, have tried to introduce the concept of the 'patient journey'. This includes three prompts around religion, spirituality and guiding values in the section on present social circumstances. Timing is the responsibility of the care coordinator, who sees that the assessment process is focused particularly on patients' strengths and ensures that the patient collaborates as fully as possible in the planning of appropriate, helpful interventions towards recovery and the meeting of his or her spiritual needs. The care coordinator is also responsible for documenting the assessment, agreed plans, reassessments and outcomes.

To introduce spiritual assessments in these ways should not have significant implications for resources. However, a new paradigm is involved (Schermer, 2003) that requires a culture shift throughout mental healthcare. Where in the past only the physical, biological, psychological and social dimensions of patients' experience have been assessed and needs catered for, now the spiritual dimension must routinely be included as well. The implications of this for the NHS are discussed further in chapter 10.

After the assessment, what next?

Formulation

The process of interpreting, organising, integrating with theory and making meaningful the information gathered through assessment is referred to as 'formulation'. The term is used in psychiatry for summarising and making sense of information gathered and observations made while taking a history, examining the physical and mental state of the patient, and conducting specific biophysical and psychological tests. Formulation is not a goal or end-point; its primary aim is to help the patient. This skilled process helps clarify where an assessment is incomplete and what information remains to be gathered. Most formulations are, therefore, provisional and should be revised regularly as observations continue and information develops.

Diagnostic formulation

The simplest type of formulation is the diagnostic formulation. Once the diagnosis is reasonably established, short-term treatment plans can be devised and implemented. Depending upon their outcome and other developments, medium- and long-term treatment plans follow. Some refer to this diagnosis–treatment approach as invoking the medical model of mental healthcare.

Bio-psychosocial formulation

A more comprehensive and thus preferable approach is the bio-psychosocial formulation, in which problems and their solutions are sought in three dimensions of human experience (biological, psychological and social). Such an approach, considering the symptoms and problems in the context of the whole person, and the person in the context of family, community and culture, is a big step towards holism. Including a spiritual history allows this process to be completed, through what may be referred to as a bio-psychosocio-spiritual formulation (the terms psycho-spiritual, person-centred and holistic are also used).

The primary purpose of the bio-psychosocio-spiritual formulation serves the well-being of the patient, acting as a guide to clinicians' planning and execution of helpful interventions.

How may taking a spiritual history and completing a bio-psychosocio-spiritual formulation contribute to patient welfare?

Better rapport

Clinicians regularly discover that taking a spiritual history – enquiring attentively about patients' primary concerns and motivating factors – deepens rapport between them and their patients and improves its quality. Feeling valued as individuals, patients often relax and invest further trust in the doctor, thus improving the therapeutic alliance.

Clarifying psychotic symptoms

Taking a spiritual history can help clarify psychotic symptoms in two main ways. First, it helps distinguish 'spiritual emergence' from psychosis.

Originally called 'spiritual emergency', this refers to a destabilising period of rapid spiritual growth (Vega, 1989; Grof, 2000; Slade, 2004).

Second, existential questions such as 'What is the purpose of my life?' are conundrums that become problematic for many. Religious grandiosity of delusional strength may be a powerful but immature defence against meaningless insignificance. As part of a psychotic reaction, these symptoms may be common in those feeling particularly unworthy or unloved. The religious content thus hints at a spiritual solution. Pastoral or spiritual support and spiritual practices may both appropriately be recommended in such cases. For further discussion, readers are referred to the relevant sections of chapters 3, 8 and 11.

Psychoneuroses

Anxiety and depression are key elements in a range of non-psychotic psychiatric disorders, particularly the psychoneuroses. In addition to the important but difficult questions and problems referred to in the previous paragraph, another universally experienced existential problem derives from emotional attachments. As soon as these are formed, they render people vulnerable to the threat of loss and to loss itself. Such emotions as anxiety, bewilderment and doubt are associated with the threat of loss, whereas anger, the emotion of resistance, arises as loss becomes more likely or imminent. Depressive emotions – shame, guilt and sadness – emerge when a loss increasingly becomes an acknowledged reality (Culliford, 2007b).

Assessing a patient's spiritual needs involves enquiry about their primary attachments, whether to a spiritual reality, to family and loved ones, to places and objects, or to ideas and ideals. Identifying the major attachments and the spectrum of emotions arising in response to threatened and actual loss encourages emotional flow towards acceptance and resolution. Taking a spiritual history is therefore intrinsically therapeutic. It helps to clarify to the patient that these emotions are normal and healthy, part of their pathway to psychological growth and maturity through the acceptance of losses and resolution of the emotional healing process (Culliford, 2007b). This reflects another principle of spirituality, that personal growth results more often through facing and enduring adversity, rather than from trying to avoid it.

In some cases of severe anxiety and/or depression, there is a profound sense of meaninglessness and personal insignificance, comparable with that experienced in psychosis. Spiritual advice and support may again appropriately be recommended, and spiritual practices may be found helpful.

Addictions

The value of a spiritual approach is specifically acknowledged by those who advocate and follow the 12-step method of dealing with addiction. The best known organisations to use this approach are Alcoholics Anonymous (where it originated), Narcotics Anonymous and Gamblers Anonymous. Narcotics Anonymous, for example, describes itself as 'a non-religious fellowship, encouraging each member to cultivate an individual understanding, religious or not, of a spiritual awakening' (www.ukna.org).

The heart of a programme of personal recovery is contained in 12 steps that describe the experience of the first members of Alcoholics Anonymous (www.alcoholics-anonymous.org.uk/geninfo/05steps.htm). Newcomers are not required to accept or follow the 12 steps in their entirety, if they feel unwilling or unable to do so. The key step for addicts is to recognise and respect some form of spiritual reality, manifest particularly as a higher power: 'We came to believe that a power greater than ourselves could restore us to a normal way of thinking and living' (Gamblers Anonymous, http://www.gamblersanonymous.org.uk/about).

Other disorders

Psychiatrists see individuals with a number of other conditions that may have a spiritual element in their aetiology. Absence or removal of meaning and sense of purpose affect drive and motivation. Having a damaged sense of belonging impairs self-esteem and a person's true and healthy sense of identity. These elements may occur, for instance, in personality disorder, eating disorder and chronic fatigue syndrome, as well as in disorders already mentioned here. Persistent psychological resistance to loss may express itself in the form of intense anger, often denied and either subconsciously repressed or consciously suppressed. Enquiry into these central and vital aspects of a person's life is part of a spiritual needs assessment, and it offers an important opportunity to reframe the problem in terms that may lead to reintegration and healing.

Involving chaplaincy services

Sensitive enquiry is in itself helpful for patients whose needs and problems have a spiritual dimension, and it may allow them to fulfil their needs and find their own solutions with greater clarity and efficacy. However, some patients may seek spiritual support and guidance, and therefore be in need of pastoral care. Referral to a chaplain or pastoral care adviser is often appropriate. Such a referral may also be necessary if more complex issues such as being possessed by a spirit are encountered.

After psychiatric staff have assessed a patient's spiritual needs by taking a spiritual history, a well-informed and experienced chaplain, prepared to see and further assess the patient, should be available for consultation and advice. Mental healthcare trusts and service providers should maintain a multi-faith chaplaincy service with adequate staffing levels. Voluntary part-time, as well as paid full- or part-time chaplains and pastoral care staff will be required.

Chaplains and spiritual advisors are increasingly valued as contributors to the multidisciplinary mental health services, taking on the status of 'expert clinician' in the field of spirituality and mental healthcare. Any chaplain working clinically should receive appropriate training in mental health matters. In return, chaplains may increasingly be expected to advise when more complex assessment methods are appropriate. They should also establish good relations with local clergy and faith communities and provide a knowledge base on local religious groups, their traditions and practices. They should be alert to situations in which religious beliefs and activities may prove harmful to individuals or groups. Suitably trained chaplains should also be available for advice on controversial issues such as spirit possession and exorcism (the latter now referred to in many Christian denominations as the ministry of deliverance).

Conclusion

To quote the Australian writer David Tacey,

> Enlightened people everywhere live according to the light of reason and logos, but we all also need a mythos, a spiritual belonging, to make life meaningful and bearable. Mythos provides a goal, offers dignity, and establishes a relationship to past, present and future [Tacey, 2006: pp. 7–10].

To assess people's spirituality regularly, particularly by taking systematic and detailed spiritual histories, will enable practitioners to rekindle *mythos* in medicine and put the psyche back into psychiatry. The psyche being, of course, our soul.

References

Anandarajah, G. & Hight, E. (2001) Spirituality and medical practice: using the HOPE questions as a practical tool for spiritual assessment. *American Family Physician*, **63**, 81–92.

Buckley, M. (1987) *At the Origins of Modern Atheism*. Yale University Press.

Carey, G. (1997) Towards wholeness: the barriers between religion and psychiatry. *British Journal of Psychiatry*, **170**, 396–397.

Cobb, M. (1998) Assessing spiritual need: an examination of practice. In *The Spiritual Challenge of Health Care* (eds M. Cobb & V. Renshaw). Churchill Livingston.

Culliford, L. (2002*a*) Spirituality and clinical care. *BMJ*, **325**, 1434–1435.

Culliford, L. (2002*b*) Spiritual care and psychiatric treatment: an introduction. *Advances in Psychiatric Treatment*, **8**, 249–261.

Culliford, L. (2007*a*) Taking a spiritual history. *Advances in Psychiatric Treatment*, **13**, 212–219.

Culliford, L. (2007*b*) *Love, Healing and Happiness: Spiritual Wisdom for Secular Times*. O Books.

Culliford, L. (2009) Teaching spirituality and health care to third-year medical students. *The Clinical Teacher*, **6**, 22–27.

Dagi, T. (1995) Prayer, piety, and professional propriety: limits on religious expression in hospitals. *Journal of Clinical Ethics*, **6**, 274–279.

Department of Health (2006) *From Values to Action: the Chief Nursing Officer's Review of Mental Health Nursing*. Department of Health.

Eagger, S. (2006) *A Short Guide to the Assessment of Spiritual Concerns in Mental Healthcare*. Royal College of Psychiatrists (http://www.rcpsych.ac.uk/PDF/DrSEaggeGuide.pdf).

Egan, M. & DeLaat, D. (1997) The implicit spirituality of occupational therapy practice. *Canadian Journal of Occupational Therapy*, **64**, 115–121.

Ellison, C. W. (1983) Spiritual well-being: conceptualization and measurement. *Journal of Psychology and Theology*, **11**, 4.

Ellison, C. G. & Levin, J. (1998) The religion–health connection: evidence, theory and future directions. *Health Education and Behavior*, **25**, 700–720.

Faulkner, A. (1997) *Knowing Our Own Minds: a Survey of How People in Emotional Distress Take Control of Their Lives*. Mental health Foundation.

Fetzer Institute/National Institute on Ageing Working Group (1999) *Multidimensional Measurement of Religiousness/Spirituality for Use in Health Research*. Fetzer Institute.

Fitchett, G. (1993) The 7 × 7 model for spiritual assessment. In *Assessing Spiritual Needs: a Guide for Caregivers* (ed. J. Hemenway). Augsburg Fortress.

Fontana, D. (2003) *Psychology, Religion and Spirituality*. BPS Blackwell.

Fowler, J. (1981) *Stages of Faith*. Harper and Row.

Govier, I. (2000) Spiritual care in nursing: a systematic approach. *Nursing Standard*, **14**, 32–36.

Greasley, P., Chiu, L. F. & Gartland, Rev. M. (2001) The concept of spiritual care in mental health nursing. *Journal of Advanced Nursing*, **33**, 629–637.

Grof, S. (2000) *Psychology of the Future: Lessons from Modern Consciousness Research*. State University of New York Press.

Hall, T. W. & Edwards, K. J. (1996) The initial development and factor analysis of the Spiritual Assessment Inventory. *Journal of Psychology and Theology*, **24**, 233–246.

Hatch, R. M., Burg, M. A., Naberhaus, D. S., *et al* (1998) The Spiritual Involvement and Beliefs Scale: development and testing of a new instrument. *Journal of Family Practice*, **46**, 476–486.

Hay, D. & Hunt, K. (2000) *Understanding the Spirituality of People Who Don't Go to Church: a Report on the Findings of the Adults' Spirituality Project*. University of Nottingham.

Hill, P. & Hood, R. Jr (1999) *Measures of Religiosity*. Religious Education Press.

Hodge, D. (2000) Spiritual ecomaps: a new diagrammatic tool for assessing marital and family spirituality. *Journal of Marital and Family Therapy*, **26**, 229–240.

Hodge, D. (2001*a*) Spiritual assessment: a review of major qualitative methods and a new framework for assessing spirituality. *Social Work*, **46**, 203–214.

Hodge, D. (2001*b*) Spiritual genograms: a generational approach to assessing spirituality. *Families in Society*, **82**, 35–48.

Hodge, D. (2004) Spirituality and people with mental illness: developing spiritual competency in assessment and intervention. *Families in Society*, **85**, 36–44.

Hodge, D. (2005) Spiritual lifemaps: a client-centred pictorial instrument for spiritual assessment, planning and intervention. *Social Work*, **50**, 77–87.

King, M., Speck, P. & Thomas, A. (1995) The Royal Free interview for religious and spiritual beliefs: development and standardisation. *Psychological Medicine*, **25**, 1125–1134.

Koenig, H., McCullough, M. E. & Larson, D. B. (2001) *Handbook of Religion and Health*. Oxford University Press.

Koenig, H. (2002) *Spirituality in Patient Care: Why, How, When and What*. Templeton Foundation Press.

Levin, J. (2001) *God, Faith and Health*. John Wiley & Sons.

Maugans, T. A. (1996) The SPIRITual history. *Archives of Family Medicine*, **5**, 11–16.

McSherry, W. (2000) *Making Sense of Spirituality in Nursing Practice*. An Interactive Approach. Churchill Livingstone.

McSherry, W. (2001) Spiritual crisis? Call a nurse. In *Spirituality in Healthcare Contexts* (ed. H. Orchard). Jessica Kingsley.

Meaden, A. & Farmer, A. (2006) A comprehensive approach to assessment in rehabilitation settings. In *Enabling Recovery: the Principles and Practice of Rehabilitation Psychiatry* (eds G. Roberts, S. Davenport, F. Holloway, *et al*). Gaskell.

Narayanasamy, A. (2001) Spiritual needs with prompt questions. In *Spiritual Care: A Practical Guide for Nurses and Healthcare Practitioners*. Quay Books.

Nathan, M. M. (1997) *A Study of Spiritual Care in Mental Health Practice: Patients' and Nurses' Perceptions* (MSc thesis). Middlesex University.

Neelman, J. & King, M. (1993) Psychiatrists' religious attitudes in relation to their clinical practice: a survey of 231 psychiatrists. *Acta Psychiatrica Scandinavica*, **88**, 420–424.

Nolan, P. & Crawford, P. (1997) Towards a rhetoric of spirituality in mental health care. *Journal of Advanced Nursing*, **26**, 289–294.

Plante, T. & Thoresen, C. (eds) (2007) *Spirit, Science and Health: How the Spiritual Mind Fuels Physical Wellness*. Praeger.

Poole, R. & Higgo, R. (2006) *Psychiatric Interviewing and Assessment*. Cambridge University Press.

Post, S. G., Puchalski, C. M. & Larson, D. B. (2000) Physicians and patient spirituality: professional boundaries, competency and ethics. *Annals of Internal Medicine*, **132**, 578–583.

Puchalski, C. & Larson, D. (1998) Developing curricula in spirituality and medicine. *Academic Medicine*, **73**, 970–974.

Puchalski, C. & Romer, A. (2000) Taking a spiritual history allows clinicians to understand patients more fully. *Journal of Palliative Medicine*, **3**, 129–137.

Rauch, J. (1993) *Assessment: a Sourcebook for Social Work Practice*. Families International.

Reed, P. (1992) An emerging paradigm for the investigation of spirituality in nursing. *Research in Nursing and Health*, **15**, 349–357.

Ross, L. (1998) The nurse's role in spiritual care. In *The Spiritual Challenge of Healthcare* (eds M. Cobb & V. Robshaw). Churchill Livingstone.

Royal College of Psychiatrists (2006) *Spirituality and Mental Health* (*Help is at Hand Series* leaflet). Royal College of Psychiatrists.

Schermer, V. L. (2003) *Spirit and Psyche: A New Paradigm for Psychology, Psychoanalysis and Psychotherapy*. Jessica Kingsley Publishers.

Slade, N. (2004) Heavenbound. In *Spirituality and Mental Health: Breakthrough* (eds P. Barker & P. Buchanan-Barker). Whurr.

Swinton, J. (2001) *Spirituality and Mental Health Care: Rediscovering a Forgotten Dimension*. Jessica Kingsley.

Tacey, D. (2006) Spirituality and the future of health. *Journal of the Scientific and Medical Network*, **91**, 7–10.

Thoresen, C. (1999) Spirituality and Health: is there a relationship? *Journal of Health Psychology*, **4**, 291–300.

Vega, S. (1989) *Spiritual Emergence or Psychosis?* Spirit Moving (http://www.spiritmoving. com/papers/SpiritPsychosis.htm).

White, G. (2006) *Talking about Spirituality in Healthcare Practice*. Jessica Kingsley.

Useful websites

AA 12 Steps: http://www.alcoholics-anonymous.org.uk/geninfo/05steps.htm

Alcoholics Anonymous: http://www.alcoholics-anonymous.org.uk/

American Academy of Family Physicians, HOPE Questionnaire: http://www.aafp.org/afp/20010101/81.html

Gamblers Anonymous: http://www.gamblersanonymous.org.uk/

George Washington Institute for Spirituality and Health: http://www.gwish.org/

Janki Foundation 'Values in Healthcare' programme: http://www.rcpsych.ac.uk/pdf/JankiValue.pdf and http://www.jankifoundation.org/ values_healthcare/index.php

Narcotics Anonymous: http://www.ukna.org/

Royal College of Psychiatrists Spirituality and Psychiatry Special Interest Group: http://www.rcpsych.ac.uk/college/specialinterestgroups/spirituality.aspx

Spiritual Competency and Resource Centre:
http://www.spiritualcompetency.com/assess_spirit/ASrshx.asp

The University of Minnesota's Center for Spirituality and Healing (online learning about spirituality in healthcare and a module on taking a spiritual history): http://www.csh.umn.edu/modules/index.html

CHAPTER 3

Psychosis

Susan Mitchell and Glenn Roberts

My mind fills me.

The Madwoman of Cork, Patrick Galvin (1996)

Both spirituality and psychosis stretch reason to its limits. They share a sense of mystery and each is notoriously difficult to define. Yet, although psychosis lies at the heart of psychiatry, psychiatrists have often dismissed or regarded with distrust spirituality that is valued by many of their patients. Every psychiatrist practising in general adult, forensic or rehabilitation specialties will be familiar with the daily struggle to make sense of, and progress with, people who have psychosis and to support their personal journeys towards recovery. We will consider how spiritual perspectives may be relevant to this clinical work.

Models of health, disease and recovery

Psychiatry as a medical discipline is sometimes pejoratively regarded as 'hostage' to a medical model that regards all illnesses as somatic, caused at some level by bodily malfunction and giving pre-eminence to biological and drug remedies. In trying to understand the relationship between spirituality and psychosis, such categorical explanatory models can be misleading as they tend either to ignore the spiritual or to see it as an addition to other aspects. Although a more balanced and holistic bio-psychosocial approach has evolved, this may still leave little place for the spirit and indeed can itself be hard to uphold. 'We have allowed the bio-psychosocial model to become the bio-bio-bio model' (Sharfstein, 2005).

Cullberg (2006) argues cogently that a humanistic view is compatible with a biological approach and there is now an increasing understanding of trauma, environment and social isolation – things that may adversely affect the spirit – as playing part both in the aetiology and management of psychosis (Read *et al*, 2004; Cullberg, 2006). In the UK, a number of agencies, the National Institute for Mental Health (2003), Rethink (2005), the Mental Health Foundation (2006), the user movement and a vanguard of mental health professionals with personal experience of psychosis have all contributed to raising awareness of spiritual issues in psychosis. Spirituality is also important within the growing international recovery movement (Care Services Improvement Partnership *et al*, 2007; Lukoff, 2007*b*); this includes the New Zealand Mental Health Commission's recognition that in Maori culture spirituality is considered the most essential requirement for health, and the incorporation of a holistic assessment which includes spirituality in the clinical practice of Maori services (the Te Whare Tapa Wha model, Durie, 2001).

Making sense of spirituality and psychosis

> Man lives in three dimensions: the somatic, the mental, and spiritual. The spiritual dimension cannot be ignored, for it is what makes us human.

> Victor Frankl (1973)

Man is a social being with complex relationships within family, groups, culture and environment; we see all of these as interrelated and traversed by the human spirit. Whatever we believe its substance to be, the spirit energises, connects and searches for meaning and purpose in life. Spirituality is the expression of that energy – the inner workings of the spirit. We trust that our view of spirituality is not confined to any particular tradition but that it is broadly inclusive.

Early heroic fables and religious myths speak of gods, spirits and 'madness' as both fate and punishment – humankind, powerless before incomprehensible forces, saw madness in spiritual terms, a mystery explained by a mystery. Equally old are the fears and suspicions that surround madness, both a fear of the mad and a fear of becoming mad oneself.

How do we understand psychosis now? As a thought experiment we might apply the definition of spirituality presented in chapter 1 (p. 4) to psychosis:

> [Psychosis] is a distinctive, potentially creative and universal dimension of human experience arising ... within the inner subjective awareness of individuals. It may be experienced as relationship with that which is intimately 'inner', immanent and personal, within the self and others, and/ or as relationship with that which is wholly 'other', transcendent and beyond the self. It is experienced as being of fundamental or ultimate importance and is thus concerned with matters of meaning and purpose in life, truth and values.

We do not, however, suggest that spirituality and psychosis are the same thing. The immanent nature of spirituality is such that you may not 'notice' it, both within yourself and others, unless you first allow for the possibility that it exists, whereas it is hard to ignore psychosis with its external confusion and distress, quiet private turmoil or self-satisfied grandiosity. In both the form and content there may be many overlaps and phenomenological equivalences but in terms of consequences spirituality and psychosis are different. Our exercise does, however, help to underline that in psychosis (madness) and in spirituality we are considering human experiences that contain elements of mystery.

What do we mean by spirituality?

The Tao that can be named is not the eternal Tao
The name that can be named is not the eternal name

Lao-Tzu (*c.* 604–531 BC)

These opening lines from the *Tao Te Ching* ('The Book of the Way') capture the difficulty of defining the ineffable quality of spirituality. There is in all beings something (a spiritual quality) that goes beyond what we can measure or define – an aspect that is an awareness of the transcendental or the 'divine'. For many people spirituality is reflected in their religious practice, for others it may be in something else such as music, poetry, nature or art. Wittgenstein, a devastating critic of conventional religious language, nevertheless recognised the mystic sense as the sense of the totality. 'I am not a religious man but I cannot help seeing every problem from a religious point of view' (in Drury, 1981: p. 94). This spiritual quality is as valid for the psychiatric patients as it is for us doctors.

Spirituality need not be the preserve of religion. Our understanding is that the spiritual – the sense of the totality – is pre-eminent and inclusive and that the guiding purpose of all religions is to connect us to the spiritual (Remen, 1993). Some find a 'spiritual home' in organised religion. For others, it is oppressive and may have a negative connotation or be linked with abusive experiences. Even for those committed to religion, its organised form may have negative as well as positive aspects; the person may feel guilt that they need something more than their faith to sustain them or may experience their religious group as stigmatising or rejecting. Thus, service user accounts of recovery confirm the importance of a safe and satisfactory spiritual home.

What is a psychotic experience?

Patients' narratives of the experience of psychosis (Lukoff, 1991; Chadwick, 2001; May, 2004) as well as accounts by psychiatrists (Jaspers, 1963; Hinshelwood, 2004; Cullberg, 2006) give good descriptions from both subjective and objective perspectives and are recommended reading for all who want to understand their patients and the inner world of psychosis. If an individual has never personally experienced psychosis, then the closest they may get to this is probably in dreams (Cullberg, 2006: p. 34).

Delusions, either well-formed or of a more fleeting nature, are characteristic of psychosis. They are usually accompanied by fear, generated both by the experience and because the person is afraid he or she may not be believed, if they share their beliefs with others, whether family members or professionals. Madness can appear as a perplexing constellation of odd experiences, perceptions and beliefs, developing over time through a number of steps and stages and susceptible to many influences. In practice, much of the prodromal stage is concealed from view and other stages will be repeated as the process continues. Accounts of this earliest phase that marks the transition between having a firm grip on consensual reality and the beginning of delusional and hallucinatory experiences, have been described as a breakdown of gestalt perception (Cutting, 1989).

Matters of meaning and purpose – a sense of coherence

> Man needs a faith, a hope and a purpose to live by and to give meaning and dignity to his existence.
>
> Theodosius Dobzhansky (1967)

'[Spirituality] is experienced as being of fundamental or ultimate importance and is thus concerned with matters of meaning and purpose in life, truth and values' (Cook, 2004), the very elements at the core of the psychotic experience (Jaspers, 1963). Psychosis often arises in adolescence or early adult life, when the individual is developing a sense of self (schizophrenia has been called the 'sickness of the self'; Cullberg, 2006: p. 127), questioning established certainties, myths and beliefs; exploring or experimenting with new ones and seeking their own sense of purpose and meaning; grappling with the conflicting demands of external expectations and opportunities while at the same time trying to fathom the internal world. Psychosis is also found disproportionally in both first- and second-generation migrants (Hutchinson & Haasen, 2004), who often find themselves in a new and challenging external reality in terms of language, culture and social support.

In psychosis, meaning and purpose may become distorted. The elaboration of delusional beliefs into systems, in which it is possible for the person to reconfigure their identity, is often significantly accompanied by a subjective experience of meaning and purpose – the 'comforts of madness'(Roberts, 1991). A person with grandiose delusions of a divine nature (being the Messiah or the Buddha) may, in their search for meaning, have interpreted a belief that there is 'that of' the Christ or the Buddha in everyone in a concrete and personal way so that they now believe themselves an incarnation of that divinity (Lukoff, 1991) (case study 3.1).

Case study 3.1

Alan, a friendless man living in poverty, believed himself to be an un-empowered Messiah and was waiting to be called forward as the Second Coming. He attended church each week, staying near the altar so as to receive the genuflections of communicants as worship. He believed that the many tourists that filled his town in the summer were his pilgrims.

People can develop beliefs woven out of their psychotic experiences that amount to a form of fundamentalism; they have become believers in a 'religion' of their own making and for which they are the only adherent. These beliefs can be tenaciously sustained in the face of all kinds of disconfirming information and experiences that such individuals find a way of transmuting into confirmation (case study 3.2).

Case study 3.2

Michael, a musician, struggling to get a tune out of the ward piano, believes that 'they' must have broken his fingers when he was 'in captivity'. He complains that as a consequence he can no longer reach the keys. He does not recognise that he is hopelessly out of practice, anxious and distracted, and continues to feel traumatised by his sojourn in the police station prior to admission.

Creating extreme certainty and purpose

> Survival in extreme circumstances depends upon one's being able to find a meaning in one's suffering.
>
> Irvin Yalom (1980: p. 446)

In the early stage of psychosis, the turmoil of the disintegrative experience – 'pre-psychotic panic' – is extremely unpleasant. It is accompanied by the fracturing of previously accepted patterns of meaning and an uncanny sense of strangeness and significance known as 'delusional mood'. This state of distressing perplexity then begins to resolve with the emergence of delusions as the new meanings attributed to the changed view of the world. At this point in the development of psychosis, a person's perception of his or her world can be turned 'inside out' – 'from a neglected, peripheral person without any power to make an impression on the world, that person suddenly becomes its centre', to which Cullberg (2006: p. 52) applies 'Conrad's picturesque label of the *Copernican revolution*', as vividly described in Peter Chadwick's personal account of his psychotic crisis (Chadwick, 2007).

Delusions and hallucinations that were frightening and destructive in the pre-psychotic phase can become central within a changed 'perspectival world' (Cox & Theilgaard, 1994). The person can have a tenuous but committed sense of 'I know what is going on' – a conviction not easily rescinded. For some, these are brief or temporary states and for others these initial delusional constructions are elaborated and developed into whole systems of belief, which can become complex and provide a basis for progressive reconstruction of the individual's identity, meaning and purpose. Understanding this confusing and contradictory process is important not only in approaches to early intervention in psychosis but

43

also in the later stages of recovery; as a patient caught in this confusion of perspectives explains:

> There are days when I wonder if it might not be more humane to leave the schizophrenic patient to his world of unreality, not to make him go through the pain it takes to become part of humanity. These are the days when the pain is so great. I think I might prefer the craziness until I remember the immobilising terror and the distance and isolation that keeps the world so far away and out of focus. It is not an easily resolved dilemma [Anonymous, 1986: p. 70].

The idea that paranoid delusions may be defensive or protective for the individual against the turmoil of their inner chaos is not new (Cullberg, 2006). It was first discussed by early psychoanalysts (Tausk, 1933) and more recently by behavioural psychologists. Bentall (2004) has described how, in the face of adversity, repeated resort to external personal attributions can lead to a paranoid world view, yet may also preserve self-esteem. The desperate attempts of a paranoid young man to maintain his delusional system, resisting all attempts by parents and doctors to break this down, now become more understandable. Breaking down his belief structure would expose him to renewed internal chaos. In clinical practice it is not unusual for a person to become depressed in the early stages of recovery, when giving up the certainty of firmly held beliefs to embrace the uncertainty of a more realistic world view. This could be seen as reconnecting in a spiritual sense; facing, accepting, owning and reconciling to reality and finding a true and wholesome place in the real world through relationships and interaction (Randall *et al*, 2003).

When, as part of a research study, 17 people with long-standing complex systems of delusional belief were asked to imagine what it would be like to recover or 'go sane', 14 gave a range of strongly felt negative answers and collectively they considered the prospective loss of their beliefs as very threatening (Roberts, 1991). Eight people said they would have nothing to live for or that they would be destroyed, for eight others the prospect was 'terrible', 'depressing' or 'frightening', five anticipated feeling futility, emptiness, bleakness or becoming inert or destitute, three felt that they would be cut off from others and two believed they would go 'mad'.

This paradoxical finding of meaning and purpose in delusional belief (illness) and anticipation of emptiness and futility on recovery is consistent with Jaspers' warning about the predicament of the very mad, whose world has changed and whose existential fulfilment is in their beliefs, 'so that a changed knowledge of reality so rules and pervades it that any correction would mean a collapse of Being itself, in as far as it is for him his actual awareness of existence' (1963: p. 105). Sims expressed a compassionate concern for people in a process of awakening to reality:

> As the delusions fade, the patient may gain insight and regard them as false beliefs 'due to the illness'. Such a person needs help in accepting himself as a fit repository for his own self-confidence once more. He may feel himself to be damaged, vulnerable and untrustworthy and suffer a massive loss of self-esteem [2003: p. 142].

Such 'awakening' on the threshold of 'going sane' may be a necessary preliminary to true recovery – and is supported by a belief in the person (even if not by an assent to their beliefs). It is an important spiritual principle to uphold a sense of value and significance for people during a crisis of losing faith with their psychosis.

Understanding the religious or spiritual delusion – a search for meaning?

> Men have lost their reason in nothing so much as in their religion.
>
> Sir Thomas Browne (1658)

The language and form of spirituality and religion are endemic in expressions of psychosis. Many patients present with delusions of a religious nature (even if they themselves do not practise a religion) and religious patients when they develop psychosis are very likely to express themselves through the language and imagery of their beliefs. We must beware of making assumptions about religious beliefs. The psychiatrist, like a good detective, barrister or journalist needs to be prepared to investigate background relevant to each individual case (perhaps including research of a religious text). An understanding of different cultures, myths and symbols, narrative and story-making and a capacity to work in metaphor are all helpful. The complex delusional system built up by a patient born on 6 June 1966 may make some sense, if the doctor is familiar with the New Testament (Book of Revelation) and the significance of the Number of the Beast (Revelation 13:18). Similarly, the act of cutting off his own feet by a Muslim becomes more understandable with some knowledge of the Qur'an (5:33).

Many scholars, Freud (1927) and Dawkins (2006) included, have regarded religious beliefs as delusions, on the basis that religion is inherently fabricated and therefore beliefs associated with it are also false. But current psychiatric convention is that beliefs shared by people with a similar religious or cultural background are not delusions, although they may be accompanied by the same phenomenological characteristics as delusion – 'a belief firmly held on inadequate grounds ... not arrived at through normal processes of logical thinking' (Gelder et al, 1996: p. 9). Delusion is the cardinal symptom of insanity; the great majority of religious believers with their creeds and congregations are recognisably different from people with psychotic illness who are alone with their idiosyncratic and isolating beliefs. The mad and the religious may share some properties in both the content and the process by which they hold their beliefs but that does not make them the same.

In the case of psychotic religious delusions, the beliefs are not generally shared with the religious or cultural group. Particular difficulties may arise, however, where the origin and resolution of the delusional beliefs held by an individual and their religious community are in conflict with conventional psychiatric practice and will need sensitive handling (case study 3.3).

Case study 3.3

Anna, a taxi driver, was admitted to a psychiatric unit, having driven her car through a hedge and down a steep bank, fortunately without injury. Her explanation was that she had swerved to avoid 'an evil nun' walking across the road in the twilight. She had become increasingly depressed in response to various life difficulties and the experience of fleeting robed 'presences' that continued on the ward distressed and puzzled her. She had no explanation of what those 'presences' were or why they had come to her but was convinced they were evil. She sought support from the hospital chaplain, who was also the bishop's advisor on health and healing. He suggested prayers for deliverance. The patient was keen to pursue this and after careful thought the clinical team were willing to work alongside this wish. They sat with Anna through a quiet and respectful service of spiritual deliverance. To the patient's relief and the staff's surprise, it worked; she felt better and reported that the 'evil nuns' had left. She remained well and was able to leave hospital. A few weeks later, however, these experiences had returned, as had other symptoms of psychotic depression, all of which this time responded to conventional psychiatric treatments.

Malevolent spirits, devils and evil: the dark side to the spirit

Much of the current interest in spirituality in mental health relates to the benefit that attention to spiritual matters can bring. Yet, our clinical practice brings us into contact with people who are distressed by their psychosis and those for whom spiritual experiences are not positive. The certainties of the psychotic world may be ruled by devils and evil spirits. In times past, the association of madness with evil led to harmful and inhumane treatment. Are we any clearer in the way we deal with this issue now?

The Church of England's present policy on exorcism explicitly requires those licensed by their bishops to conduct such rites to consider the possibility of mental disorder and first seek appropriate professional advice. This cautious practice arose from the consequences of naively attributing supernatural causes to mental disorder and of embarking on spiritual remedies with someone who was mentally ill, to the detriment of their condition. Delusional assertions may be understandable in terms of the individual's past life experience, but that is a different matter to simply regarding one as caused by the other (Roberts, 2006).

It is wholly unjustifiable to identify all evil in the world with any specific psychiatric symptom or complaint – even if a person with psychosis is disposed to so identify themselves. To collude with such self-attributions is of itself a form of inhumanity and abuse. Besides, the great majority of both perpetrators and victims of 'evil' do not go on to experience severe mental illness.

If we accept that for many people organised religion can be a relatively safe container or channel for their spirituality, it is also reasonable to ask whether some forms of religion are more likely to promote harmful rather than beneficial spirituality. Pathological spirituality will be considered in more detail in chapter 13, but some issues merit consideration here. Is there a link between less tolerant and more dogmatic forms of religion and malign manifestations of spirituality? In a cult the person may be subjected to a high degree of control by a leader who prevents any contact with the outside world. The drive of 'true belief' (rather than the seeming uncertainty of compassion) may lead to various kinds of cruelty and operate as a justification for stigma, discrimination and subsequent measures against the 'others'. Conversely, the *Intentional Peer Support* (Mead, 2005) for people with severe mental health problems enquires how people become separated, stigmatised and subject to the destructive beliefs of those with power, a process described as being 'othered'.

Impact of psychosis on the spirit: the discomforts of madness

We have touched on some of the confirming, compensatory or consoling aspects of psychotic experience as 'the comforts of madness', but more commonly psychosis is a state of disruption and disturbance with a negative impact on the spirit – characterised by immobilising terror, distance and isolation. The isolation that the psychotic experience can bring is too often compounded by the way in which mental health services are delivered. This can have a negative impact on the spiritual life of both the patient and their family or carers.

Diagnosis and discernment – spiritual considerations

The process of reaching a diagnosis is one of discernment (perceiving and knowing apart) – the doctor, student or teacher brings to his or her meeting with the patient a diagnostic framework and a set of working definitions to guide and help his or her thinking. Even so, in psychosis there remains the challenge of making some sense of the symptoms (psychopathology) in order to reach a diagnosis (concept of illness) that corresponds to the pragmatic structure and classification adopted both in the teaching and training of psychiatry and in the worldwide collection of data, as set out in the DSM–IV (American Psychiatric Association, 1994) and the ICD–10 (World Health Organization, 1992), anthologies of internationally agreed names and patterns.

How should we construe and respond to psychosis? How does our response to psychosis condition how we construe it? Here is the dilemma: as soon as we construe psychosis (part of the individual's experience) as an 'it', we risk losing connection with the person, ceasing to see them as an individual in their own existential context (Buber, 1923; Laing, 1959). This should not be confused with an important mediator of recovery – the patient's ability to gain a sense of personal identity separate from their own illness (Strauss, 1994).

47

Both clinicians and spiritual advisors need the humility to give value to the unusual experiences of others, holding concepts and conceptualisations tentatively while allowing for new information to arise and patterns and attributions to shift. We should consider the possibility that a person might be having both a spiritual and a psychotic experience or the possibility that in psychosis, at the limits of reason, there may be a crack that lets the light in.[1] Jaspers (1963: p. 108) comments that 'religious experience remains what it is whether it occurs in saint or psychotic or whether the person in whom it occurs is both at once'.

The work of David Lukoff (Lukoff *et al*, 1998), a psychologist who himself had a psychotic experience, has been important in promoting awareness of spiritual issues in the USA, both by providing training and by helping to clarify some diagnostic problems (see Spiritual Competency Resource Centre website, www.spiritualcompetency.com). In 1985, he proposed a diagnostic category of 'mystical experience with psychotic features' for intense spiritual experiences that present as psychotic-like episodes (Lukoff, 1985*b*). Mystical experience with psychotic features was proposed as a V-code, denoting that this was a 'normal reaction', analogous to uncomplicated bereavement. It was eventually included in DSM–IV as religious or spiritual problem (V62.89), a non-pathological category which 'can be used when the focus of clinical attention is a religious or spiritual problem'. Examples include distressing experiences that involve loss or questioning of faith, problems associated with conversion to a new faith, or questioning of other spiritual values which may not necessarily be related to an organised church or religious institution (American Psychiatric Association 1994: p. 685). This allows for the recognition of spiritual problems without having to pathologise them. In ICD–10, the diagnostic manual used in the UK, there is only a pathological category (F44.3) for trance and possession disorders as a subsidiary category of dissociative disorders, formerly called hysteria. These are classified as disorders in which 'there is a temporary loss of both the sense of personal identity and full awareness of the surroundings'; in some instances the individual acts as if taken over by another personality, spirit, deity or 'force' but includes only trance disorders 'that are involuntary or unwanted, and which intrude into ordinary activities by occurring outside (or being a prolongation of) religious or other culturally accepted situations' (World Health Organization, 1992).

'Spiritual practice-related experiences' with psychotic features are included as one category of visionary spiritual experience by Lukoff *et al* (1998) and it seems possible that those who engage in New Age spiritual practices without a supportive structure may be more vulnerable to psychotic breakdown (Lukoff, 2007*a*).

---

1   The Baptist Minister, John Martin, proclaimed that if Blake was 'cracked', 'his is a crack that lets in the Light' (Bentley, 2001).

Madness as a spiritual journey?

Mysticism and the characteristics of mystical experiences have been defined in chapter 1. Mystics of different religious faiths have long been known to have psychotic experiences; this neither confirms nor invalidates their spiritual standing. James (1902: p. 29) observes that 'a religious life exclusively pursued, does tend to make the person exceptional and eccentric … religious geniuses have often shown symptoms of nervous instability … subject to abnormal psychical visitations'. Mystical experiences are not uncommon in the population and they may be reported more frequently by people with certain abnormalities of personality, notably schizotypy (Day & Peters, 1999; Jackson, 2001).

Are there any phenomenological differences between the voices and visions of the mystic and the psychotic that would unequivocally distinguish one from the other? A number of studies (Greenberg *et al*, 1992; Jackson & Fulford, 1997; Saver & Rabin, 1997) have found it impossible to differentiate between mystical experiences and psychosis solely on the basis of phenomenological description. Peters (2001) concludes that the overall findings of these and other studies support the idea of a continuum from normality to psychosis and the need to consider the multidimensionality of delusional beliefs. In general, little difference is found between the beliefs and experiences of a person with psychosis and a spiritual person in form or content but it is the way in which the experiences are evaluated that distinguishes them. We share the view that there are no clear phenomenological differences that distinguish the psychotic experience from the spiritual one, but that they differ in terms of life consequence. The important issue is therefore the way in which the psychotic phenomena are embedded in the individual values and beliefs: 'it is not what you believe but how you believe it' (Peters, 2001: p. 207).

Jackson & Fulford (2002) acknowledge the limitations of traditional descriptive diagnostic criteria in distinguishing pathological from non-pathological psychotic experiences. They stress the need for an additional evaluative criterion, one that will distinguish medical value from values of other kinds. Buckley (1981), who compared autobiographical accounts of acute mystical experience and schizophrenia, found that the appearance of a powerful sense of noesis, heightening of perception, feelings of communion with 'the divine', and exultation may be common to both states. Distress and unwanted preoccupations characterise psychosis, whereas spiritual experiences may be sought after and are more often associated with positive life changes (Lukoff 1985*a*; Greenberg *et al*, 1992). Jackson, however, observes that the distinction based on whether the experience is life-enhancing or overwhelming and isolating becomes blurred in the longer term; many people see their psychosis 'as part of a process through which they reached, from their perspective, a constructive spiritual reorientation' (Jackson, 2001: p. 183). The kinship and difference between mystical and psychotic states is captured in essence here by Jelaluddin Rumi, a 13th-century Persian Sufi (Barks, 1993):

> The mystic dances in the sun,
> hearing music others don't.
> 'Insanity', they say, those others.
> If so, it's a very gentle,
> nourishing sort.
>
> Rumi

Spiritual elements in therapeutic approaches to psychosis

If the validity of spirituality is affirmed by the growth of such qualities as compassion, humility, patience, goodness and kindness, it is clear that these are not just present in extreme experiences and for the most part develop quietly without them. John of the Cross, a 16th-century Spanish visionary, wrote in what may well be a personal exercise in humility:

> 'it must be noted that all visions, revelations and feelings coming from Heaven, and any thoughts that may proceed from these, are of less worth than the least act of humility. And humility is one of the effects of charity, which esteems not its own things nor strives to attain them; nor thinks evil, save of itself; nor thinks any good thing of itself, but only of others. It is well, therefore, that these supernatural apprehensions should not attract men's eyes, but that they should strive to forget them in order that they may be free' [Peers, 1943: p. 245].

Each of these positive expressions of spirituality (patience, kindness, compassion, humility and goodness) is reflected in all aspects of life; if we provide truly humane care, it will have a spiritual aspect. Spiritual care has been described as 'practical wisdom' (Swinton, 2001). It is not something extra that we do but the application of insight and understanding to all that we do. It is as much a way of being as a way of doing. Therapeutic approaches that enhance creativity, connection and communication for the individual have been shown to improve self-esteem and well-being. Fallot (2001) describes several ways in which spiritual and religious concerns may be integrated into psychosocial rehabilitation services: conducting spiritual assessments; offering spiritually-informed discussion groups; incorporating spiritual dimensions of psychotherapy; and facilitating links to faith communities and spiritual resources.

Every form of therapy has the potential to be spiritual. 'Spirituality' is not a special form of treatment; there are no technical routines that are inherently spiritual. It is the way in which the work is carried out that imparts the spiritual quality. Nonetheless, some treatments come from spiritual or religious enlightenment. Paul Chadwick (2006) has adapted mindfulness within person-based cognitive therapy for people with distressing psychosis – an approach that integrates cognitive therapy, Rogerian person-centred therapy and mindfulness. In small group studies this has shown encouraging reduction in levels of distress (Chadwick, 2005) and further research is in process.

One important aspect of spirituality is transcendence that can be reached through creativity, music or contact with nature. Vincent Van Gogh, writing to his brother Theo, declared: 'I can very well do without God both in my life and in my painting, but I cannot, ill as I am, do without something which is greater than I, which is my life – the power to create' (Van Gogh in Roskill, 1963). The opportunities we offer patients to explore this dimension should remain 'live' and not become just 'therapy' or 'occupation', important as these are. Murray Cox's initiative in bringing Shakespeare, 'this great and amazing libertarian ... shaking his spear at ignorance and talking about spiritual things but in such an open way that you can take it as you like it' (Cox, 1992: p. 32) to offender patients in Broadmoor is an excellent example. Ferris, a forensic psychiatrist at Broadmoor, writes that the process of diagnosing and deciding about treatment 'actively avoids the spiritual aspects or dimensions which something like the play (*Hamlet*) taps' (in Cox, 1992: p. 33).

Narrative therapy – storytelling, being listened to, and gaining new understanding in the process of telling and listening – is important to patients in the process of recovery and to us as physicians. Through this process, meaning and coherence can be regained. Language and meaning, point of view or frame of reference are all important in this. A New Zealand Mental Health Commissioner Julie Liebrich (2002), writes:

> Yes, of *course* I sometimes ask myself am I having a mystical experience or going nuts? Am I walking towards the light or into the dark? But it is *my* question. Not someone else's. And it's *my* answer. Does that matter? Of course it does, because if someone else is defining your personal experience, your status can change overnight from valid to invalid (in-valid). That is very dangerous because then the very *ways* in which you heal might be interpreted as sick too. And no longer available to you' [p. 154].

For a clinician in discussion with Julie Liebrich there are important questions to listen for (or accept as implicit): 'Are you willing to work with or within my frame of reference?' 'Are you willing to understand me on my terms?' 'Will you believe in me, even if you do not agree with me?'

Implications for clinical practice – practical spirituality

Spirituality is often central to mental health service users but usually only peripherally to mental health professionals; indeed, some studies show a bias against spirituality among psychiatrists, psychologists and mental health nurses (Fry, 1998; King & Dein, 1998). Psychiatrists have been viewed as either ignoring or pathologising spiritual experiences and failing to recognise the positive aspects of spirituality (Lukoff *et al*, 1992). Some patients, particularly those with psychosis, report being afraid to discuss spiritual issues with psychiatrists. A recent study (Dinniss *et al*, 2007) suggests that there may be a relationship between the stage of the patient's recovery and the importance they place on spirituality in their lives. Those who are so unwell as to be subject to compulsory care and treatment may be at that stage, in a Maslowian sense, when other matters might appear more important than spiritual ones. Dinniss's study also illustrates some of the difficulties with enquiries about spirituality, depending on how the questions are put. Yet we must be careful about generalisations in dealing with an experience that is so personal (case study 3.4).

Finding out about patients' religious and spiritual background may help us to avoid making premature assumptions (case study 3.5). What is important here is not so much 'taking a history' as reaching a shared understanding; being aware of the difference between 'my story of you' and 'your story of you', with all the complex overtones of author-ity (whose meanings count?) (see Hunter, 1991 for a fuller discussion). For the therapist it is important to keep in mind three questions: 'What is your inner world like?', 'What sustains you?', 'What has your life been like?' And then, together with the patient, to explore how each can be understood in the context of the other (Roberts, 2006).

This collaborative exploration of the religious and spiritual is a dynamic process; meanings may change depending on the severity or stage of the disorder. Yet it can be difficult to maintain this collaboration in the company of a person in the confusion of their psychotic reality and in the pressurised 'unreal' setting of a psychiatric ward. It may be difficult to have any sense of the person's whole psychological reality and only too easy to fall back on

---

Case study 3.4

James, a middle-aged man, had a strong sense of religious vocation and liked to attend mass each day, often acting as acolyte. He believed that divine healing was more important than medication and psychological therapy, which he felt were only half the story. Yet he regularly relapsed severely into a catatonic state either when medication was reduced or if he became an informal patient and stopped taking medication on his own initiative. During relapse his religious beliefs took on an intense delusional quality.

This situation led to tension within the clinical team. Some team members saw his religious beliefs as part of his illness and concluded that he should be medicated and prevented from attending mass (or that it should at least be limited to Sundays). Some wished to facilitate his attendance at mass because they acknowledged his spiritual needs and respected his view that spiritual healing could play a part in his recovery. The tension was resolved by the team agreeing that he needed help in developing and maintaining a balance in his life in order to remain well. The team, having contacted his minister, now help to validate the patient's religious experience and his need for communication with his congregation, while also encouraging other interests that have a more practical, grounding spiritual element (such as gardening, which he has found helpful).

Case study 3.5

During her first pregnancy, Julie, a young lawyer, suffered a recurrence of an earlier depression; she was anxious, fearful and gave up work. As her pregnancy continued, her mood worsened and she began psychotherapy. Before her child was born an interpretation was made in therapy that she was having murderous thoughts towards her unborn child. Her condition deteriorated with the emergence of paranoid delusions that she was being poisoned, which progressed to a serious puerperal psychosis. She had been brought up as a Roman Catholic and, as she later explained, had been taught that thoughts could have the moral culpability of actions. She believed that she had killed her unborn child. Once she recovered she was very apprehensive about further psychotherapy and believed that the therapist had not taken enough time to find out about her religious beliefs.

a checklist style of interviewing, not really listening (Jackson & Williams, 1994). Fear may make it hard to communicate; there may be aspects of the experience for which there are no words (or for which it is difficult to find words). Hence we may need other 'languages', such as drama, art, literature (especially poetry) and music; some way for the person to turn their pathology round 'in a productive and creative direction' and to 'give oneself over to something bigger and more important than oneself' (Chadwick, 2008: p. 52).

Connection with the non-psychotic, 'sane' aspect of a person when their way of presenting themselves is unfathomable or unacceptable is a key issue in rehabilitation psychiatry and recovery. It is no casual issue that rehabilitation psychiatry and recovery trace their roots back to the pioneering work begun at the Retreat in York in 1796, underpinned by the concept that there is 'that of God' in everyone, irrespective of their degree of sanity. The Retreat began as a place where Quakers could be cared for by fellow Quakers. This element of common values of patients and therapists – a continuity of spiritual dimension – may well have been one of the important factors that created this unique and successful form of what Samuel Tuke (1813), the grandson of the founder William Tuke, termed 'moral treatment', an approach that continues to be reappraised (Thomas & Bracken, 2005).

Exploring the relevance of the controversial concept of 'moral treatment' to contemporary mental health services, Borthwick et al (2001) identified seven basic principles, including a spiritual perspective. These principles highlight the relevance of this perspective especially to the training of professionals and to mental health legislation. Spiritual perspective adds 'an important philosophical and creative aspect to mental health work that invites us to step outside the conventional paradigms to consider the 'larger meanings' of what we experience as human beings' (p. 438).

Spiritual support for journeys in recovery

> Somewhat, to hope for,
> Be it ne'er so far
> Is Capital against Despair –
> Emily Dickinson (1865)

Peter Chadwick (2007) believes that his psychotic crisis 'definitely kindled spiritual sensitivities'. Personal accounts of recovery from serious mental illness regularly refer to the importance of spiritual factors (Leibrich, 1999), from the healing aspects of the psychosis itself to relationships, connections, creativity and storytelling, the things that foster hope and support resilience on the journey to recovery. This could include involvement in a community, whether explicitly spiritual or not, participation in spiritual and religious practices, and having a therapist who is alive to spiritual values. Chadwick (2007) refers to the spiritual dimension of his illness as reinvigorating and enriching of creative and emotional life and states that 'the recognition of the spiritual side of my illness and the taking of it seriously by clinicians and social workers were extremely important in my recovery' (Chadwick, 2001).

A service needs to work with the service users to support their own story and values so that their resilience is strengthened, and that they, rather than the professionals, retain control. 'Personal recovery involves much more than losing symptoms. It involves becoming a person again, regaining a personal life that has some value and meaning' (Whitwell, 2005: p. 158). The impact of a psychotic illness on the life of the individual and their families can be devastating. The disorder can take over and redefine the person (and their family members). The qualities that keep a sense of humanity alive are challenged and often overwhelmed; there is a loss of meaning and purpose, loss of relationships and place in the family, work and society. Unfamiliar and frightening emotions can lead to discomfort and withdrawal, and mental health institutions can be desolate and friendless places. In this situation, 'hope is not just a nice sounding euphemism. It is a matter of life or death' (Deegan, 1996: p. 3). Deegan talks of the importance of relationships in keeping hope alive. Perkins (2006: p. 119), too, acknowledges the importance of relationships – 'hope does not exist in a vacuum' – and emphasises the value of 'hope-inspiring relationships', which include allowing expression of a spiritual dimension.

Patte Randall, a rehabilitation psychiatrist who has herself had psychotic episodes, felt stigmatised and rejected by her profession. She puts it like this:

> I have really questioned, *am I credible, am I worth listening to?* And I think you need to recover that in a relationship, you need someone to enable you to experience again that you have validity and value. You're not an invalid. You're not invalid. You have worth, value, validity, credibility. You mean something to someone else. I don't think you can discover that except in a relationship [Randal, 1999: p. 142].

Cullberg also acknowledges the importance of relationships at the 'turning-point' in recovery.

> In a positive sense to tire of dependence on inner destructive forces and to decide to depend on one's own potential is a process that sometimes bears a resemblance to Christian parables of conversion. Often the event is conveyed through a personal relationship with a carer, a partner or someone who believes in the person's potential and who does it at the right time [Cullberg, 2006: p. 166–167].

Relationships offer vital spiritual support for practitioners as well as for service users. Mental health professionals may sometimes find relationships with their psychotic patients difficult to sustain. It is important that professionals can draw on appropriate support from an individual colleague or from the team to look after their own spiritual well-being.

Spirituality as experienced by the professional faced with psychosis

When working with a group of patients who have been ill and in hospital for many years, and who may have long ago given up hope or any sense of agency for themselves, it is not uncommon for staff members to be affected by the patient's state (case study 3.6). Trying to make the unbearable bearable and sustain the spirit is a practical task (Clever, 1999).

> Mental health professionals also need to maintain and sometimes recover the sense of meaning and fulfilment in their work, the humanity and compassion that first brought them into the field. The day-to-day work in settings that are pressured from many directions can lead to self-protective defences such as emotional detachment, reductive labelling, them-and-us blaming, and retreat to the paperwork [Kennard *et al*, 2007: p. 207].

Despair as well as hope is contagious. Psychiatrists (physicians of the psyche) need to be able to develop the capacity to witness and endure the distress of those with psychosis and to travel the long and complex road to recovery with them, while sustaining an attitude of hope.

'Understanding or Thought is not natural to Man; it is acquir'd by means of Suffering & Distress i.e. Experience' (Blake, 1789, quoted in

---

Case study 3.6

An experienced nurse told the consultant that he was finding it extremely difficult to look after one of his patients. 'I can't go there with her.' What he meant was that the degree of this woman's depression was so profound, so palpable in its pain and distress that it touched on his own past periods of depression too keenly. He was afraid of being dragged down too. Within the team staff members were each struggling to hold on to hope on behalf of this woman who had lost all her own. They were able to share this sense of hopelessness in the staff support group and in so doing regained some hope for her.

Frankl, 1984), as Victor Frankl, Austrian psychotherapist and survivor of Auschwitz, exemplified and described in *Man's Search for Meaning* (1984). Frankl's 'logotherapy' was developed from what he learnt through his own experience of suffering and loss. Too often we do not use our experience to support our colleagues; we grow to accept burnout as a condition of our work (Roberts, 1997).

Teaching, listening and learning

> The lyf so short, the craft so long to lerne

> Geoffrey Chaucer (1380)

Our professional training focuses on valuable technical knowledge, skills and experience, all of which are essential if we are to think clearly about how to help our patients. But we must also have the care and compassion or, as Hebrew Scriptures guide, we must 'do justice, love kindness and walk humbly' (Micah 6:8). Jaspers implied that this range of attributes was the empathic basis of understanding: 'We can have no psychological understanding without empathy into the content (symbols, forms, images ideas) and without seeing the *expression* and sharing the *experienced phenomena*. All these spheres of meaningful objective facts and subjective experience form the matter for understanding' (Jaspers, 1963: p. 311). Empathy, like all our deeper art and communication, includes a spiritual dimension.

From history we learn the things that can de-humanise, that lack spirit and so limit recovery (Cullberg, 2006). We know that isolation, lack of trust and fractured or intensely critical relationships worsen psychotic states. In-patient and community services need to avoid these dangers. An individual is a person, not a diagnosis – their spiritual needs do not change just because a diagnosis has been made (Strauss, 1994). Recovery is about helping the person re-emerge and gain a sense of personal identity separate from their illness.

Conclusion

For working well with people who are struggling with the confusion and suffering of psychosis, we believe in a practical, grounded, 'recovery-oriented' spirituality that incorporates humanity and compassion while accepting the integrity of personal experience. This should be more a matter of:

- values than visions
- love, compassion and kindness than beliefs
- humility and tolerance than knowingness
- spiritual life than religious conformity
- the pursuit of wellness than possessing 'the truth'
- the deep experience of common humanity than allowing unusual experience to separate us.

We have indicated only some of the complexities encountered in the problematic relationship between spirituality and psychosis. We hope we have encouraged our readers to enquire further and to seek answers for themselves to the questions we have raised. The importance of having an awareness of the spiritual in psychiatric practice and our understanding of psychosis will find resonance in other parts of this book. As clinicians who believe that all good medical practice is founded on values that include compassion, honesty and humility, we hope that we have offered some support for a practical spirituality, which will be of help in caring for people with psychosis.

References

American Psychiatric Association (1994) *Diagnostic and Statistical Manual of Mental Disorders* (4th edn) (DSM–IV). APA.

Anonymous (1986) 'Can we talk?' The schizophrenic patient in psychotherapy. *American Journal of Psychiatry*, **143**, 68–70.

Barks, C. (1993) *Rumi. Birdsong: Fifty-three Short Poems* (trans. C. Barks), p. 24. Maypop Books.

Bentall, R. P. (2004) Abandoning the concept of schizophrenia; the cognitive psychology of delusions and hallucinations. In *Models of Madness: Psychological, Social and Biological Approaches to Schizophrenia* (eds J. Read, L. Mosher & R. Bentall), pp. 195–208. Brunner-Routledge.

Bentley, G. E. Jr. (2001) *The Stranger from Paradise: a Biography of William Blake*. Yale University Press.

Blake, W. (1789) Annotations to Swedenborg's Wisdom of Angels concerning divine love and divine wisdom. In *Blake Complete Writings* (1969) (ed. G. Keynes), p. 89. Oxford University Press.

Borthwick, A., Holman, C., Kennard, D., *et al* (2001) The relevance of moral treatment to contemporary mental healthcare. *Journal of Mental Health*, **10**, 427–439.

Browne, Sir T. (1658) Hydriotaphia: Urne Buriall. In *Religio Medici and Other Works* (1964) (ed. L. C. Martin), p. 113. Clarendon Press.

Buber, M. (1923) *I and Thou* (1996) (trans. W. Kaufmann). Simon and Schuster.

Buckley, P. (1981) Mystical experience and schizophrenia. *Schizophrenia Bulletin*, **7**, 516–521.

Care Services Improvement Partnership, Royal College of Psychiatrists & Social Care Institute for Excellence (2007) *A Common Purpose: Recovery in Future Mental Health Services*. SCIE.

Chadwick, P. K. (2001) Sanity to supersanity to insanity: a personal journey. In *Psychosis and Spirituality: Exploring the New Frontier* (ed. I. Clarke), pp. 75–89. Whurr.

Chadwick, P. (2005) Mindfulness groups for people with psychosis. *Behavioural and Cognitive Psychotherapy*, **33**, 351–359.

Chadwick, P. (2006) *Person-Based Cognitive Therapy for Distressing Psychosis*. Wiley & Sons.

Chadwick, P. K. (2007) Peer-professional first-person account: schizophrenia from the inside; phenomenology and the integration of causes and meanings. *Schizophrenia Bulletin*, **33**, 166–173.

Chadwick, P. K. (2008) *Schizophrenia: the Positive Perspective. Explorations at the Outer Reaches of Human Experience* (2nd edn). Routledge.

Chaucer, G. (1380) The parliament of fowls. In *The Works of Geoffrey Chaucer* (1957) (ed. F. N. Robinson), p. 310. Oxford University Press.

Clever, L. (1999) A call to renew: doctors who feel ground down can renew their spirits and their values. *BMJ*, **319**, 1587–1588.

Cook, C. C. H. (2004) Addiction and spirituality. *Addiction*, **99**, 539–551.

Cox, M. (1992) *Shakespeare comes to Broadmoor*. Jessica Kingsley.

Cox, M. & Theilgaard, A. (1994) *Shakespeare as Prompter*. p. 182. Jessica Kingsley.

Cullberg, J. (2006) *Psychoses: an Integrative Perspective*. Routledge.

Cutting, J. (1989) Gestalt theory and psychiatry: discussion paper. *Journal of Royal Society of Medicine*, **82**, 429–431.

Dawkins, R. (2006) *The God Delusion*. Bantam Press.

Day, S. & Peters, E. R. (1999) The incidence of schizotypy in new religious movements. *Personality and Individual Differences*, **27**, 55–67.

Deegan, P. (1996) *Recovery and the Conspiracy of Hope* (conference paper). Pat Deegan & Associates, LLC (http://www.patdeegan.com/pdfs/articles_hope.pdf).

Dickinson, E. (1865) Poem 1041. In *The Complete Poems of Emily Dickinson* (1988) (ed. T. H. Johnson), p. 476. Little, Brown & Co.

Dinniss, S., Roberts, G., Hubbard, C., *et al* (2007) User-led assessment of a recovery service using DREEM. *Psychiatric Bulletin*, **31**, 124–127.

Dobzhansky, T. G. (1967) *The Biology of Ultimate Concern*. New American Library.

Drury, M. O'C. (1981) Some notes on conversations with Wittgenstein. In *Ludwig Wittgenstein, Personal Recollections* (ed. R. Rhees). Blackwell.

Durie, M. (2001) *The Dynamics of Maori Mental Health*. Oxford University Press

Fallot, R. D. (2001) Spirituality and religion in psychiatric rehabilitation and recovery from mental illness. *International Review of Psychiatry*, **13**, 110–116.

Frankl, V. E. (1973) *The Doctor and the Soul: from Psychotherapy to Logotherapy* (trans. R. Winston & C. Winston). Vintage Books.

Frankl, V. E. (1984) *Man's Search for Meaning*. Washington Square Books.

Freud, S. (1927) The future of an illusion. In *The Complete works of Sigmund Freud* (eds J. Strachey & A. Freud). Hogarth Press.

Fry, A. (1998) Spirituality, communication and mental health nursing: the tacit interdiction. *Australian and New Zealand Journal of Mental Health Nursing*, **7**, 25–32.

Galvin, P. (1996) The madwoman of Cork. In *New and Selected Poems of Patrick Galvin*. Cork University Press.

Gelder, M., Gath, D., Mayou, P., *et al* (1996) *Oxford Textbook of Psychiatry* (3rd edn). Oxford University Press.

Greenberg, D., Witztum, E. & Buchbinder, J. T. (1992) Mysticism and psychosis: the fate of Ben Zoma. *British Journal of Medical Psychology*, **65**, 223–235.

Hinshelwood, R. D. (2004) What's it like? Psychoanalytic theories of schizophrenia. In *Suffering Insanity: Psychoanalytic Essays on Psychosis*, pp. 47–105. Brunner-Routledge.

Hunter, K. M. (1991) *Doctors Stories: the Narrative Structure of Medical Knowledge*. Princeton University Press.

Hutchinson, G. & Haasen, C. (2004) Migration and schizophrenia. *Social Psychiatry and Psychiatric Epidemiology*, **39**, 350–357.

Jackson, M. (2001) Psychotic and spiritual experience: a case study comparison. In *Psychosis and Spirituality: Exploring the New Frontier* (ed. I. Clarke), pp. 165–190. Whurr Publishers.

Jackson, M. & Fulford, K. W. M. (1997) Spiritual experience and psychopathology. *Philosophy, Psychiatry & Psychology*, **4**, 41–65.

Jackson, M. & Fulford, K. W. M. (2002) Psychosis good and bad: values-based practice and the distinction between pathological and non-pathological forms of psychotic experience. *Philosophy, Psychiatry and Psychology*, **9**, 387–394.

Jackson, M. & Williams, P. (1994) *Unimaginable Storms: A Search for Meaning in Psychosis*. p. 178. Karnac Books.

James, W. (1902) *The Varieties of Religious Experience (1960)*. Collins Fontana Library.

Jaspers, K. (1963) *General Psychopathology* (trans. J. Hoenig & J. W. Hamilton). Manchester University Press & the University of Chicago Press.

Kennard, D., Fagin, L., Hardcastle, M., *et al* (2007) Things you can do to make in-patient care a better experience. In *Experiences of Mental Health In-Patient Care: Narratives from*

Service Users, Carers and Professionals (eds M. Hardcastle, D. Kennard, S. Grandison, *et al*), pp. 205–207. Routledge.

King, M. B. & Dein, S. (1998) The spiritual variable in psychiatric research. *Psychological Medicine*, **28**, 1259–1262.

Laing, R. D. (1959) *The Divided Self: an Existential Study in Sanity and Madness*. Tavistock Publications.

Lao-Tzu (1988) *Tao Te Ching: the Book of the Way* (trans. S. Mitchell). Kyle Cathie.

Liebrich, J. (1999) *A Gift of Stories: Discovering How to Deal with Mental Illness*. University of Otago Press.

Liebrich, J. (2002) Making space, spirituality and mental health. *Mental Health, Religion and Culture*, **5**, 143–162.

Lukoff, D. (1985a) Transpersonal perspectives on manic psychosis: creative visionary and mystical states. *Journal of Transpersonal Psychology*, **20**, 111–139.

Lukoff, D. (1985b) The diagnosis of mystical experiences with psychotic features. *Journal of Transpersonal Psychology*, **17**, 155–181.

Lukoff, D. (1991) Divine madness: shamanistic initiatory crisis and psychosis. *Shaman's Drum*, **22**, 24–29.

Lukoff, D. (2007a) Visionary spiritual experiences. *Southern Medical Journal*, **100**, 635–641.

Lukoff, D. (2007b) Spirituality in the recovery from persistent mental disorders. *Southern Medical Journal*, **100**, 642–646.

Lukoff, D., Lu, F. & Turner, R. (1992) Towards a more culturally sensitive DSM–IV: psycho-religious and psycho-spiritual problems. *Journal of Nervous and Mental Disease*, **180**, 673–682.

Lukoff, D., Lu, F. & Turner, R. (1998) From spiritual emergency to spiritual problem: the transpersonal roots of the new DSM–IV category. *Journal of Humanistic Psychology*, **38**, 21–50.

May, R. (2004) Making sense of psychotic experiences and working towards recovery. In *Psychological Interventions in Early Psychosis* (eds J. Gleeson & P. McGorry), pp. 245–260. Wiley.

Mead, S. (2005) *Intentional Peer Support: an Alternative Approach*. Shery Mead Consulting.

Mental Health Foundation (2006) *The Impact of Spirituality on Mental Health: a Review of the Literature*. Mental Health Foundation.

National Institute of Mental Health (2003) *Inspiring Hope: Recognising the Importance of Spirituality in a Whole Person Approach to Mental Health*. Care Services Improvement Partnership (http://www.abdn.ac.uk/cshad/documents/spirituality.pdf).

Peers, E. A. (1943) John [De Yepes] of the Cross: the ascent of Mount Carmel, book I, chapter IX. In *The Complete Works*. Burns, Oates & Washbourne.

Perkins, R. (2006) First person: 'you need hope to cope'. In *Enabling Recovery: the Principles and Practice of Rehabilitation Psychiatry* (eds G. Roberts, S. Davenport, F. Holloway, *et al*), pp. 112–124. Gaskell.

Peters, E. (2001) Are delusions on a continuum? The case of religious and delusional beliefs. In *Psychosis and Spirituality: Exploring the New Frontier* (ed. I. Clarke), pp. 191–207. Whurr.

Randall, P. (1999) Loving relationship is at the root of recovery. In *A Gift Of Stories: Discovering How to Deal with Mental Illness* (ed. J. Liebrich). University of Otago Press.

Randall, P., Simpson, A. I. F. & Laidlaw, T. (2003) Can recovery-focused multimodal psychotherapy facilitate symptom and function improvement in people with treatment-resistant psychotic illness? A comparative study. *Australian and New Zealand Journal of Psychiatry*, **37**, 720–727.

Read, J., Goodman, L., Morrison, A., *et al* (2004) Childhood trauma, loss and stress. In *Models of Madness: Psychological, Social and Biological Approaches to Schizophrenia* (eds. J. Read, L. Mosher & R. Bentall), pp. 9–20. Brunner-Routledge.

Remen, N. (1993) On defining spirit. *Noetic Sciences Review*, **27**, 40.

Rethink (2005) *Spirituality and Mental Illness* [factsheet]. Rethink (http://www.mentalhealthshop.org/products/rethink_publications/spirituality_and_men.html).

Roberts, G. A. (1991) Delusional belief systems and meaning in life: a preferred reality? *British Journal of Psychiatry*, **159** (suppl. 14), 19–28.

Roberts, G. A. (1997) Prevention of burn-out. *Advances in Psychiatric Treatment*, **3**, 282–289.

Roberts, G. A. (2006) Understanding madness. In *Enabling recovery: the Principles and Practice of Rehabilitation Psychiatry* (eds G. Roberts, S. Davenport, F. Holloway, *et al*), pp. 93–111. Gaskell.

Saver, J. L. & Rabin, J. (1997) The neural substrates of religious experience. *Journal of Neuropsychiatry and Clinical Neurosciences*, **9**, 495–510.

Sharfstein, S. (2005) Big Pharma and American psychiatry: the good, the bad, and the ugly. *Psychiatric News*, **40**, 3.

Sims, A. (2003) *Symptoms in the Mind: an Introduction to Descriptive Psychopathology* (3rd edn). Elsevier Science.

Strauss, J. (1994) The person with schizophrenia as a person. *British Journal of Psychiatry*, **164** (suppl. 23), 103–107.

Swinton, J. (2001) *Spirituality and Mental Healthcare*. Jessica Kingsley.

Tausk, V. (1933) On the origin of the influencing machine in schizophrenia. *Psychoanalytic Quarterly*, **2**, 519–556. Reprinted in *Essential Papers on Psychosis* (1988) (ed. P. Buckley). New York University Press.

Thomas, P. & Bracken, P. (2005) *Postpsychiatry: Mental Health in a Postmodern World (International Perspectives in Philosophy & Psychiatry)*. Oxford University Press.

Tuke, S. (1813) *Description of the Retreat, an Institution near York for Insane Persons of the Society of Friends*. Reprinted 1996. Process Press.

Van Gogh, V. (1888) Letter to Theo. In *The Letters of Vincent Van Gogh* (1963) (ed. M. Roskill), p. 286. Collins.

Whitwell, D. (2005) *Recovery Beyond Psychiatry*. Free Association Books.

World Health Organization (1992) *The ICD–10 Classification of Mental and Behavioural Disorders*. WHO .

Yalom, L. (1980) *Existential Psychotherapy*. Basic Books.

CHAPTER 4

Suicide

Cherrie Coghlan and Imran Ali

The understanding and management of suicide is a critical part of the practice of psychiatry. Spirituality is concerned with life, death and meaning, and so it may be said that it is concerned with the understanding of suicide. We will approach this vast subject by considering: membership of faith communities and spiritual practices, attitudes to suicide in faith traditions, spirituality and mental anguish, suicide in literature, the question of the meaning of life, spiritual issues in the clinical management of people who have suicidal thoughts, physician-assisted suicide, and the impact of suicide on survivors.

From the legal perspective, suicide was considered in the UK to be a crime, insofar as it was deemed to constitute self-murder. It followed that attempted suicide was attempted murder, which could result in the tragic irony of individuals being punished by death for trying to kill themselves (an example is cited in Alvarez, 2002: p. 63). The law changed in 1961; suicide is now seen as an issue for the helping professions rather than the law.

Religious attitudes to suicide have generally underpinned the legal position and used to be similarly condemnatory. However, these have become more humane over time and the emphasis has shifted to one of compassion for the deceased and support of the bereaved.

The effect of spiritual practices and membership of faith communities on suicide

Émile Durkheim (1858–1917) remains one of the most quoted authors on suicide. He approached it from a social rather than an individual perspective, seeing it as dependent upon factors external to the individual, such as the level of social integration. This was defined along two dimensions: the individual's sense of community and the community's control over the individual, disturbance to the balance of these two factors increasing the chance of suicide. Durkheim described four states that can threaten the equilibrium between the individual and the community: where the bond between the two is too strong, leading to either altruism or fatalism, and where the bond is too weak, resulting in egoism or anomie (Bille-Brahe, 2000).

Durkheim also observed that suicide rates were lower for Catholics than for Protestants and ascribed this to a difference in religious emphasis between the certainty of dogma and the individual conscience. However, Stack (1980) has noted that over recent years those rates have converged. Durkheim found that Judaism, although valuing freedom of thought, was not associated with high suicide rate. He attributed this to the solidarity within Jewish communities, which could come under threat from the wider society.

Masaryk has suggested that a decline in religious practice in the 20th century was associated with higher suicide rates (Masaryk, 1970). This hypothesis has been further explored (Neeleman & Lewis, 1999; Clarke et al, 2003). Neeleman and Lewis postulate that a factor protective in one society may not be so in another, so that cross-cultural studies considering both individual and 'ecological' factors are required to ascertain whether they act separately or together to affect risk, and to consider any interaction between them. They examined a large sample of data from 26 countries from the 'Judeo-Christian' tradition from the point of view of individuals and populations, looking at religiosity (personal beliefs and practices) and church attendance. They found a protective effect of religiosity that was stronger in less religious countries, and that was stronger than church attendance. However, when they further examined other variables such as birth rate, education, divorce and unemployment, religiosity was no longer protective for men except in the least religious countries, although it still was for women. A population study by Clarke et al (2003) in Ireland also found religiosity to have a more protective effect for women than for men. Higher suicide rates were demonstrated in rural than in urban populations, despite their greater religious observance. Belief in a personal God, however, was similar across urban and rural groups despite the decline in religious practice in the urban group. The rate of male suicide was lower in areas of greater religious observance. This finding may reflect community support and/or reduced tolerance of suicidal behaviour.

Neeleman et al (1997) tested whether the negative association between suicide and religion in individuals and countries is mediated by the degree to which death by suicide is tolerated. They considered tolerance against church attendance and socio-demographic factors and found that suicide tolerance was inversely related to all religious beliefs and practices. Religiosity was found to be the key factor affecting suicide rates, and tolerance was only significant as a mediating link between them. Contrary to the findings of Durkheim, Neeleman et al found religiosity to be more important than communal religious observances.

Other studies focus on different traditions. Kohn et al (1997) found generally low rates of suicide among young people in Israel comprising Jewish, Druze, Muslim Arab and Christian Arab groups. Religious affiliation is associated with ethnicity in this study and religiosity is not considered separately. Kamal & Loewenthal (2002), using the Reasons for Living Inventory (Linehan *et al*, 1983), compared small samples of British Hindus and Muslims and found that Hindus endorsed reasons for living less strongly than Muslims. This may be attributable to scriptural differences between the faiths in attitudes to suicide. Despite this finding, there were no significant differences in suicidal thoughts, plans or behaviour between the groups.

Among studies looking at Islam, Simpson & Conklin (1989) in a large-scale study involving an aggregate of suicide rates from 71 countries found a negative correlation between suicide rates and adherence to Islam. Controlling for economic, social and demographic factors, they attribute this to the influence of the religion at an individual and communal level. Cheng & Lee (2000) have suggested that the low suicide rates in Muslim countries could be linked with suicide being viewed as homicide in Islam. Ineichen (1998) also suggested that it may reflect stigma resulting from sinfulness associated with suicide in this religion. Studying suicide rates in Singapore, Peng (1992) noted lower rates for Muslim Malays than for Singaporeans of Chinese and Indian ethnicity. He related this to the Muslim group being less preoccupied by material concerns and more accepting of fate. It is worth noting that in large population studies generally, some degree of bias may possibly result from concealment and under-reporting of suicide.

Koenig *et al* (2001) have examined quantitatively the relationship between suicide and religion. Religious involvement has been measured by frequency of prayer, frequency of religious attendance and the extent of religious salience. Of the 68 studies that examined suicide rate/attitude by religious involvement, 57 (84%) found fewer deaths by suicide and more negative attitudes towards suicide in the more religious, 9 demonstrated no relationship and 2 revealed mixed results. The authors cite a study by Stack considering the benefits of religious commitment, suggesting that it may aid suicide prevention by promoting beliefs in the afterlife and in a loving God, conveying purpose and self-esteem, providing role models for coping with crisis and stress, and development of resources to help with life's difficulties. This is in addition to social support and lower divorce rates in religious individuals.

Faith communities can be involved in government initiatives to prevent suicide. An example of this is the Scottish Choose Life Strategy (The Scottish Executive, 2002), which aims to substantially reduce suicide rates, and which is incorporating work on the training needs of faith communities and religious leaders in responding to death by suicide and suicidal behaviour. Mowat *et al* (2006), also in Scotland, have developed a parish nursing movement (based on an earlier American model by Westberg, in Westberg & McNamara, 1990), in which a specialist nurse is employed by the congregation of which he or she is a member. So far this work has been confined to Christian groups, and research is needed on other faith communities.

Spiritual practice and experience is not confined to religious traditions despite often having historical roots within them. Prayer and meditation are widespread spiritual practices, not exclusive to faith communities, from which people who have depression and suicidal thoughts may benefit. Tacey (2004) writes of the importance of recognising spiritual yearning in young people who do not always relate to conventional religion:

> The problem of youth suicide is intimately connected with the spiritual side of youth experience, and when meaning or truth cannot be found, lives can be broken or lost by the terrible discovery that the spiritual vacuum in society has not been filled by a personal encounter with meaning [Tacey, 2004: p. 179].

Tacey recommends openness of leaders and educators to the value of alternative forms of spirituality, such as those associated with the New Age movement and ecological concern that can resonate more for young people than traditional forms. In a moving single case study, Holt (2004) describes the positive impact of meditation on a physically ill man who had made a determined suicide attempt. Birnbaum & Birnbaum (2004) have also shown that meditation can be a powerful resource for therapists and their clients, with suicidal intentions or otherwise, regardless of whether beneficial insights are experienced as coming from a deeper part of the self or from an external source.

People who have depression and suicidal thoughts have been noted to have a generalised autobiographical memory with less access to specific useful memories that would show them how they have coped with adversity in the past (Williams & Pollock, 2001). Mindfulness-Based Cognitive Therapy (MBCT), developed by Segal, Williams and Teasdale (2002), combines key elements of cognitive therapy with mindfulness training. The latter derives from the work of Kabat-Zinn (1994), which in turn has roots in Buddhism, Taoism and yoga. The mindfulness component of MBCT involves a focus on moment-to-moment experience, appreciating the thought as simply a mental event and observing it with an attitude of non-judgement, while maintaining an awareness of bodily sensation and breathing to which the mind can return. The aim is to reduce the reactivation of destructive patterns of thought by equipping people experiencing depression and suicidal ideation with the skill to observe such thoughts with acceptance but without identification ('I am not my thoughts') and thereby escape from a downward spiral. For people with suicidal thoughts, Williams has suggested an increased emphasis on externally focused mindfulness practices to provide grounding in times of crisis when internal affects can overwhelm. Research on MBCT and suicide continues (Williams *et al*, 2006).

Attitudes to suicide in religious traditions

Despite generally condemnatory views of suicide in religious moral teachings, there is heterogeneity within and between traditions, and mental disorder is usually seen as a mitigating factor.

Suicide in the ancient world

In ancient Greece, there was a taboo against death by suicide, resulting in the corpse being buried outside the city with the hands cut off and buried separately. Alvarez (2002) sees this as a logical extension of a taboo against killing members of one's own family. Pythagoras regarded humans as the chattels of gods who would be angered by the self-destruction of their creation, whereas Aristotle took the more pragmatic view that suicide robs the state of economic contributions.

Plato's account of the death of Socrates suggests that Socrates was opposed to suicide on both these grounds (Holland, 1969; Alvarez, 2002). Although he died by his own hand, it is arguable that Socrates' death was not suicide but a courageous acceptance of the death penalty. He did not choose to die, but neither did he choose to run away. He considered it appropriate to desire death, but not to bring it about deliberately. Unlike his contemporaries, Socrates did not believe that captivity resulted in dishonour, but rather in indignity, and that suffering only implied dishonour if brought about by one's own evil deeds (Holland, 1969). Socrates did not see death as a way of escape from anything: 'if it were, it would indeed be a boon to the wicked' (Holland, 1969: p. 76). He did argue that a life without opportunity for critical thinking was not worth living, and Bille-Brahe (2000) suggests that his ideas about the blessedness of death inspired others to die by suicide.

In ancient Rome, suicide was considered honourable for private citizens and military leaders facing defeat. It was forbidden for ordinary soldiers and for slaves who were the property of their masters.

Suicide in the Judaic and Christian traditions

In studies of biblical suicides, Barraclough (1992) and Koch (2005) describe up to eleven deaths by suicide and possible suicides. The most famous among those who died by or attempted suicide were King Saul, Samson (both in the Old Testament) and Judas Iscariot (in the New Testament). King Saul, defeated in battle and facing humiliation, asked his servant to kill him. One account (1 Samuel 31:1–4)[1] suggests that the servant refused and Saul killed himself; another (2 Samuel 1:1–10) suggests that he was killed by a soldier on request. Samson, who was held captive, blinded and humiliated, pushed against the pillars of the temple, causing the building to collapse, killing himself and his Philistine captors. There are two accounts of Judas's death. In the first (Matthew 27:3–5) he hangs himself; in another (Acts 1:18) he falls to the ground with his abdomen bursting open. In the former account Judas returns the money given for betraying Jesus to the authorities, before hanging himself in anguish and remorse.

The Bible does not specifically condemn suicide (Alvarez, 2002; Koch, 2005), but it is implicitly condemned in the sixth commandment, 'You

---

1   Quotations are from the Bible, New Revised Standard Version.

shall not murder' (Exodus 20:13), and in Genesis 9:5, 'For your lifeblood I will surely require a reckoning'. Both Alvarez and Koch note that actual and possible deaths by suicide are recorded in Hebrew and Christian scriptures in a factual way that neither praises nor condemns the act. The context is generally one of personal crisis and only in the case of Saul is there also evidence of prior mood swings (Barraclough, 1992). Koch (2005) notes that those expressing suicidal ideas are treated with compassion; for example, Sarah is comforted by thoughts of her family and prayer (Tobit 3: pp. 10–16).

The former UK Chief Rabbi, Lord Jakobovits (1988), has written of Judaism's uncompromising attribution of value to human life.

> In Jewish thought and law, human life enjoys an absolute, intrinsic and infinite value. Man is not the owner of his body but merely its custodian, charged to preserve it from any physical harm and to promote its health where this has been impaired [p. 5].

Condemnation of suicide is found most notably in the post-Talmudic tractate of Semachot, which denies formal funeral rites for those who 'destroy themselves' *lada-at*, meaning wittingly (Kaplan & Schoeneberg, 1988). In Judaism, the right to take away life belongs to God alone; to kill oneself is to usurp the divine priority. Suicide also deprives the community. Kaplan & Schoeneberg emphasise that Jewish Law (*Halacha*) is very rigorous in defining suicide. There has to be clear indication that the person acted wittingly. Not only mental illness but behavioural abnormalities and the influence of substances serve to reduce responsibility; what is classified as death by suicide in secular law may therefore not be regarded as such in Jewish law.

In Jewish history, mass suicide at the fort of Masada in AD 70 was seen as a heroic act whereby the entire population under siege by the Romans put themselves to death rather than submit to the absolute destruction of their way of life. During the Second World War, when Europe's Jews suffered decimation in the Holocaust, 'suicide was the conscious decision to end the unendurable: to refuse to remain at the whim of tormentors whose cruelties were sadistically drawn out: to die at one's chosen moment' (Gilbert, 1987: p. 322). When incarcerated, the psychiatrist and Auschwitz survivor Victor Frankl, together with another medical prisoner, set up emergency therapeutic teams to prevent recently arrived fellow prisoners from dying by suicide through shock and despair. The focus was on aiding individuals to find personal or spiritual meaning (Frankl, 1967).

In the Christian tradition, Augustine of Hippo (AD 354–438) first pronounced clearly on the issue of suicide, considering it to be a violation of the sixth commandment. He clashed with the heretical Donatists, who sought death for the glory of martyrdom. In the Christian Church, it has additionally been important to distinguish between martyrdom and suicide. 'Discussions of the morality of suicide are often confused by a failure to distinguish between the willing surrender of one's life and the deliberate taking of it' (Wood, 1986: p. 609).

Augustine's views influenced future scholars, most notably Thomas Aquinas in the 13th century (Alvarez, 2002). Aquinas believed that the act of suicide was a mortal sin, as the final repentance had not been undertaken. Echoing Plato and Aristotle, he argued first that suicide was unnatural, second, that it damaged social community, and third, that life was a gift of God not to be squandered by man, securing the Church's official stance against suicide.

Harsh condemnation of suicide as a sin by the Church was prevalent throughout the Middle Ages. This view influenced the legal status of suicide as a crime. There were, however, exceptions and variations across denominations. An early example of this is John Donne, who did not see suicide as always sinful, but deserving of understanding (Stengel, 1965).

From the age of Enlightenment onwards, Christian attitudes began to change and to question why people die by suicide. The Christian teaching to care for one's neighbour led to an emphasis on prevention, as well as feelings of guilt about failing to prevent suicide (Bille-Brahe, 2000). More recently in England, the Church had a leading role in reform of the law on suicide, following a committee set up by the Archbishop of Canterbury in 1959. Among its recommendations were that suicide should no longer be considered a crime and that the clergy should take a pastoral interest in people with suicidal thoughts (Stengel, 1965). An example of the positive influence of the Christian Church in suicide prevention was the founding in 1953 of Samaritans by the Anglican priest, the Reverend Chad Varah.

Suicide and Islam

The Qur'an and Hadith (sayings and actions of the Prophet Muhammad) are more explicit than other scriptures: 'Do not kill yourselves. Surely Allah is ever Compassionate to you' (Qur'an 4:29)[2]. Among the many bounties Allah (the Muslim name for God) has bestowed upon mankind, the most precious is life. In the 'Maqasid al-Shari'ah' or the goals and objectives of Islamic law, one of its five principles is protection and preservation of life. The Islamic view is that people who die by suicide will be deprived of Allah's blessings and mercy in the life hereafter. An exception to this is someone who has an impairment of his mind, caused by a mental disorder.

It is recorded in Hadith that the Prophet Muhammad said:

> A man was inflicted with wounds and he committed suicide, and so Allah said: 'My slave has caused death on himself hurriedly, so I forbid Paradise for him' [al-Bukhari, 1971a: verse 445].

This Hadith makes it clear that blessings of Paradise will not be bestowed upon those who die by suicide.

In another recording it is stated:

---

2   All quotations from the Qur'an are from the 2007 translation by Zafar Ishaq Ansari.

> None of you should long for death, for if he is a good man, he may increase his good deeds, and if he is an evil-doer, he may stop the evil deeds and repent [al-Bukhari, 1971b: verse 341].

Muslims should not desire death as an option in difficult times:

> None of you should make a request for death because of the trouble in which he is involved, but if there is no other help to it, then say: 'O Allah, keep me alive as long as there is goodness in life for me and bring death to me when there is goodness in death for me' [Muslim, 1990].

The Qur'an states that during the journey of experience in which man will be tested, there will be no burden that he cannot cope with; therefore during periods of difficulty one should walk away from despair: 'Allah does not lay a responsibility on anyone beyond his capacity' (Qur'an 2:286). Patience and prayer is a constant theme through the Islamic teaching and scriptural quotations such as the above can be used to help people come through difficult times.

Suicide in Eastern faith traditions

Buddhism and Hinduism have a more ambiguous attitude to suicide than the Western faiths. There is less condemnation of suicide and the idea of eternal damnation is not found in Buddhism and Hinduism. This relates to a central doctrinal difference between Eastern and Western traditions:

> In contrast with the Judeo-Christian religions, one theme dominates the world view of both Hinduism and Buddhism, the doctrine of rebirth. According to this doctrine the individual is subject to repeated cycles of birth and death before he arrives at the ultimate salvation of Nirvana [Bhugra, 2004: p. 13].

Buddhism and suicide

In Buddhism, death by suicide is usually considered regrettable, since the potential for spiritual development that a human life represents is being squandered (Harvey, 2000). The act may cause harm to others as well as depriving them of the good that one could do. Life entails suffering, but it is a distorted state of mind that leads one to take this personally (Harvey, 2000; Bhugra, 2004). Reflection on impermanence and karma is recommended to enable more patient living, as is the practice of loving-kindness towards the self. Longing for something better may not bring it about and dying in an agitated state of mind may damage the transition into the next life. 'Suicide from despair has been seen in Buddhism as a prudential error since, given their unresolved karma, suicides will just be reborn in situations similar to those they were seeking to escape from' (Perret, 1996: p. 312).

Heroic and altruistic suicides can be revered, as in the case of certain Bodhisattvas, or monks who burned themselves in protest at the Vietnam

War. The person's state of mind and intentions at the time of death influence the view adopted by Buddhism and cultures influenced by Buddhism (Keown, 1996; Becker, 1990).

Suicide in Hinduism

Bhugra (2004) reviews suicide in several different religious traditions. In the Hindu tradition, he notes that Ayurveda (a subsection of one of the four Vedas that are traditional sources of wisdom in Hinduism) is literally translated as 'knowledge of long life', and within the Ayurvedic system 'the cognitive triad for well-being includes desire for self-preservation, wealth and a happy future' (Bhugra, 2004: p.10). There is some condemnation of suicide in the Hindu tradition, such that individuals who hanged themselves could be denied funeral rites. Yet, there are accounts of deaths by suicide in the Hindu scriptures, including the deaths of Rama and Sita, which are not condemned (Bhugra, 2004: p. 26–27).

The Hindu practice of *sati*, in which the devoted wife offers herself to be burned to death in her husband's funeral pyre, was once widely practised in India. When a widow elected to join her husband in death, *sati* conferred blessing on the couple, their families and the congregation in the next life (Cheng & Lee, 2000; Bhugra, 2004). Political and cultural change, including women's rights, is likely to have contributed to the abolition and cessation of *sati*, which was legally abolished by the British in 1829 and has since been generally discarded by Indian society, although sporadic cases are still reported (Chadda *et al*, 1991).

Mental anguish, spirituality and psychotherapy

Suicide is associated with serious mental anguish that may manifest in a variety of themes, some of which may be:

- anger, violence, rage, conflict, envy, rejection, abandonment
- despair, isolation, meaninglessness, void, annihilation, nihilism
- contrast between inner and outer worlds, perfectionism
- option, autonomy, choice, control, 'last way out', regression
- destiny, sacrifice, gamble/ordeal
- afterlife, heaven/paradise, hell, escape, oblivion, rest
- reunion with deceased loved one(s), union with God/nature, mother
- judgement, courage, altruism, political or religious ideals
- transformation.

Anger and despair are often mixed. Where one of these is the predominant subjective experience, the other may be denied, having impact on others through projection. 'Negative' emotions like anger and despair can be simplistically viewed as feelings to be got rid of, even at the cost of physical damage or death. Spirituality and psychoanalytic understanding can overlap creatively in valuing the components of both the 'dark' and the 'light' in the human psyche.

Religious language is rich with this theme. Both light and darkness are necessary for balance and harmony, as exemplified by the yin and yang symbol of Taoism. Light may shine in darkness, but if there is no darkness, light may be blinding (the abolition of darkness by continual artificial light is used in torture situations, as in the ironically named Ministry of Love in George Orwell's *Nineteen Eighty Four* (Orwell, 1949)). A person who has depression may have a heightened need for darkness, just as a bereaved person may need to cry.

In Freud's instinct theory, Eros and Thanatos – the life and death instincts – exist in a dynamic tension (Freud, 1932, reprinted 2001). Melanie Klein built on this in stressing the importance for healthy infant development of reaching the 'depressive position', in which good and bad experiences are experienced as coming from the same source (mother) so that ambivalence and empathy are enabled (Klein, 1997). In analytic psychology, recognising and owning the 'shadow', or disowned darker aspects of the self, is valued as vital to the attainment of personal integration and wholeness (Jacobi, 1973).

Thomas Moore, a psychotherapist and former monk, and James Hillman (1997), a Jungian analyst, both write about the care of the soul, using the word 'soul' in a broad sense that incorporates psychological and spiritual dimensions. Moore's *Dark Nights of the Soul* (2004), which takes its title from the writings of the Spanish poet and mystic St John of the Cross, aims to help the reader to value the insights that can emerge from difficult times and might otherwise feel hopeless and destructive. During such times, even for religious people, the experience of a sustaining God may be absent. Religious mystics and psychotherapists alike recognise the potentially transformative value of darkness – periods of 'stuckness' and intense uncertainty, when waiting may be more appropriate than prayer or overtly therapeutic activity. Moore suggests that the experience of darkness can be conceived of as a symbolic womb, a gestation period, or a chrysalis stage from which something new may emerge.

Suicide in literature

The theme of suicide is frequently explored in works of literature, including the famous soliloquy from Shakespeare's Hamlet beginning 'To be or not to be', wherein uncertainty is a disincentive to suicide (Shakespeare, reprinted 2003, Act 3, Scene 1, line 56).

In another soliloquy, Hamlet expresses the wish that suicide was not religiously condemned:

> ... that the Everlasting had not fixed
> his canon 'gainst self-slaughter

Act 1, Scene 2, lines 131–132

In *Ode to a Nightingale*, Keats expresses a passive death wish. He is 'half in love with easeful Death' and longs for the release it represents:

Now more than ever seems it rich to die,
To cease upon the midnight with no pain'
While thou art pouring forth thy soul abroad
In such an ecstasy!

[Keats 1819, reprinted 1998: pp. 174–177]

He goes on to reflect, however, that if he were dead he would no longer be able to hear and enjoy the song of the nightingale.

Many creative people in literature and the arts have been afflicted by mental illness and serious personal anguish, and the struggle with the dark side of personal experience may be manifest in their work. Jamison (1993) has made a detailed study of writers, artists and musicians with affective disorders, indicating those who attempted or died by suicide.

Spiritual issues in the clinical management of people with suicidal thoughts

There is a professional and social expectation that psychiatrists have a duty to prevent suicide, which reflects moral and religious views about the wrongness of suicide. Such pressures can inhibit the freedom of the interaction with the person who may be thinking of or has attempted dying by suicide. Furthermore, if not able to be creatively contained, the pressures can result in anger being focused on the doctor or the system rather than permitting exploration of the particular crisis or illness.

Death by suicide and attempted suicide may raise questions about faith, hope and the meaning of life (case studies 4.1–4.4). The experience of loss of faith may emerge from a life crisis or may itself be a symptom of illness, bearing in mind that Beck's cognitive triad for depression includes a negative view of the self, the future and the outside world (Beck *et al*, 1987). In the case of illness, diagnosis and assurance of treatment may bring some relief.

Religious thought content may be problematic, arising from illness, religious background, or both. If it is purely symptomatic, assurance can be given that treatment will help: if it is based on personal beliefs, then open questions about the person's faith may aid understanding and referral to a chaplain may help. Distorted religious ideas about sin and having to be perfect can feed into depression and scruples. Even valuing and caring for the self as a spiritual aim may be denigrated as 'selfish'. By gently encouraging questioning of these issues, mental health professionals and chaplains can help to release people from tyrannical religious views.

Self-criticism and self-loathing may be depressive symptoms or a narcissistic preoccupation with an unrealistic idea of how one should be. Spiritual understanding can aid psychiatric management, in so far as death can be looked at symbolically as 'dying' to self-destructive ways of living and the subsequent 'birth' of a more life-affirming direction. The professional challenge is to free the person from the concrete intention to

---

Case study 4.1

Mr Smith, a 58-year-old confirmed atheist, was estranged from his family of origin. He had one confiding relationship with his wife. When she suddenly left, he became seriously depressed. He had access to a gun. He didn't shoot himself, but he killed his dog. In the following months he regularly went to church, where he sat thinking and crying, thus arousing a priest's concern. He decided to learn to sail, a decision that eventually led to solitary voyages during which he felt both challenged and sustained by the forces of nature. He entered a new relationship with a friend who was spiritually inclined.

Case study 4.2

Martin, a young Jewish man, feared he might be homosexual. He tried to convince himself that he could marry, yet all his fantasies were of men. He was sure his parents could never accept him as gay. Within his religious community suicide seemed preferable to the shame of 'coming out'. After psychotherapy, he managed to have a general discussion with his father, which revealed that the parental attitude was not what he had feared. At the end of his treatment he could accept being homosexual and began browsing a website about how to be Jewish and gay.

Case study 4.3

Geraldine, a young woman with a history of sexual abuse and a borderline personality disorder, was habitually preoccupied with suicide and took frequent serious overdoses. She became aware that suicide attracted her partly as revenge on her abuser, who had never been brought to justice, and on her parents who had not believed her. She happened to read a book about the afterlife which cast doubt on the value of suicide as punishment for the living, who would eventually meet their own karma. The book also suggested that the deceased person would still have problems to contend with in the afterlife. Reading this book did not altogether stop Geraldine from self-harming, but provided a focus for therapeutic dialogue about her motives, feelings and plans.

Case study 4.4

Mrs Foster, a devout Christian who had a personal history of abandonment, took a serious overdose when her son moved to Canada. Her daughter had previously moved to a war-torn part of Africa where she was working as a missionary, taking her children with her. While an in-patient, Mrs Foster had depression with psychotic features, believing that God was condemning her for her anger with her children. In addition to her medical treatment, the team worked together with the chaplain to encourage a healthier spiritual attitude of self-acceptance and freedom to be angry.

---

find release through destruction of the body and instead begin a journey of transformation, helped by emphasis on the unity of body, mind and spirit.

The need for revenge can be a motivating factor, as in the case of Geraldine (case study 4.3), with a fantasy of watching one's funeral, and the expressions of anguish, regret and love that were never acknowledged in life. This can be explored by enquiring into the person's ideas about life after death. If appropriate, *in vivo* meetings with relatives may also be arranged, enabling the psychological work to be more grounded in life in the here and now.

Experiencing the call of a dead person to join them in the afterlife may result from unresolved grief, illness or personal anguish about unmet needs, as well as underlying illness. In grief, it is important not to inhibit the process with inappropriate medication but to respect the need to experience painful emotions before being able to 'let go'. Counselling, therapy and spiritual support may help the person to develop an inner dialogue with the deceased, find peace and move on. Where there are long-term unmet needs, a sense of belonging and a deepening attachment to a faith community may offer befriending outside the mental health service setting.

The question of the meaning of life

People who have attempted suicide or have suicidal thoughts commonly experience feelings of meaninglessness and futility. Writers and philosophers have considered this from the religious and secular standpoint. In mid-life Tolstoy suffered a crisis of meaning. At a time when everything in his life was going well in terms of family, prosperity and success, he was increasingly assailed by questions such as: 'What will come of what I am doing today and will do tomorrow? What will come of my whole life? Is there in my life a meaning which would not be destroyed by my inevitable, imminent death?' (Tolstoy, 1905: p. 14).

These questions prompted intellectual pursuit of a solution, but just reinforced the idea that life was meaningless. While Tolstoy's preoccupation with futility could be conceptualised as a depressive symptom, his crisis lasted 15 years. He continued with his work, but as the preoccupation increased, he found that before attending to ordinary concerns, he needed constantly to know why he was doing so. His views at the time echo the biblical passage in Ecclesiastes: 'All is vanity. What do people gain from all the toil at which they toil under the sun?' (Ecclesiastes 1: 2–3). The ground on which Tolstoy stood had given way and there was now a serious risk of suicide: 'I arrived at the conclusion that I could not live, and, fearing death, I had to use cunning against myself in order that I might not take my life' (Tolstoy, 1905: p. 11).

Tolstoy reasoned that if one lived according to an aim, then once this was achieved, another needed to be found to sustain a reason for living. This was particularly difficult once he had reached the peak of his achievements. Looking ahead, he could only see more of the same for succeeding generations. This idea is given powerful expression in the Greek myth of Sisyphus, described by the existential writer Albert Camus (1975). Sisyphus was condemned by the gods to an eternal round of rolling a stone up a hill, only for it to fall back down just before he reached the summit and for the toil to have to be repeated. Tolstoy found no satisfying answer to his dilemma in science and philosophy, eventually concluding that it was not right to look for an answer in rational knowledge but rather in the realm of faith with its 'irrational knowledge'.

Other writers have reached different conclusions that do not rely on religious faith and are not threatened by reason. Baier (1981) argues that although the traditional Christian, raised to believe him- or herself the offspring of a loving parent God, created for a divine purpose, may feel that the scientific world view strips life of its meaning, the purpose of the Creator and the Created may not be one and the same. After the initial shock of the loss of a particular kind of faith, there may be new freedom in redefining purpose for oneself. Baier sees inherent qualities, such as beauty, as having value independent of purpose.

If this life is to be endured merely in preparation for the reward of Paradise, then its meaning and value are reduced by failing to appreciate the present. For Camus, the tragedy of Sisyphus lies in his consciousness of his infinite drudgery, when there is the possibility of experiencing joy in doing his activity and so of transcending the drudgery. As the Taoist tradition advises, wisdom lies in the existence of the present moment, unselfconsciously imbuing it with meaning. Taylor (1970) also considers the state of mind to be more important than goal-directedness, writing: 'The point of ... living is simply to be living ... The meaning of life is from within us, it is not bestowed from without, and it far exceeds in both its beauty and permanence any heaven of which men have ever dreamed or yearned for' (p. 48).

Suicide in terminal illness and physician-assisted suicide

Longing for death as a way of ending pain applies to individuals who are both in mental and physical anguish and much attention has been given to this in the context of terminal illness. The most recent debate on the subject in the UK Parliament was a Bill introduced by Lord Joffe (2005), framed to allow persons with terminal illness undergoing unbearable suffering and with mental capacity to request assisted dying, also known as physician-assisted suicide. In the event, the Bill was defeated by a relatively small margin in the House of Lords in May 2006.

Representatives of religious organisations traditionally oppose euthanasia and physician-assisted suicide. The issues are complex, however, and religious faith is not incompatible with condoning physician-assisted suicide in some circumstances. There are non-religious arguments against it too, seeing the sanctity of life as a spiritual value that does not require adherence to a faith tradition. Compassion, as a spiritual value, can be seen on both sides of the debate that centres on the relative importance of personal autonomy and the sanctity of life. Support for the legalisation of physician-assisted suicide may reflect the increasing secularisation of Western society. Personal autonomy is currently highly valued in the West and reflected in general empowerment of the individual in other areas of healthcare. The debate has implications for society, family relationships, trust in role of the doctor and the wider community.

If such a Bill is ever passed, psychiatrists are likely to be involved in the ascertainment of capacity. Although provision would doubtless be made for opting out of this role for conscientious reasons, it would represent an enormous challenge for psychiatrists and their patients, especially in liaison psychiatry. Unbearable suffering has a subjective dimension and depression, which may be treatable, commonly complicates serious physical illness. These and other considerations led the Royal College of Psychiatrists (2006) to conclude its formal response to Lord Joffe's Bill with the view that it is 'deeply worried about these likely effects of the Assisted Dying for the Terminally Ill Bill if it were to be enacted.'

The hospice movement advanced in the UK by Dame Cicely Saunders has pioneered incorporating spiritual care into the care of the dying. Its general philosophy stresses dying as an important experience for the individual and family, where pain can be minimised and a peaceful state of mind can be researched. The debate around physician-assisted suicide acknowledges the importance of palliative care, and Lord Joffe's Bill proposed that this be offered in the assessment process for those requesting physician-assisted suicide.

The impact of suicide on survivors

Suicide always occurs in a social context and will have a considerable impact on those left behind (sometimes called the survivors). In reviewing the impact of suicide on the bereaved, Clark & Goldney (2000) have estimated that 6 million people worldwide are affected annually by suicide. They review a number of studies, indicating that families bereaved by suicide are a vulnerable group. The support they receive is vital, as they are at risk of depression and death by suicide themselves. However, they may be reluctant to access support because of stigma and because they may mistrust the mental health services, whom they may see as having failed to help the deceased person. Among their difficulties are shock, anger, guilt, blame, stigma, unfinished business, rejection, questions of 'how' and 'why', and confusion about their own beliefs and values. There may be concern about God, the afterlife and the spiritual state of the deceased, regardless of religious belief (Clark & Goldney, 2000).

The funeral may be a healing opportunity, allowing for the reality of the person's death to dawn and for the celebration of the positive attributes of their life so that these are not eclipsed by the manner of death. It can provide support for mourners and opportunity for those outside the immediate family to experience their grief. When sensitively conducted, the funeral can allow safe expression of difficult emotions, bring the family together and enable 'letting go'. The memory of a beautiful funeral may help to balance the negative impact of the event (Wertheimer, 2001). Viewing the body also allows an encounter with the reality of death and generally aids the grieving process.

Undertakers and ministers of religion have an important role to play when in contact with survivors, and can convey acceptance, information and a non-judgmental atmosphere. Hawton (2003) suggests that specialised training for them may help the bereaved. Survivors may be concerned about the officiant's attitude to suicide. What families are seeking is not a theological discussion but an assurance that the deceased is no longer suffering and is 'at peace' (Wertheimer, 1991).

One hospital chaplain (Christian, 2007, personal communication) suggests that each mourner will have particular views about the circumstances behind the act, leading to blame and self-criticism. It is never possible to know the whole story of what led the person to that point. Christian suggests that this is a reason not to persist with guilt and blame. In better moments the deceased would have wanted the bereaved to get on with their lives, and this is something the chaplain can remind them about before, during and after the funeral. This type of intervention could be helpful to mental healthcare professionals in communicating with the bereaved, as well as in dealing with their own emotional reactions to suicide.

Recovery may take years and the sense of loss may be enduring. Psychiatrists should not expect 'closure' but support adaptation to the circumstances of continuing life. Most bereaved persons eventually find an adjustment, although some may continue to experience depression and relationship difficulties. Others are relieved that the deceased person is no longer suffering. Many find a new, inner relationship with the deceased person and a new purpose or direction (Clark & Goldney, 2000).

Mental health professionals' attitudes towards suicide

Suicide is controversial. It has variously been viewed as honourable, a sin and a human right. In clinical experience, it is hard to escape the underlying mixture of anger and despair that may be experienced as a personal or professional attack, and an attack on life itself. The severity with which suicide has sometimes been condemned reflects the threat it poses and the abhorrence it can evoke. Such attitudes may be culturally denied, but they persist at some level and can be encountered by people who attempt or die by suicide and their families. In the general hospital setting, for example, some nurses and doctors show negative attitudes to people who self-harm (Hawton, 2000: p. 526). That both mental health professionals and non-clinical carers may experience self-harm as an attack upon themselves and their efforts to help the person may need to be addressed in the therapeutic relationship.

Inquiries following suicide, although necessary, may feel threatening, and a culture of blame can be difficult for institutions to transcend. Psychological debriefing may help. A spiritual attitude can help those involved in the aftermath of suicide to move on from the facts of the case and to begin enabling acceptance and forgiveness of self and others. This in turn may free the professional to learn more from the experience.

Some psychiatrists may hold strong moral views about suicide. It is important to put aside these opinions while relating to the individual, in order to appreciate the uniqueness of his or her situation. Additionally, the medical imperative to 'do no harm' and medical concern with prevention (Hillman, 1997) can get in the way of understanding the personal meaning of suicide; the idea 'where there's life there's hope' can induce an excess of medical zeal. A different kind of hope may be called for – the hope for something different. In acute mental illness and where there is substantial immediate risk of a person attempting suicide, the imperative to prevent may seem obvious; for chronically ill people who long for an end to their suffering, it may be less so.

People contemplating suicide may express spiritual concerns that may be useful to explore, noting how they may have changed with time and circumstance. Where spiritual practices such as prayer and meditation have helped in the past but have now been discarded, the person may implicitly seek encouragement to resume them. However, it is unwise and presumptive to try to provide answers to another individual's spiritual quest. Compassion and human acceptance are spiritual values that overlap with therapeutic ones and respectful listening may offer a lifeline in the course of treatment.

It is possible to see suicide as a choice against life. The psychoanalyst Symington (1994) observed that his patients who are diagnosed with narcissism are repeatedly presented with crises and opportunities for change, only to repeatedly make choices that amount to a refusal of 'the Life Giver'. Change is very difficult, perhaps because it means loss of the known inner world to which the person is deeply, if painfully, attached. The challenge echoes a passage from Hebrew scripture: 'I have set before you life and death, blessings and curses. Choose life so that you and your descendants may live' (Deuteronomy 20: 19). In general psychiatry, it is worth remembering that a life-denying course of action may not feel like a choice to the person involved.

People may respond to questions about suicide by saying that they would do it, if they had the courage. In the authors' experience this and concern for family members are the most common reasons presented for desisting; both deserve respect. Concern about family implies a capacity for empathy and love which, in time, may be applied to the self. It can be useful to comment on the courage required to remain alive and struggle with adversity, as the person may not have considered this before. Paul Tillich, a theologian, has written of 'the courage to accept acceptance' (Tillich, 2000: pp. 163–171). Low self-esteem and past deprivations may make it very hard for people to 'accept acceptance', such that they may feel threatened by the goodness of the therapist or the mental health team sufficiently to need (unconsciously) to try to subvert their treatment by acting out destructively, thus reasserting the familiar experience of rejection and neglect.

Conclusion

Spirituality has profoundly contributed to prevailing cultural views about suicide. Different religious traditions have variously condemned the act to a greater or lesser degree, yet shown compassion to those involved. The act of suicide has moral and existential implications for the individual and society. Spiritual beliefs and practices can have a positive impact on mental health and suicide prevention. Furthermore, recognition of the spiritual dimension of mental healthcare is likely to improve the understanding and support available to patients, carers and professionals.

References

al-Bukhari, M. I. I. (1971a) *The Translation of the Meanings of Sahih al-Bukhari by Muhammad Mushin Khan, Vol 2, Book 23, no. 445*. Hilal Publishing House.

al-Bukhari, M. I. I. (1971b) *The Translation of the Meanings of Sahih al-Bukhari by Muhammad Mushin Khan, Vol 9, Book 90, no. 341*. Hilal Publishing House.

Alvarez, A. (2002) *The Savage God*. Bloomsbury.

Ansari, Z. I. (2007) *Towards Understanding The Qur'an: Abridged Version of Tafhim al-Qur'an by Sayyid Abdul A'la Mawdudi*. Islamic Foundation.

Baier, K. (1981) The Purpose of Man's Existence. In *Life and Meaning* (ed. O. Hanfling), pp. 20–33. Blackwell in association with the Open University.

Barraclough, B. M. (1992) The Bible Suicides. *Acta Psychiatrica Scandinavica*, **86**, 64–69.

Beck, A. T., John Rush, A., Shaw, B. F., *et al* (1987) *Cognitive Therapy of Depression*. Guilford.

Becker, C. (1990) Buddhist views of suicide and euthanasia. *Philosophy East and West*, **40**, 543–555.

Bhugra, D. (2004) *Culture and Self-Harm: Attempted Suicide in South Asians in London*. Maudsley monograph 46. Psychology Press.

Holy Bible with Apocrypha: New Revised Standard Version (anglicised edn) (1995). Oxford University Press.

Bille-Brahe, U. (2000) Sociology and suicidal behaviour. In *The International Handbook of Suicide and Attempted Suicide* (eds K. Hawton & K. van Heeringen), pp. 193–207. John Wiley.

Birnbaum, L. & Birnbaum, A. (2004) In search of inner wisdom: guided mindfulness meditation in the context of suicide. *Scientific World Journal*, **March 18**, 4, 216–227.

Camus, A. (1975) *The Myth of Sisyphus* (trans. J. O'Brien). Penguin.

Chadda, R. K., Shome, S. & Bhatia, M. S. (1991) Suicide in Indian women (letter). *British Journal of Psychiatry*, **158**, 434.

Cheng, A. & Lee, C. (2000) Suicide in Asia and the Far East. In *The International Handbook of Suicide and Attempted Suicide* (eds K. Hawton & K. van Heeringen), pp. 29–48. John Wiley.

Clark, S. & Goldney, R. (2000) The impact of suicide on relatives and friends. In *The International Handbook of Suicide and Attempted Suicide* (eds K. Hawton & K. van Heeringen), pp. 476–484. John Wiley.

Clarke, C. S., Bannon, F. J. & Dennihan, A. (2003) Suicide and religiosity – Masaryk's theory revisited. *Social Psychiatry and Psychiatric Epidemiology*, **38**, 502–506.

Frankl, V. E. (1967) Group psychotherapeutic experiences in a concentration camp. In *Psychotherapy and Existentialism*, pp. 95–104. Penguin.

Freud, S. (2001) The ego and the id and other works. In *Standard Edition of the Complete Works of Sigmund Freud*, Vol. XIX (1923–1925). Vintage.

Gilbert, M. (1987) The Holocaust. Fontana Press.

Harvey, P. (2000) *An Introduction to Buddhist Ethics*. Cambridge University Press.

Hawton, K. (2000) General hospital management of suicide attempters. In *The International Handbook of Suicide and Attempted Suicide* (eds K. Hawton & K. van Heeringen), pp. 519–537. John Wiley.

Hawton, K. (2003) Helping people bereaved by suicide. *BMJ*, **327**, 177–178.

Hillman, J. (1997) *Suicide and the Soul* (new edn). Spring Publications.

Holland, R. F. (1969) Suicide. In *Talk of God*, pp. 72–85. Royal Institute of Philosophy Lectures, 1967–1968. Macmillan.

Holt, J. (2004) Psychiatry and spirituality at the end of life: a case report. *Practical Geriatrics*, **55**, 618–622.

Ineichen, B. (1998) The influence of religion on the suicide rate. *Mental Health, Religion and Culture*, **1**, 31–36.

Jacobi, J. (1973) *The Psychology of C. G. Jung* (English edn). Yale University Press.

Jakobovits, I. (1988) Some modern responses on medico–moral problems. *ASSIA – Jewish Medical Ethics*, **1**, 5–10.

Jamison, K. R. (1993) *Touched with Fire*, pp. 63–71, 267–270. Free Press Paperback.

Joffe, Lord (2005) *Assisted Dying for the Terminally Bill (HL)*. TSO (The Stationery Office).

Kabat-Zinn, J. (1994) *Wherever You Go, There You Are*. Piatkus.

Kamal, Z. & Loewenthal, K. M. (2002) Suicide beliefs and behaviours among young Muslims and Hindus in the UK. *Mental Health, Religion and Culture*, **5**, 111–118.

Kaplan, S. & Schoeneberg, L. (1988) Defining suicide: importance and implications for Judaism. *Journal of Religion and Health*, **27**, 154–156.

Keats, J. (1819) Ode to a Nightingale. In *John Keats, Selected Poetry* (1998), pp. 174–177. Oxford University Press.

Keown, D. (1996) Buddhism and suicide – the case of Chana. *Journal of Buddhist Ethics*, **3**, 8–31.

Klein, M. (1997) *Envy and Gratitude and Other Works*. Vintage.

Koch, H. J. (2005) Suicide and suicide ideation in the Bible: an empirical study. *Acta Psychiatrica Scandinavica*, **112**, 167–172.

Koenig, H. G., Mc Cullough, M. E. & Larson, D. B. (2001) *Handbook of Religion and Health*. Oxford University Press.

Kohn, R., Levav, I., Chang, B., *et al* (1997) Epidemiology of youth suicide in Israel. *Journal of the American Academy of Child and Adolescent Psychiatry*, **79**, 468–473.

Linehan, M. M., Goodstein, J. L., Nielsen, S. L., *et al* (1983) Reasons for staying alive when you are thinking of killing yourself: the Reasons for Living Inventory. *Journal of Consulting and Clinical Psychology*, **51**, 276–286.

Masaryk, T. G. (1970) *Der Selbsmord als sociale Massenerscheinung der modernen Zivilisation* [Suicide and the meaning of civilisation]. University of Chicago Press.

Moore, T. (2004) *Dark Nights of the Soul* (UK edn). Piatkus.

Mowat, H., Cameron, S., Swinton J., *et al* (2006) Religion and suicide: exploring the role of the Church in deaths by suicide in Highland Scotland. *Scottish Journal of Healthcare Chaplaincy*, **9**, 3–7.

Muslim, A. H. (1990) *Sahih Muslim* (transl. A. H. Siddiqi). Book 35, Chapter 4. Sh. Muhammad Ashraf Publishers.

Neeleman, J. & Lewis, G. (1999) Suicide, religion and socioeconomic conditions: an ecological study in 26 countries, 1990. *Journal of Epidemiology and Community Health*, **53**, 204–210.

Neeleman, J., Halpern, D., Leon, D., *et al* (1997) Tolerance of suicide, religion and suicide rates: an ecological and individual study in 19 Western countries. *Psychological Medicine*, **27**, 1165–1171.

Orwell, G. (1949) *Nineteen Eighty Four*. Reprinted 1996 (revised paperback edn). Penguin.

Peng, K. L. (1992) Suicidal behaviour in Singapore. In *Suicidal Behaviour in the Asia–Pacific Region* (eds K. L. Peng & W. S. Tseng), pp. 176–198. Singapore University Press.

Perret, R. W. (1996) Buddhism, euthanasia and the sanctity of life. *Journal of Medical Ethics*, **22**, 309–314.

Royal College of Psychiatrists (2006) *Statement from the Royal College of Psychiatrists on physician assisted suicide*. Royal College of Psychiatrists (http://www.rcpsych.ac.uk/pressparliament/collegeresponses/physicianassistedsuicide.aspx).

Segal, Z. V., Williams, J. M. G. & Teasdale, J. D. (2002) *Mindfulness-Based Cognitive Therapy for Depression: a New Approach to Preventing Relapse*. Guilford Press.

Shakespeare, W. (2003) *Hamlet, Prince of Denmark*. Reprinted (2003) *The New Cambridge Shakespeare* (ed. P. Edwards). Cambridge University Press.

Simpson, M. E. & Conklin, G. H. (1989) Socioeconomic development, suicide and religion. *Social Forces*, **67**, 945–964.

Stack, S. (1980) Religion and suicide: a re-analysis. *Social Psychiatry*, **15**, 65–70.

Stengel, E. (1965) *Suicide and Attempted Suicide*. Bristol. Macgibbon & Kee.

Symington, N. (1994) *Emotion and Spirit*. Karnac.

Tacey, D. (2004) *The Spirituality Revolution: the Emergence of Contemporary Spirituality*. Routledge.

Taylor, R. (1970) The meaning of life. In *Life and Meaning* (ed. O. Hanfling), pp. 39–48. Blackwell in association with the Open University.

The Scottish Executive (2002) *Choose Life: A National Strategy and Action Plan to Prevent Suicide in Scotland*. TSO (The Stationery Office).

Tillich, P. (2000) *The Courage to Be* (2nd edn). Yale University Press.

Tolstoy, L. (1905) My confession. In *Life and Meaning* (ed. O. Hanfling), pp. 9–19. Blackwell in association with the Open University.

Wertheimer, A (2001) *A Special Scar*. Brunner-Routledge.

Westberg, G. E. & McNamara, J. W. (1990) *The Parish Nurse: Providing a Minister of Health for Your Congregation*. Augsburg Fortress.

Williams, J. M. & Pollock, L. R. (2001) Psychological aspects of the suicidal process. In *Understanding Suicidal Behaviour: the Suicidal Process Approach to Research, Treatment and Prevention* (ed. K. van Heeringen), pp. 76–93. John Wiley.

Williams, J. M., Duggan, D. S., Crane, C., *et al* (2006) Mindfulness-based cognitive therapy for prevention of recurrence of suicidal behaviour. *Journal of Clinical Psychology*, **62**, 201–210.

Wood, T. (1986) Suicide. In *A New Dictionary of Christian Ethics* (eds J. Macquarrie & J. Childress), pp. 609–610. SCM Press.

CHAPTER 5

Child and adolescent psychiatry

Mike Shooter

How many loved your moments of glad grace,
And loved your beauty with love false or true;
But one man loved the pilgrim soul in you,
And loved the sorrows of your changing face.

W. B. Yeats (1893)

Every child has a story to tell; some are joyous, some painful, most a mixture of the two. It is the psychiatrist's privilege to listen to that story and to help the child retell it, without excuses, to whoever it concerns.

Robert Coles, the great paediatrician-turned-psychotherapist, spent years listening to the stories of children across the world, in schools, homes and all their private places. In *The Spiritual Life of Children* (Coles, 1990: p. xvi), he describes them as 'seekers … young pilgrims well aware that life is a finite journey and as anxious to make sense of it as those of us who are farther along in the time allotted to us'. The concept of life as a journey was one that Liam understood (case study 5.1), but it has many implications. What sort of a journey is it and what goal is the pilgrim child journeying towards? What blessings and hardships might he or she encounter along the way? What outside influences might be brought to bear and how might a therapist be called upon to help? This chapter is an attempt to explore those questions and to work out what they might mean in the triangle between children like Liam, the therapist and the outside world.

What sort of a journey is life and what are its goals?

The study of spiritual development in childhood was frustrated for decades by its association with religion and the attitudes of psychoanalysts who took their cue from Sigmund Freud's dismissal of it as an obsessional neurosis derived from infantile wishes. True, Carl Jung thought that religion could be an aid towards personal and social moral values and the object relations school saw it as a transitional bridge from self to others via 'god images'. Even Freud's own concept of Weltanschauung (Freud, 1933) – a world view that addresses the most basic questions of origin, purpose, suffering and

Case study 5.1

Liam was a 15-year-old with chronic renal failure since early childhood. A history of non-adherence to his treatment regimen had led to two rejected kidney transplants and a return to dialysis by the ward team who had looked after him, through thick and thin, for over a decade. The staff were appalled when he told them that he had had enough, that he wanted no more treatment and wished to be left alone to die. The child psychiatrist attached to the team was asked to advise on whether Liam was 'in his right mind'.

Liam's parents had separated soon after the birth, his father having left for a succession of other partners. The mother struggled to bring up Liam on her own but he had spent several periods in local authority care because of his behaviour. He had little formal schooling. Liam's contact with his father was sporadic and explosive, usually ending in rows between the parents over his illness. His father often accused his mother of causing Liam's kidney failure by not looking after him properly. His mother had met a new partner a year ago and was now 6 months pregnant.

The psychiatrist's assessment showed Liam to be rational and determined. He had thought through his options carefully and was well aware of the consequences of his wish to end treatment. It was a decision that the psychiatrist thought should be respected. Though 'Gillick competence' applied only to the right of a child to opt into treatment against adult wishes, not out of it, he felt that Liam showed the same capacity to decide for himself. Forcing treatment upon him, under the Mental Health Act, would not be legally, ethically or practically appropriate. Liam should be allowed to die.

The staff were split by this advice into those who felt it their responsibility to save Liam at all costs and those who had no wish to prolong the suffering they had seen him go through over the years. Liam's mother was in favour of withdrawing treatment; the father reappeared and accused the mother of wanting to clear Liam out of the way so she could start a new life with her partner and their baby. He threatened to take the hospital to court if they obeyed Liam's wishes and to expose their 'incompetence' to the press.

The psychiatrist continued to talk with Liam. Despite his lack of education, Liam had a vivid turn of phrase, describing his life as a journey with lots of ups and downs, 'like a roller-coaster ride'. He had often been angry with his illness, with his need for treatment and with everyone involved in it; but since coming to his decision he had 'found peace of mind'. He wanted to say sorry to his mother for causing her so much trouble and wish her well with the partner he had initially resented. He realised that his decision had upset the nurses close to him and wanted them to know that dying was sometimes the best way out, not the worst. Above all, he wanted to tell his father not to feel so guilty about walking out on him when he was little.

The team came together to offer Liam palliative care while trying to persuade him to accept further treatment – to no avail. His parents reached a fragile agreement to bury their differences for Liam's final months and he died, peacefully and painlessly, on the ward. All were left both astounded and deeply affected by Liam's decision and the wisdom he had shown since making it.

what constitutes the good life – is a little more sympathetic. But all this is a long way from Coles' (1990) idea of spirituality as the sort of life-changing force that Liam had so clearly experienced. In such a conceptual climate, spirituality was virtually ignored in the West.

The explosion of the literature on spirituality in Europe (Reich et al, 1999) and in the USA (Roehlkepartain et al, 2006) was made possible by its separation from religion (see chapter 1), although in America the two have remained entangled in both positive and negative ways. Religion is seen as a formally structured framework of ritual and theology that is traditional and socially bound; spirituality is a more subjective, experiential and personal sensitivity but it needs the religious framework in which to flourish. 'Finding moral guidelines that help define the boundaries of acceptable behaviour for their children can be a challenge for parents' (Josephson & Dell, 2004: p. 13). Religious parents and children have a sense of purpose. Secular families flounder in 'a swamp of circumstance'. Religion and spirituality are seen as bound together in a common search for the sacred.

For others, the pendulum has swung to the opposite extreme and spirituality is seen as 'good' in contrast to 'bad' religion that is 'tainted by an incriminating record of injustice, tribalism, violence and the violation of fundamental human rights' (King, 2001: p. 2) in which young people too often find themselves at the centre of conflict as refugees, physical victims or boy soldiers (Iweala, 2005). The violence around them is a challenge to their spirituality (Garbarino & Bedard, 1996). What seems to 'save' children in such circumstances in South Africa, Cambodia and Northern Ireland is not adherence to the religion that is so often part of the conflict, but an active, personal and hard-questioning political morality of their own (Coles, 1986). In his own battle with chronic illness, Liam came to a spiritual peace of mind in a family with no shred of a religious framework of any kind in which to find structure or to react against.

So what is spiritual development, if it is a concept in its own right, independent of religious structure? The key elements may be said to be the growth of self-awareness, sympathy with the views of others and transcendence over both to a universal consciousness of values and purpose. Liam had certainly reached a settled view of himself and his illness and was deeply concerned for the feelings of others around him. His decision to end treatment transcended his own initial earthly hopes and those of his parents and the treatment team. In all of that he was most certainly in his 'right mind' in a spiritual as well as legal sense. The concept remains vague and some would have it remain that way, believing that too rigid a definition would cripple its complexity. Spirituality may be compared to the wind; though it might be experienced, observed and described, it cannot be captured (Nye, 1999). But that is little help to the child psychiatrist struggling to understand a child's spiritual world just as they would any other aspect of development.

Some have tried to link spirituality with cognitive development (Johnson & Boyatzis, 2006), attachment theory (Granqvist & Dickie, 2006) and even

83

with essential brain functions (Newberg & Newberg, 2006). It was left to James Fowler to attempt to plot the seven stages on the way to 'self-hood' that claim to be broader than any religious faith, universal in application and giving coherence and direction to life. In the process he echoes both Eriksonian concepts of trust (e.g. Erikson, 1959) and the cognitive stages of Piaget (e.g. Piaget, 1952), namely:

- primal faith (in infancy): a pre-language trust forming in the two-way relationship of a child with its caregivers that offsets the anxiety of repeated separations and is increasingly rich in the awareness of others in the world about;
- intuitive–protective faith (in early childhood) in which the child's imagination, stimulated by stories, gestures and symbols and not yet controlled by logical reasoning of cause and effect, combines with perceptions and feelings to create long-lasting images of both protective and threatening powers;
- mythic–literal faith (in later childhood): a developing ability to think logically helps the child to order the world more consistently, to enter into the perspective of others, and to capture life's texture and meaning in stories;
- synthetic–conventional faith (adolescence and beyond) in which cognitive abilities allow the adolescent to integrate diverse self-images into a coherent synthesis of beliefs and values that form a personal identity, on the basis of which he or she is able to exchange perspectives with people of a different identity and make compromises with the world (Fowler & Dell, 2004).

All this leads to three further stages of development into the mature spiritual outlook of the adult:

- individuative–reflective faith (young adulthood), an increasing understanding of one's responsibilities as part of the social system;
- conjunctive faith (early mid-life), a more sophisticated appreciation of different views of truth and reality;
- universalising faith (mid-life and beyond), emergence from the limits of self into oneness with a deity, a state rarely reached.

In other words, in an 'ideal trajectory' we are born with a natural urge to spirituality. In childhood, we imbibe spiritual meaning from the world around us. In adolescence, we establish our own spirituality. In early adulthood, we develop that in our relationship with others and in late life we achieve a universal consciousness (Miller & Kelley, 2006).

Critics of this scheme would say that, like all stage-based theories, it is too chronologically rigid. It is possible for an adult to be mature in many ways but spiritually naïve, while a young adolescent like Liam seems to have found a maturity of spirituality way beyond his own age and that of most of the adults around him. Development is a multidimensional process rather than a series of discontinuous jumps (MacDonald, 2000). The critics might also say that Fowler's stages of faith are too introspective and that spiritual development is at least a two-way interaction with other people in the child's world rather than an individual quest. At its most complicated, the particular nature of the child at the centre of it all influences and is influenced by: inherited myths, narratives and interpretative frameworks of what is good, important and real; significant life experiences in both history and lifespan; the social context of family, school, peer group and public; and the language, customs, norms and symbols of culture in a multi-girdered 'spiritual architecture' (Benson, 2006).

Since many of these factors will differ from family to family (Boyatzis *et al*, 2006), from culture to culture (Mattis *et al*, 2006) and from social grouping to social grouping (Schwartz *et al*, 2006), perhaps we should talk not of a universal process but of an 'ecology' of spiritual development that will vary enormously from the world of a Muslim child on the streets of London (Roehlkepartain & Patel, 2006) to that of West African adolescents from the Beng culture of the Ivory Coast (Gottlieb, 2006).

Whatever the criticisms that might be made of it, Fowler's stage theory does at least provide a framework for understanding where a child might be in his or her spiritual development, what particular spiritual tasks he or she might be expected to be tackling at that time and how that might be impinged upon by what is going on around about. But the therapist must always be ready for surprises. In Liam's case we have to ask how it is that a lad of 15 could emerge with such wisdom from a family where early separation might have destroyed his basic trust in relationships, where his cognitive development would have been compromised by metabolic imbalance and lack of schooling, where he was isolated by the demands of treatment from peer group and other social interactions, and where the illness itself might have undermincd his sense of self-mastery and encouraged a paranoid and persecutory view of the world.

To fully understand a child's spirituality we need 'conversation' across all the domains of development as the spiritual realm intertwines with the material realm, the social realm and others in creating what might be called our human nature (Bloom, 2004). Indeed, some would see it as organising those domains into one whole while being independent of all of them and capable of remarkable maturity in the most hostile of environments. This raises issues of both risk and resilience.

What are the blessings and hardships along the way?

Cognitive ability, physical health, emotional stability and the capacity to make relationships are not ends in themselves but vehicles through which the developing child is better able to negotiate the world and its demands. And so it is with spirituality. The therapist's task is to interpret the child's level of spiritual development from his or her everyday behaviour, but here the body of outcome research is woefully thin. It is largely limited to older adolescents rather that children; it struggles with complex constructs, uncertain definitions and multiple variables; and it is still hooked onto religious indices (Mabe & Josephson, 2004). Some of it seems little more than a prescription for an all-American, healthy lifestyle. This could, of course, mean acceptance of coercive discipline, ideological repression and abusive relationships that would require spiritual repair in later life (Rossetti, 1995).

Drawing on youth development models, claims are made that spirituality induces a sense of well-being in which adolescents are better able to wrestle with all the tasks of identity formation (King & Benson, 2006) and that even 'macho' Australian boys can come to a more spiritual expression of their masculinity (Engebretson, 2006). There are claims that healthy spiritual development and physical health might be linked in some way (Oman & Thoresen, 2006), perhaps through better prenatal and early parental care, though this comes perilously close to a *mens sana in corpore sano* philosophy!

More specifically, mature spirituality is said to reduce rates of depression and self-harm in adolescents (Mabe & Josephson, 2004), though there are such huge inconsistencies across gender and culture as to make this almost meaningless. When it comes to sexual activity, alcohol and drugs, it is clear that the criterion for a successful outcome of spiritual development is seen as the abstinence of all three in a religious context (Stewart, 2000). There are more balanced views of drug taking as a reflection of the spiritual need for a more fulfilling life as described by 15-year-olds and parents in group discussions (Mallick & Watts, 1999), of spirituality as a critical component of recovery for substance-abusing parents and their maltreated children (DiLorenzo *et al*, 2001) and of the 'spiritual hunger' behind some aspects of eating disorders (Anderson, 1998).

Some adolescents see spirituality as protective against mental health problems in general (Sveidqvist, 2003) and there is much theoretical discussion about this protective relationship. Ken Wilber (1999) would see a 'dislocation' of spiritual development as the basis of mental disorder on several different levels – at the pre-personal level, leading to personality disorder and psychosis and needing directive and supportive restructuring; at the personal level, leading to affective disorders and concern over life events, needing dynamic or cognitive therapy; and at a transpersonal level, leading to spiritual suffering (the dark night of the soul), needing contemplative spiritual practice. This is not difficult to plot onto Fowler's stages of spiritual development which thus become the essential core of mental well-being rather than the surface fingerprint of cognitive, physical, emotional and social components. In this sense, spirituality is not just one form of development but the glue that holds everything together. Things fall apart into mental disorder if that glue comes unstuck. This approach echoes Eastern philosophy, in which a flourishing spiritual life leads to mental health and its eclipse to mental illness (Dalai Lama, 2001).

Interestingly for Liam's history, claims have been made both for spiritual development leading to decreased rates of delinquency and delinquent behaviour itself being a search for spiritual and moral meaning (Blakeney & Blakeney, 2006). Looking again at Liam's early aggression, the family relationships that led to his periods in local authority care, and his non-adherence to hospital treatment that led to his loss of two kidney transplants, one could see an analogy here. True, his disturbance could be seen as his anger towards his parents; but it could also be seen as a search for the boundaries they had so conspicuously failed to provide. Equally, while his failure to take his immunosuppressants could be seen as his way of expressing his anger with his illness, it could also be seen as a testing out of the reality of his kidney failure and the necessity for treatment in the first place. In both cases, the delinquency of his behaviour would be a stage through which he had healthily to pass in order to achieve his later calm.

Liam's spiritual development was tempered in the fire of adversity and, in turn, buttressed him against it. And it is this aspect of research that has been most productive – the concept of resilience in general (Crawford *et al*, 2006), of children coping with family violence, divorce, poverty and abuse (Casado, 2000), children struggling with serious illnesses such as poliomyelitis in the 1950s (Coles, 1986) or cystic fibrosis in modern times (Pendelton, 2002) and especially children confronting death (Stuber & Houskamp, 2004).

The early writers on spiritual development highlighted the spiritual needs of dying children (Sommer, 1989) and their search for meaning: the stand we take towards fate (Frankl, 2000). Once again, the contrast is drawn for many writers between negative aspects of religious coping, with a lack of fit between the child's expectations of the world and the horrors in which it finds itself, and the positive aspects of spirituality. Thus concepts like guilt ('the world is just, so I must have done something wrong to have deserved this illness'), anger ('the world is not fair, so whoever is in charge of it is either not fair to me or not in control') and helplessness ('this event is random and justice is irrelevant') (Stuber & Houskamp, 2004) could be seen as a religious and passive acceptance of the child's fate – whether that springs from Catholic ideas of confession and forgiveness or Protestant faith in a dictatorial God. Spirituality, on the other hand, could be seen to encourage the child to challenge that lack of fit, as Liam could be said to have done. In the hands of a skilled therapist, such a child could be helped to shed the sense of guilt, have his anger validated, and turn helplessness into an active hope for reconciliation in relationships, as a first move towards a more successful treatment or, in Liam's case, a better death.

All this is agony for everyone involved – for the child at the centre of the adversity, for the family around him or her and for the wider 'family' of school, peer group friendships and the healthcare system. This brings us to the therapist's role and how he or she might be called upon to help.

The therapist's role in the child's spiritual development

The therapist's relationship with the child lies at the centre of concentric rings of influence (involving family, friends, the healthcare system, society).

The attitudes, emotions and behaviours in each one may reflect and reinforce those in any other, further damaging or helping to heal them in the process. Splits within the paediatric team echoed the rival views of Liam's parents, which in turn may have mirrored his own initial ambivalence towards his future prospects. More positively, Liam's final resolve could be seen to have brought together both parents and team in his terminal, palliative care.

Any therapist wishing to help must therefore take account not only of individual work with the child, but of the systemic context, both to free relationships of negative influences and to make proper use of the positives. To that extent, systems theory is applicable not only to the way we must draw on many different streams of study to understand a child's spiritual development, but also to the multilayered approach necessary for help (Lerner *et al*, 2006).

Social context

Those layers begin with the conflict-ridden social system within which we all live and work. On the one hand, most countries would sign up to the philosophy behind the United Nations' Convention on the Rights of the Child, even to the 'spiritual rights' of children over and above their more prosaic reflections (Bradford, 1994), but little seems to find its way into practice. Recent reports suggest that the gap between the haves and have-nots in UK society has widened (Dorling *et al*, 2007), to the extent that of all the 21 most developed nations, it is now the unhappiest place for a child to be brought up (UNICEF, 2007). Some groups of young people with strong cultural or ethnic identities may survive the chaos around them, such as young Asian women (Kassam, 1997) or inner-city Black girls (West Stevens, 2002). Others at least find a sense of purpose and belonging in ways which adults may deem pathological. It is no good castigating young boys for their gang culture or young girls for teenage pregnancy, if all society has to give them to show their self-worth is a flick-knife to wave or a pram to push down the street.

Again, we have to ask why it is that someone like Liam, from a wind-swept housing estate in which family breakdown, child abuse, drug and alcohol addiction, crime and school drop-out are rife, may yet grow up with such a powerful spirituality intact. Social resilience is just one of the many mysteries still to be addressed in research which as yet seems to have had little impact on social and civic policy (Hornberger *et al*, 2006).

Educational context

Not surprisingly, a similar ambivalence is reflected in the many service contexts in which a developing child like Liam might find him- or herself. Thus, government policy has stressed the links between school and home in a child's spiritual and moral development for over a decade (National Curriculum Council, 1993), backed up by a succession of inspectorate reports (Office for Standards in Education, 1994; 1999; 2004). There is much research into school-based values (Halstead & Taylor, 2000) and outline responses from individual schools (Farrer, 2000), authorities (Kent County Council Education Services, 1994) and chief executives (Tate, 1996). There are guidelines on spiritual education for particular faith schools – Catholic (Diocesan Department of Religious Education, 2001), Muslim (The Islamic Academy, 1991) and various Christian denominations (Peacocke, 1993) – but there are huge gaps between the perspectives of inspectors and teachers (Sokanovic & Miller, 1999). This is hardly surprising in a context where teachers are told one minute that they are to be judged solely on their pupils' academic performance and the next that they are central to a holistic view of child development (Department for Education and Skills, 2004), especially when most pastoral skills have been eradicated from their training. Admittedly, there are many guides that a child psychiatrist working with teachers may use, particularly in the early years (Dowling, 2005; Eaude, 2005) but it may be difficult to find room for such approaches within the pressure cooker atmosphere of secondary schools or in the units for children with special educational needs (Brown, 1998) or emotional and behavioural disturbance (Cole & Visser, 1998).

Someone like Liam, in and out of school in his early years and increasingly distant from any formal schooling in adolescence, would receive no such guidance at all. His maturity is testimony again to the fact that spiritual development is influenced by what happens around a child, but is ultimately dependent on neither innate cognitive abilities nor what education makes of them.

Care system

Arguably, it is the responsibility of all of us to promote the spiritual well-being of children in everyday life (Crompton, 2001), but that must be particularly true of those who have children as deprived as Liam in their statutory care. This has been recognised in Children Act legislation (Bradford, 1995) and in the provision of training packs for social workers (Crompton, 1998). There are compendia of youth-work projects on spirituality (Nacif, 2005) and individual accounts of efforts to make a difference for Black and minority ethnic communities (Blueprint Project, 2004). Four areas have been identified for spiritual social work: gift giving (unconditional generosity towards cared-for children without expectation of reward); taking their suffering seriously (including behavioural manifestations of emotional pain); forgiveness of their behaviour; and the creation of new choices (different ways of expressing feelings that free the children's lives from old battles) (Scott & Magnuson, 2006).

All that is easier said than done. Strong doubts have been expressed about whether the care services are upholding young people's rights to spiritual development (Callaghan, 2003). Much of that may be due to the usual antipathy between those struggling at the coalface with very challenging behaviour and academics preaching at them from the safety of their ivory towers (Borgman, 2006). Much may be due to the load carried by individual social workers and residential care staff who are simply too ground down by statutory tasks, responsibilities and the anxieties associated with them to spend quality time with any one child on their books. But much might also be a defence against absorbing the pain of children by care workers who are aware of their own unhappiness, lurking just beneath the surface of their working life – an 'intentional strategy of avoidance' (Anglin, 2002: p. 108).

The child psychiatrist wanting to help children like Liam when they are in local authority care might first have to give more support to the staff before they are able, in turn, to approach the behaviour of the children with that most difficult but important message of good parenting – 'I don't like what you have done but it doesn't affect my love for you'.

Health service

The technology of healthcare has advanced to such a degree that transition has become one of its hottest topics – how to transfer patients who would once have died in childhood or adolescence from paediatric to adult services. The emotions involved for staff trying to let go of a child that they may have looked after for years, through all stages of development, may echo those of parents who are proud of their child's growing independence while aware that it will carry him or her further and further away from their care. But for many children, of course, transition is not an option because their illness cannot be cured. Staff may be plunged into a bereavement process almost as keen as that of the child's family itself. How that process is handled by medical professionals may have a dramatic effect on how the family handles its own grief in turn. Where staff are open and mutually supportive, so are the family more likely to be, with each other and with their child. Conversely, where staff are closed off and coldly professional, so parents may be too, condemning each other and their child to a lonely death, trapped in denial. Repeated pleas have been made for a sensitive honesty at all levels, but there is a strong argument from liaison child psychiatrists and other professionals for the need for staff support before that could happen (Shooter, 2005).

When to let go

Nowhere is this more fraught than when an active decision is made to withhold or withdraw treatment. The number of deaths in neonatal intensive therapy units due to withdrawal rose nearly five-fold in the 1990s as the ability to save lives, it seems, was matched by increasing recognition of how little relief it may have to offer the severely, multiply-disabled child. When the quality of a baby's life is poor, the quality of its death might be more important (Shooter, 1998). There are professional guidelines to help implement such a decision and ethics committees are available in many hospitals to act as a forum for debate (Watson, 1999). But most staff and parents come to their decision bravely together, being careful to act in the best interest of the child, taking time to respect every viewpoint, trying to achieve consensus and to avoid landing one person (parent, consultant or manager) with the whole burden of the decision, offering palliative care and support to all, and recognising, albeit painfully, that they can only make the best decision they see fit. There are no ideal solutions (Shooter & Watson, 2000).

Such ethical decisions may shake the religious faith of anyone. They may also represent a spiritual challenge in a much broader sense, about the sanctity of life and the balance to be struck with suffering. Where the law becomes involved in a decision not to treat a baby, often in the glare of media publicity, spiritual strengths may be severely stressed. Where the patient is an adolescent like Liam, making the decision to withdraw from treatment on his own account, they may be stretched to breaking point. To hold the situation together, to contain the distress of everyone while healing processes are at work in child, family and hospital team, may be the most difficult but vital task the liaison child psychiatrist can perform.

Family

Within these envelopes, the family meets the influences of those around them with their own structural and systemic dynamics. To understand the child's family and to work successfully with them, the child psychiatrist must grasp something of their relationships, both positive and negative, that are mutually dependent and may bind the members together emotionally, even though, as in Liam's case, the parents may have long since separated. Built upon those relationships, the psychiatrist needs to know what roles each family member performs (who does what) and what rulebook the family obeys (how we do it). Is this a family that shares its joys and upsets openly together or is it a family that keeps secrets? Is it a family where everyone shoulders their share of responsibilities or is it one in which one person or one relationship carries the can for everybody? Above all, the psychiatrist needs to know what body of tradition, what 'mythology', has been handed down in the family from one generation to another. This may be very different from the psychiatrist's own way of doing things but he or she must work within it, initially at least, if he or she is to engage them in therapy. What, for example, is the meaning of illness in this family? With Liam's parents, the implications were only too obvious as his kidney failure became yet another battleground in the continuing war of guilt between his mother and father. Liam's decision to take responsibility for his own prognosis must have been a devastating shock to their perception of blame and counter-blame. No wonder it was impossible for them, at first, to come to terms with it.

Unlike childhood research, there are well-authenticated indices for the assessment of individual, adult spiritual development, such as the

Spiritual Well-Being Scale (SWBS), Index of Core Spiritual Experience (INSPIRIT), Spirituality Assessment Scale (SAS) and Religious Coping Styles Questionnaire (RCOPE) (Houskamp *et al*, 2004). Still, the family may have a spirituality as a whole, of greater or lesser maturity, that can be plotted across generations in 'spiritual genograms' (Hodge, 2001). All aspects of the family's spiritual functions that may help or hinder their child's spiritual development must be assessed (Boyatzis *et al*, 2006). Rough guides have been laid down to help, such as BELIEF:

- What is the family's Belief system?
- What Ethical values does it adhere to?
- What Lifestyle does it practise?
- What Involvement does it have in any constructive or destructive spiritual communities?
- What Education has it received in spiritual issues that it may have passed on to its members?
- What attitudes does it have to Future family issues? (McEvoy, 2003).

It is easy here for therapists to slip into a high moral tone: 'associated childhood emotional and behavioural problems have increased at an alarming rate ... married people are healthier, happier and live longer ... children from homes with married parents tend to fare better ... and are at less risk of pathology and disruptive family life events' (Moncher & Josephson, 2004: p. 50). Whether the research shows all that to be true or not, such judgements are unlikely to get the therapist very far in working with a family like Liam's, and would miss the surprise of discovering a child of such spiritual maturity from entirely the 'wrong' sort of background. Clinicians have contact with families at life's most critical transition points; the therapist's job is to draw upon whatever resources there are for change, and to facilitate the family's growth rather that thrust the therapist's own values upon them.

Child–psychiatrist relationship

And so to the very heart of those concentric layers – the spirituality of the child and the part the child psychiatrist might have in its development. Extravagant claims have been made for the importance of that relationship and the disastrous consequences of shirking responsibility for it.

> By ignoring spiritual development in times of suffering and transition, the therapist is fostering (in the child) an understanding of the world that does not embrace or validate the sacred dimension of human experience ... [the child] is left with depleted ways of coping, connecting, and ultimately evolving. From a spiritual perspective a therapist unwilling to address the highest potential within the child can divert an individual from his or her life's work and may perpetuate suffering by disavowing the client's inherent dialogue with the universe [Miller & Kelley, 2006: p. 426].

One has to ask why practitioners used to dealing with every other aspect of child development should be loath to tackle spirituality (Plotnikoff,

1997; Pfund, 2000). Some seem wary of intruding into what is seen as the child's and the family's private world. Some are anxious about the enormity of the issues they might uncover there and their inability to provide answers. Some doubt their capacity to hold onto their own opinions and to avoid proselytising in their approach. Some may still not understand the significance of spiritual development or, if they do, have no idea how and to what end to assess and work with it.

There are no IQ scores for measuring a young person's spirituality. As in most unexplored territory, the therapist must fall back on a qualitative feel for the stage of development the child's spirituality has reached, plotted against a schema such as Fowler's (see p. 84) and its appropriateness in a child of such age and circumstances. With adolescents of even moderate verbal ability, this might be relatively easily achievable by open-ended questioning. Once enough trust has been secured, most adolescents are only too willing to explore their identity, what they stand for, what their calling might be and how successful or frustrated they are in expressing it in their life. Given time, respect and privacy, Liam's spirituality had a drive of its own. The therapist's task was to support it and watch 'with proper awe' the course of its trajectory (Miller & Kelley, 2006).

Younger children may be limited cognitively but this should be no barrier to spiritual assessment through skilled observation and play. A study of sixty 3 to 6-year-olds (Champagne, 2003) identified three 'modes of being', covering all aspects of the child's spirituality:

1   The sensitive mode (perceptions and expressions, as evident in their screaming, laughing, crying, running and physical gestures).
2   The relational mode (interactions with others, as evident in affectionate or distant behaviour, the need for affirmation, participating with caregivers or peers in play or resolving problem situations).
3   The existential mode (participation in the moment through games, imagination and symbols with which they explore the world in the here and now).

In other words, spirituality is a child's basic dimension of being and is open to discovery by the therapist prepared to seize the moment through any medium available (Sexson, 2004) – drawing, toys, stories, conversation and the natural world, being alive to their metaphorical as well as their literal meaning.

Help lies not in imposing spiritual truths upon a child but in uncovering their natural spirituality and helping to repair it or use its strength in whatever adverse circumstances there may be. If it has been recognised at all, spiritual development has traditionally been seen as just one aspect to suffering in primary mental health problems but the new psycho-spiritual therapies operate from the assumption that there are primary spiritual factors in all mental disorders (Miller & Kelley, 2006). Problems with spirituality are the very core of those disorders rather than their surface reflection. Symptoms are 'signals of spiritual challenge' and even the pain that brings the patient to therapy is an opportunity for growth rather than something to be eradicated.

In all this, children and adolescents are seen as being more curious, aware and open to a natural understanding of the universe than adults, including therapists! They may take on board quite naturally the belief that suffering comes from living out of synchrony with their spiritual values and that such values need encouragement rather than revising, editing or flattening by those around them. Given the opportunity to explore them in the 'contemplative space' of psychotherapy (Semple *et al*, 2009), children like Liam could express them more clearly, families could be helped to hear them, and child and family together could use the crisis to shift old relationships and attitudes into new ones.

Such therapy is child-centred in every sense; but this may open up huge questions of ethics and technique for the therapist. There are, at the very least, some difficult tightropes to walk between pairs of principles perched precariously on either side. In tackling Liam's core spirituality in circumstances that amount to anticipatory grief-work, therapist and patient were bound to become very close. Issues of transference and counter-transference would have been important. It would have been easy for the therapist to have become Liam's substitute parent, pushing the real parents even further out of his life just at the point at which they needed to be reconciled to him before his death. Conversely, it would have been easy for Liam to have 'become' the therapist's child, especially if the therapist had children of a similar age, eliciting a parental desperation to save him rather than respect for his decision to die. There is something of the parent–child in every successful therapeutic relationship, and that can be examined as part of the work, but some professional distance has also to be maintained.

Similarly, risk has to be balanced with safety. It is difficult to know how a therapist could ever work with adolescents without taking risks. This is, after all, what adolescents are supposed to be doing with their lives and the good-enough parent knows that they will not develop an independent identity without being allowed to do so. Yet the parent's role is also to provide boundaries within which that experimentation can take place and against which the adolescent can have a safe rebellion. In Liam's case, the natural parents never seemed to have understood this paradox and the wider hospital 'family' were on the verge of fragmentation in the face of his impending death. Once he had established that Liam's decision was a rational one, the therapist was therefore faced with the sternest test of this balance: how to allow him the most fateful risk of all, to withdraw from treatment, within a continuing envelope of emotional, physical and spiritual support.

Normally, any therapeutic relationship would have a shape to it. There would be an initial joining period during which enough trust is established to work with such deep issues as spirituality; a middle period in which those issues can be tackled; and a final separation period in which therapist and client let go of a relationship of some intimacy. None of those periods should be hurried beyond the pace that either therapist or child can manage. But everything is telescoped by death. The urgency of Liam's situation opened a window through which the therapist had to jump lest the opportunity be lost forever. In the process, traditional clarities of role had to give way to a much greater flexibility. At one moment, Liam's therapist found himself acting as a psychiatrist assessing legal capacity, the next as therapist working with Liam to understand his needs, then as advocate for Liam's wishes to family and treatment team and finally as supporter of everyone concerned with the consequences of Liam's decision. No doubt, following Liam's death, he would have been called upon to help with the grief it left in its wake.

All these issues would be enough to keep the most skilled of therapists awake, sweating in the night, for the pain of Liam's situation would shake him or her to the core of their own spiritual self, challenging their faith in its widest sense and stirring up their own unresolved experiences. This brings with it some further balances to be struck. To avoid going under, the therapist would need support, someone with whom to share the feelings that get no easier with experience. But this could undermine the confidentiality of the therapeutic relationship, without which no adolescent would be likely to trust it.

In establishing the rules of confidentiality, therefore, the therapist must make clear three caveats:

1   'If you tell me that you are being abused, I am legally obliged to disclose it.'
2   'If you tell me that you want me to pass on a message that is too difficult to disclose yourself, I will do so.'
3   'If you tell me something so anxiety provoking that I cannot carry it alone, I may need to seek a trusted other with whom to share it.'

It may be that Liam's trust in the therapist would be reinforced, not weakened, by such a contract. Certainly, the therapist helped pass on and support Liam's wishes to the adults around him. Knowing that the therapist had his own support may well have encouraged Liam to unburden on the therapist the feelings in the face of which other adults had threatened to crumble.

Despite all these challenges, working with young people in need remains a privilege. That an adolescent approaching death, like Liam, or other children in their everyday difficulties, should trust a therapist with their spiritual story that should fill us with wonder (Hart, 2003). If the responsibility of it seems too great, if the therapist is unbalanced on any of those tightropes of technique, if the fear of making things worse prevents him or her from doing anything at all, the therapist should be led by the children themselves and the 'raw' spiritual guidance of their words (Miller & Kelley, 2006).

Like Liam's therapist, his parents and the hospital staff, all of us have the chance to learn from our child-teachers 'as they hustle their way through space and time, doing and doing and doing, but also stopping and asking and wondering, and in their own fashion declaring and affirming' (Coles, 1990: p. 351). All of us have the chance to be inspired in our own spirituality by their pilgrim soul.

References

Anderson, P. (1998) Spiritual hunger. *Nursing Times*, **94**, 34–35.

Anglin, J. P. (2002) *Pain, Normality and the Struggle for the Congruence: Re-Interpreting Residential Care for Children and Youth*. Haworth Press.

Benson, P. L. (2006) The science of child and adolescent spiritual development: definitional, theoretical, and field-building challenges. In *The Handbook of Spiritual Development in Childhood and Adolescence* (eds E. C. Roehlkepartain, P. Ebstyne King, L. Wagener, *et al*), p. 484. Sage Publications.

Blakeney, R. F. & Blakeney, C. D. (2006) Delinquency: a quest for moral and spiritual integrity? In *The Handbook of Spiritual Development in Childhood and Adolescence* (eds E. C. Roehlkepartain, P. Ebstyne King, L. Wagener, *et al*), pp. 371–383. Sage Publications.

Bloom, P. (2004) *Descartes' Baby: How the Science of Child Development Explains What Makes Us Human*. Heinemann.

Blueprint Project (2004) *The Care Experience: Through Black Eyes*. National Children's Bureau. Voice for the Child in Care.

Borgman, D. (2006) Bridging the gap: from social science to congregations, researchers to practitioners. In *The Handbook of Spiritual Development in Childhood and Adolescence* (eds E. C. Roehlkepartain, P. Ebstyne King, L. Wagener, *et al*), pp. 435–444. Sage Publications.

Boyatzis, C., Dollahite, D. C. & Marks, L. D. (2006) The family as a context for religious and spiritual development in childhood and youth. In *The Handbook of Spiritual Development in Childhood and Adolescence* (eds E. C. Roehlkepartain, P. Ebstyne King, L. Wagener, *et al*), pp. 279–309. Sage Publications.

Bradford, J. (1994) Spiritual and religious rights of children. *Children Worldwide*, **21**, 16–19.

Bradford, J. (1995) *Caring for the Whole Child: a Holistic Approach to Spirituality*. Children's Society.

Brown, E. (1998) Things of the spirit: spiritual, moral, social and cultural development. *Support for Learning*, **13**, 157–162.

Callaghan, D. (2003) Free the spirit. *Community Care*, **1469** (24 April), 28–29.

Casado, M. (2000) Coping strategies and gender differences among children who have been exposed to risk factors. *Dissertation Abstracts International*, **61**, 1305.

Champagne, E. (2003) Being a child, a spiritual child. *International Journal of Child Spirituality*, **8**, 43–53.

Cole, T. & Visser, J. (1998) How should the 'effectiveness' of schools for pupils with EBD be assessed? *Emotional and Behavioural Difficulties*, **3**, 37–43.

Coles, R. (1986) *The Political Life of Children*. Houghton Mifflin Company.

Coles, R. (1990) *The Spiritual Life of Children*. Houghton Mifflin Company.

Crawford, E., Wright, M. O. & Masten, A. S. (2006) Resilience and spirituality in youth. In *The Handbook of Spiritual Development in Childhood and Adolescence* (eds E. C. Roehlkepartain, P. Ebstyne King, L. Wagener, *et al*), pp. 355–370. Sage Publications.

Crompton, M. (1998) *Children, Spirituality, Religion and Social Work*. Ashgate.

Crompton, M. (2001) *Who am I? Promoting Children's Spiritual Well-Being in Everyday Life: A Guide for All Who Care for Children*. Barnado's.

Dalai Lama (2001) *An Open Heart: Practising Compassion in Everyday Life*. Little, Brown.

Department for Education and Skills (2004) *Every Child Matters: Next Steps*. DfES Publications.

DiLorenzo, P., Johnson, R. & Bussey, H. (2001) The role of spirituality in the recovery process. *Child Welfare*, **80**, 257–273.

Diocesan Department of Religious Education (2001) *All That I Am*. Diocesan Department of Religious Education.

Dorling, D., Rigby, J., Wheeler, B. *et al* (2007) *Poverty, Wealth and Place in Britain 1968–2005*. Policy Press for the Joseph Rowntree Foundation.

Dowling, M. (2005) All about ... spirituality. *Nursery World*, **105**, 17–24.

Eaude, T. (2005) Strangely familiar? Teachers making sense of young children's spiritual development. *Early Years*, **25**, 237–248.

Engebretson, K. (2006) Identity, masculinity and spirituality: a study of Australian teenage boys. *Journal of Youth Studies*, **9**, 91–110.

Erikson, E. H. (1959) *Identity and the Life Cycle: Selected Papers*. Psychological Issues, Monograph 1, Vol. I. International Universities Press.

Farrer, F. (2000) Words into action. *TES Primary*, **9**, 14–17.

Fowler, J. W. & Dell, M. L. (2004) Stages of faith and identity: birth to teens. *Child and Adolescent Psychiatric Clinics of North America*, **13**, 17–33.

Frankl, V. (2000) *Man's Search for Meaning*. Beacon Press.

Freud, S. (1933) The ouestion of a Weltanschauung. Reprinted 1962 in *The Standard Edition of the Complete Psychological Works of Sigmund Freud* (ed. J. Strachey), vol. 22, pp. 158–167. Hogarth Press.

Garbarino, J. & Bedard, C. (1996) Spiritual challenges to children facing violent trauma. *Childhood*, **3**, 467–478.

Gottlieb, A. (2006) Non-Western approaches to spiritual development among infants and young children: a case study from west Africa. In *The Handbook of Spiritual Development in Childhood and Adolescence* (eds E. C. Roehlkepartain, P. Ebstyne King, L. Wagener, *et al*), pp. 150–162. Sage Publications.

Granqvist, P. & Dickie, J. R. (2006) Attachment and spiritual development in childhood and adolescence. In *The Handbook of Spiritual Development in Childhood and Adolescence* (eds E. C. Roehlkepartain, P. Ebstyne King, L. Wagener, *et al*), pp. 197–210. Sage Publications.

Halstead, J. M. & Taylor, M. J. (2000) *Development of Values, Attitudes and Personal Qualities: a Review of Research*. NFER.

Hart, T. (2003) *The Secret Spiritual World of Children*. Inner Ocean.

Hodge, D. R. (2001) Spiritual genograms: a generational approach to assessing spirituality. *Family and Society*, **82**, 35–48.

Hornberger, S., Jones, R. F. & Miller, R. L. (2006) Bridging to public policy and civic society. In *The Handbook of Spiritual Development in Childhood and Adolescence* (eds E. C. Roehlkepartain, P. Ebstyne King, L. Wagener, *et al*), pp. 458–472. Sage Publications.

Houskamp, B. M., Fisher, L. A. & Stuber, M. L. (2004) Spirituality in children and adolescents: research findings and implications for clinicians and researchers. *Child and Adolescent Psychiatric Clinics of North America*, **13**, 221–230.

The Islamic Academy (1991) *Faith as the Basis of Education in a Multi-faith, Multicultural Country*. Islamic Academy.

Iweala, U. (2005) *Beasts of No Nation*. John Murray.

Johnson, C. N. & Boyatzis, C. J. (2006) Cognitive–cultural foundations of spiritual development. In *The Handbook of Spiritual Development in Childhood and Adolescence* (eds E. C. Roehlkepartain, P. Ebstyne King, L. Wagener, *et al*), pp. 211–223. Sage Publications.

Josephson, A. M. & Dell, M. L. (2004) Religion and spirituality in child and adolescent psychiatry: a new frontier. *Child and Adolescent Psychiatric Clinics of North America*, **13**, 1–15.

Kassam, N. (1997) *Telling It Like It Is: Young Asian Women Talk*. Women's Press.

Kent County Council Education Services (1994) *Starting together*. Kent County Council.

King, P. E. & Benson, P. L. (2006) Spiritual development and adolescent well-being and thriving. In *The Handbook of Spiritual Development in Childhood and Adolescence* (eds E. C. Roehlkepartain, P. Ebstyne King, L. Wagener, *et al*), pp. 384–398. Sage Publications.

King, U. (2001) Introduction: spirituality, society and the millennium – wasteland, wilderness or new vision? In *Spirituality and Society in the New Millennium*, pp. 1–13. Sussex Academic Press.

Lerner, R. M., Alberts, A. E., Anderson, P. M., *et al* (2006) On making humans human: spirituality and the promotion of positive youth development. In *The Handbook of Spiritual Development in Childhood and Adolescence* (eds E. C. Roehlkepartain, P. Ebstyne King, L. Wagener, *et al*), pp. 60–72. Sage Publications.

Mabe, P. A. & Josephson, A. (2004) Child and adolescent psychopathology: spiritual and religious perspectives. *Child and Adolescent Psychiatric Clinics of North America*, **13**, 111–125.

MacDonald, D. A. (2000) Spirituality: description, measurement. *Journal of Personality*, **68**, 157–197.

Mallick, J. & Watts, M. (1999) Spirituality and self: a case from drug education. *Early Child Development and Care*, **155**, 79–94.

Mattis, J. S., Ahluwalia, M. K., Cowie, S.-A. E., *et al* (2006) Ethnicity, culture and spiritual development. In *The Handbook of Spiritual Development in Childhood and Adolescence* (eds E. C. Roehlkepartain, P. Ebstyne King, L. Wagener, *et al*), pp. 283–297. Sage Publications.

McEvoy, M. (2003) Culture and spirituality as an integrated concept in paediatric care. *American Journal of Maternal Child Nursing*, **28**, 39–43.

Miller, L. & Kelley, B. (2006) Spiritually oriented psychotherapy with youth: a child-centred approach. In *The Handbook of Spiritual Development in Childhood and Adolescence* (eds E. C. Roehlkepartain, P. Ebstyne King, L. Wagener, *et al*), pp. 421–434. Sage Publications.

Moncher, F. J. & Josephson, A. M. (2004) Religious and spiritual aspects of family assessment. *Child and Adolescent Psychiatric Clinics of North America*, **13**, 49–70.

Nacif, A. P. (2005) A sense of self. *Young People Now*, **306**, 14–15.

National Curriculum Council (1993) *Spiritual and Moral Development (discussion paper)*. National Curriculum Council.

Newberg, A. B. & Newberg, S. K. (2006) A neuropsychological perspective on spiritual development. In *The Handbook of Spiritual Development in Childhood and Adolescence* (eds E. C. Roehlkepartain, P. Ebstyne King, L. Wagener, *et al*), pp. 183–196. Sage Publications.

Nye, R. M. (1999) Rational consciousness and the spiritual lives of children: convergence with children's theory of mind. In *Psychological Studies on Spiritual and Religious Development* (eds K. H. Reich, F. K. Oser & W. G. Scarlett), *Vol. 2: Being Human*. Pabst Science.

Office for Standards in Education (1994) *Spiritual, Moral, Social and Cultural Development: an OFSTED Discussion Paper*. OFSTED.

Office for Standards in Education (1999) *Primary Education: a Review of Primary Schools in England 1994–1998*. TSO (The Stationery Office).

Office for Standards in Education (2004) *Promoting and Evaluating Pupils' Spiritual, Moral, Social and Cultural Development*. OFSTED.

Oman, D. & Thoresen, C. E. (2006) Religion, spirituality and children's physical health. In *The Handbook of Spiritual Development in Childhood and Adolescence* (eds E. C. Roehlkepartain, P. Ebstyne King, L. Wagener, *et al*), pp. 399–416. Sage Publications.

Peacocke, R. (1993) Religious education in the early years. *Early Education*, **10**, 4–7.

Pendleton, S. M. (2002) Religious/spiritual coping in childhood cystic fibrosis. *Pediatrics*, **109**, 134–135.

Pfund, R. (2000) Nurturing a child's spirituality. *Journal of Child Health Care*, **4**, 143–145.

Piaget, J. (1952) *The Origins of Intelligence in Children*. International Universities Press.

Plotnikoff, G. (1997) Spirituality, religion and the physician: new ethical challenges in patient care. *Bioethics Forum*, **13**, 25–30.

Reich, K. H., Oser, F. K. & Scarlett, W. G. (eds) (1999) *Psychological Studies on Spiritual and Religious Development, Vol. 2: Being Human: the Case of Religion*. Pabst Science.

Roehlkepartain, E. C. & Patel, E. (2006) Congregations: unexamined crucibles for spiritual development. In *The Handbook of Spiritual Development in Childhood and Adolescence* (eds E. C. Roehlkepartain, P. Ebstyne King, L. Wagener, *et al*), pp. 324–336. Sage Publications.

Roehlkepartain, E. C., King, P. E., Wagener, L., *et al* (eds) (2006) *The Handbook of Spiritual Development in Childhood and Adolescence*. Sage Publications.

Rossetti, S. J. (1995) The impact of child sexual abuse on attitudes towards God and the Catholic Church. *Child Abuse and Neglect*, **19**, 1469–1481.

Schwartz, K. D., Bukowski, W. M. & Aoki, W. T. (2006) Mentors, friends and gurus: peer and non-parental influences on spiritual development. In *The Handbook of Spiritual Development in Childhood and Adolescence* (eds E. C. Roehlkepartain, P. Ebstyne King, L. Wagener, *et al*), pp. 310–323. Sage Publications.

Scott, D. G. & Magnuson, D. (2006) Integrating spiritual development into child and youth care programmes and institutions. In *The Handbook of Spiritual Development in Childhood and Adolescence* (eds E. C. Roehlkepartain, P. Ebstyne King, L. Wagener, *et al*), pp. 445–457. Sage Publications.

Semple, R. J., Lee, J. & Miller, L. F. (2009) Mindfulness-based cognitive therapy for children. In *Mindfulness-Based Treatment Approaches for Clinical Practitioners* (ed. R. Baer). Elsevier.

Sexson, S. B. (2004) Religious and spiritual assessment of the child and adolescent. *Child and Adolescent Psychiatric Clinics of North America*, **13**, 35–47.

Shooter, M. S. (1998) The ethics of withholding and withdrawing therapy in infants and young children. In *CAPD/CCPD in Children* (eds R. N. Fine, S. R. Alexander & B. A. Warady), pp. 433–450. Kluwer Academic Publishers.

Shooter, M. S. (2005) Children and adolescents who have chronic physical illness. In *Child and Adolescent Mental Health Services: Strategy, Planning, Delivery and Evaluation* (eds R. William & M. Kerfoot). Oxford University Press.

Shooter, M. S. & Watson, A. (2000) The ethics of withholding and withdrawing treatment in infants. *Paediatric Nephrology*, **14**, 347–351.

Sokanovic, M. & Muller, D. (1999) Professional and educational perspectives on spirituality in young children. *Pastoral Care in Education*, **17**, 9–16.

Sommer, D. (1989) Spiritual needs of dying children. *Issues in Comprehensive Paediatric Nursing*, **12**, 225–233.

Stewart, C. (2000) The influence of spirituality on substance use of college students. *Journal of Drug Education*, **31**, 343–351.

Stuber, M. L. & Houskamp, B. M. (2004) Spirituality in children confronting death. *Child and Adolescent Psychiatric Clinics of North America*, **13**, 127–136.

Sveidqvist, V. (2003) Who am I, and why am I here? Young people's perspectives on the role of spirituality in the promotion of their mental health. *International Journal of Mental Health Promotion*, **5**, 36–44.

Tate, N. (1996) The role of the school in promoting moral, spiritual and cultural values. *Education Review*, **10**, 66–70.

UNICEF (2007) *Child Poverty in Perspective: an Overview of Child Well-Being in Rich Countries*. UNICEF Innocenti Research Centre.

Watson, A. R. (1999) An ethics of clinical practice committee: should every hospital have one? *Proceedings of the Royal College of Physicians of Edinburgh*, **29**, 335–337.

West Stevens, J. (2002) *Smart and Sassy: the Strengths of Inner City Black Girls*. Oxford University Press.

Wilber, K. (1999) Spirituality and developmental lines: are there stages? *Journal of Transpersonal Psychology*, **31**, 1–10.

Yeats, W. B. (1893) When We Are Old. Reprinted (1979) in *The Collected Poems of W. B. Yeats*. Macmillan.

CHAPTER 6

Psychotherapy

Andrew Powell and Christopher MacKenna

> We live in succession, in division, in parts, in particles. Meantime within man is the soul of the whole; the wise silence; the universal beauty, to which every part and particle is equally related, the eternal ONE. And this deep power in which we exist and whose beatitude is all accessible to us, is not only self-sufficing and perfect in every hour, but the act of seeing and the thing seen, the seer and the spectacle, the subject and the object, are one. We see the world piece by piece, as the sun, the moon, the animal, the tree; but the whole, of which these are shining parts, is the soul.
>
> Ralph Waldo Emerson, 'The Over-Soul', Ninth Essay (1841)

For many doctors, let alone the general public, the relationship of psychiatry to psychotherapy is a source of confusion. When is emotional disturbance a sign of a mental illness requiring drug treatment? When is it a problem that can be resolved through discussion and discovering how it arose? When is it a mixture of the two? And what is best done about it? People seeking help are often directed to psychiatrists, psychologists, psychotherapists, or counsellors without understanding either the range of options available to them or the rationale for consulting one rather than the other.

Spiritual concerns are regarded with even less clarity. Where there is a core religious problem and the person belongs to an established faith tradition, the priest, imam, rabbi or appropriate spiritual advisor is likely to become involved. However, for people who do not belong to a religious community or faith tradition there are no guidelines; the healthcare practitioner may or may not be personally interested in the patient's spiritual reality. In addition, psychiatrists working with a medical model of mental illness are likely to see spiritual issues as beyond their competence and many psychotherapists prefer to stick specifically to psychological objectives.

Yet some psychiatrists and psychotherapists do see the importance of addressing spiritual concerns, either because they intuitively recognise this to be an essential part of treating the 'whole' person or because they have undergone training in therapy that values this dimension of human life.

101

Mapping the territory

Psychiatry is a medical discipline specialising in the treatment of mental illness; as all Western medicine, it is founded on the concept of disease and its greatest ambition is nothing less than cure. Symptoms are the signs of disease and progress is directly measured by their alleviation.

Psychotherapy, too, aims to relieve mental distress, whether or not it occurs in the presence of diagnosable mental illness. Symptom reduction is an important indicator of success, yet other subjective indices of improvement, less easily measured, such as becoming more aware of feelings, both one's own and other peoples', are also counted as important.

A working definition of spirituality has been given in chapter 1 of this book (p. 4). It is one of many such attempts to address humankind's 'quest for understanding answers to ultimate questions about life, about meaning, and about relationship with the sacred or transcendent' (Koenig *et al*, 2001). It is described elsewhere as 'the essentially human, personal and interpersonal dimension, which integrates and transcends the cultural, religious, psychological, social and emotional aspects of the person or is more specifically concerned with "soul" or "spirit"' (http://www.rcpsych.ac.uk/spirit).

The wholeness of being with which spirituality is primarily concerned can be conceived in many ways. For some, it is to be found in the majesty of the physical universe; for some, it is the expression of love on which the future of every family, nation, even our planet depends, while others seek the presence of the Divine through meditation, worship and prayer.

In contrast, the prevailing reductionist culture of science deals not with the whole but with the part. A prime value, therefore, of introducing spirituality into this discussion is in offering a framework for relating the part to the whole, indeed, one in which the whole is greater than the sum of its parts.

One coin, two sides

Just over a hundred years ago, Albert Einstein showed in his famous theory of relativity that mass and energy are exchangeable. Biological psychiatry, having taken the path of physicalist science, invests in the study of the physical brain. Psychotherapy, in contrast, is concerned with the mind, which has no mass. The psychiatrist who looks exclusively for physical explanations of mental illness, or the psychotherapist who dismisses the impact of brain chemistry, is each overlooking the other side of the coin by mistaking the part for the whole.

Einstein's vision was holistic and profoundly spiritual. Indeed, he was later to claim that 'every one who is seriously involved in the pursuit of science becomes convinced that a spirit is manifest in the laws of the Universe – a spirit vastly superior to that of man, and one in the face of which we with our modest powers must feel humble' (as quoted in Abrams

& Primack, 2000: p. 154). Einstein's groundbreaking perspective shows us the whole coin, impressing on us the complementarity of brain and mind, how they exist conjointly, how each is irreducible and yet indispensable to the other. Einstein offers us a vision of integration, which is the essence of spirituality. Applied to the psychiatric profession, it spans the divide within mental healthcare (Fig. 6.1).

Fig. 6.1 Spirit as the unifying principle

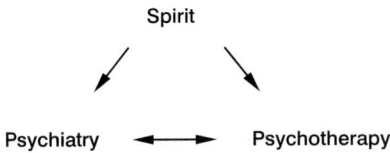

Why should such a holistic paradigm have been so tenaciously resisted? The answer lies in the human tendency to become emotionally attached to the culturally sanctioned vision of reality. Since Isaac Newton, the physicalist world view that matter is primary and mind secondary has prevailed. Yet current science, especially quantum mechanics, is making counter-intuitive demands on us that challenge common sense perception so that we may have to abandon the notion that matter comes before mind (consciousness) (Powell, 2002), and instead envisage both arising out of what astronomers call 'dark matter', now known to be swarming with unimaginable energies.

Psychiatry, like other applied sciences, has remained loyal to the physicalist world view, but research into spirituality and mental health is widening the horizon (Larson & Larson, 2001; Larson *et al*, 2001). Instruments are being developed (King & Dein, 1998) that can provide a measure of the religious and spiritual dimension and there is strong outcome research on the value of specific spiritually-informed treatment approaches such as mindfulness–meditation (Kabat-Zinn *et al*, 1992; Kabat-Zinn, 1995). Psychiatrists also need to be better informed about the science of parapsychology (Radin, 2006) and of the phenomenology of altered states of consciousness, so that they can be maximally discerning when patients are reporting anomalous events (Powell, 2004*a*,*b*).

Psychotherapy, too, is slowly waking up to the spiritual dimension, as seen in the increasing number of publications in the field (Bomford, 1999; Stein, 1999; MacKenna, 2002, 2004, 2005*a*,*b*, 2006, 2007; Schreurs, 2002; Field *et al*, 2005). Indeed, all psychological therapies have the potential to lead to spiritual development. Cognitive–behavioural approaches, which focus on changing components of behaviour, enhance a person's capacity to engage more fully with the richness of life. Of the analytical therapies, the Jungian approach has traditionally valued spiritual experience (Aziz,

1990; Singer, 1995; MacKenna, 2000; Casement & Tacey, 2006). However, within the Freudian approach, there are signs of increasing interest in spiritual and religious matters (Meissner, 1984; Symington, 1994; Klein, 2003; Black, 2006). Last, there is now a range of transpersonal therapies that seek directly to address the spiritual dimension (this will be discussed further).

The place of soul

We have highlighted the principle focus of psychiatry as identifying and treating the physical basis of mental illness, whereas psychotherapy addresses the psychopathology of mind. Further, we have used the term 'spirit' to denote that super-ordinate plane which embraces both the physical and mental worlds and which, in relation to mental healthcare, brings psychiatry and psychotherapy together in a unified field.

We will now consider the individual human being and in doing so we shall adapt our paradigm (Fig. 6.1) by substituting 'body' for psychiatry, 'mind' for psychotherapy and 'soul' for spirit (Fig. 6.2).

Fig. 6.2   Soul as the unifying principle

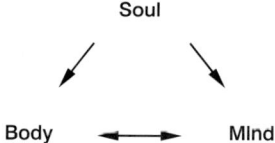

For most people the word 'soul' evokes a deep intuitive response. As we use it here, Soul describes the essence of each person, being a unique manifestation of the animating principle (Spirit) that enlivens each individual's psyche–soma. However, it reaches beyond that, for it also characterises the most elevated expression of human values, unselfish love, compassion and wisdom. Lastly, Soul conveys a sense of wholeness – of indivisibility, indestructibility and therefore, for many, eternal life.

In contrast to Soul, we are defining Mind more narrowly as the domain of the ego. Mind is identified with emotions, desires, thoughts and actions, indissolubly linked with the body and ultimately concerned with the survival of the organism.

Where the soul meets the mind there is invariably a conflict between the 'higher' and 'lower' self (in Eastern metaphysics, according to the Vedic chakras, ego-driven love yields to selfless love) (Powell, 2003). Enabling the wisdom of soul to enrich the limitations of mind is the aim of all spiritual endeavour.

Psychosomatic research has shown that disturbances of the mind can have a profound impact on the body (Shoenberg, 2007). In contrast, studies in psychoneuroimmunology show that religious and spiritual practices protect against down-regulation of the immune system, with important implications for infections and cancer (Koenig & Cohen, 2002), which we would understand as the influence of Soul on cell physiology.

What are the implications for clinical practice? The doctor–patient relationship is crucial in the success of any treatment being offered (Dixon & Sweeney, 2000). From the outset, the patient needs to feel he or she is being valued and treated as a human being – to be sympathetically received, listened to without judgement being passed and helped to make sense of what has gone wrong. The effect is to strengthen the 'the therapeutic alliance'[1], which in turn assists with relevant information-gathering, accurate diagnosis and ensuring the patient's full cooperation with the agreed treatment choices. All such therapeutic interventions, whether physical or psychological, will have the best possible effect when they are offered with sensitivity, care and concern, coming not from the self-interest of the ego but from the magnanimity of the soul.

One man's anguish

In this section we will explore the relationship of spirituality to mental health through the anguish of one particularly eloquent patient, the poet John Clare (1793–1864) (Bate, 2003). Clare was unusually well able to make the connection between his mental distress and his spiritual yearning. The poem 'I AM', which he wrote while confined to St Andrew's County Lunatic Asylum, Northampton, reveals the suffering of all humanity, for the poet's art shows us that what is the most personal is also universal.

> I AM
>
> I AM – yet what I am, none cares or knows;
> My friends forsake me like a memory lost:
> I am the self-consumer of my woes –
> They rise and vanish in oblivion's host
> Like shadows in love-frenzied stifled throes –
> And yet I am and live – like vapours tossed

The first two lines powerfully express Clare's sense of desolation and loneliness. 'I am the self-consumer of my woes' – tells us that Clare feels his misery to be beyond the reach of others. The phrase 'love-frenzied stifled throes' suggests there was once a time when his passions sought fulfilment in a relationship. Yet, now having lost contact with others, he is

---

1   The 'therapeutic alliance' is a term coined by Freud. The attributes needed in the therapist have been variously described as 'genuineness, empathy and non-possessive warmth' (Truax & Carkhuff, 1967), unconditional positive regard (Rogers, 1965) and 'the therapist's agapeistic attitude' (Lambert, 1981). (In the New Testament the Greek word *agape* is used for the love that seeks always to act in the best interest of the other.)

caught in a swirl of feelings that either parades before his eyes, or else he is painfully obliged to swallow. It is a measure both of Clare's isolation and of his genius, that he can create a poetic form strong and supple enough to give such profound expression to his distress.

Apparently, there is no one in whom Clare can confide who might, in some measure, be able to help contain his impassioned anguish. The best he is able to do is to assert, if only briefly, the fact of his existence: 'I am and live' – like vapours tossed'. But this momentary achievement rapidly unravels:

> Into the nothingness of scorn and noise,
> Into the living sea of waking dreams,
> Where there is neither sense of life or joys,
> But the vast shipwreck of my life's esteems;
> Even the dearest that I love the best
> Are strange – nay, rather stranger than the rest.

Without a sufficient sense of self, Clare is reduced to 'scorn and noise', a 'waking dream' in which there is only a sense of catastrophe (shipwreck) and estrangement from those he loved 'the best'.

Finding himself in this alienated state of mind, Clare's yearning for relationship is stripped to the most basic of mental structures. We see this in his deep longing for union with God – the desire to be cradled by the archetypes of the divine feminine, mother earth, and the divine masculine, father sky.

> I long for scenes where man hath never trod,
> A place where woman never smiled or wept,
> There to abide with my Creator, God,
> And sleep as I in childhood sweetly slept:
> Untroubling and untroubled where I lie,
> The grass below – above, the vaulted sky.

(Bate, 2004)

Given the prevalence of religious images in psychotic states of mind, from the psychiatric perspective it would be easy to discount Clare's spiritual *cri de coeur*. Equally, the psychotherapist might see in it merely the desire for regression to an infantile state.

We believe it is important neither to dismiss nor pathologise the patient's spirituality. From the spiritual standpoint, we would argue that Clare's archetypal imagery reveals the universal need for primary relatedness of self to other. Where to begin with Clare is only able to experience being in relation to himself – as the *I AM* – he then finds ontological security in his relationship with the Divine Other. The effect of this is to assuage his anxiety sufficiently for the poet to put down his pen.

Yet the suffering revealed in Clare's poem continued throughout the last 23 years of his life, all of which he spent in an asylum where he died on 20 May 1864. In such circumstances, should the psychiatrist stand by and condone suffering in the service of creativity? This ethical dilemma is all the greater because so many creative people are wary of therapeutic 'interference', be it pharmaceutical or psychological, knowing instinctively that there is an intimate relationship between their pain and their capacity to create.

The problem for the clinician is therefore to know how and when to intervene, and to what effect. Should it be simply to relieve suffering? Is it to find a way of bringing the person back into the fold of human relationships (sometimes kicking and screaming)? Or is the aim to enable the person to make sense of his or her suffering so that, while pain may not be alleviated, life can nevertheless be as rich and meaningful as possible?

In order to discover what the task may be, the psychiatrist has first to be able meaningfully to connect with the patient. How is this to be done, when someone, like Clare, has turned so emphatically away from the interpersonal world?

Finding a soul-centred response

All psychiatrists in the UK are obliged to make diagnoses in accordance with ICD–10 (World Health Organization, 1992) and detailed questioning is necessary to elucidate the signs and symptoms of the disorder. Unfortunately, this process of objectification can also have the unintended effect of denying the human reality of the individual with whom we are dealing. It is all too easy to end up by referring to someone as 'psychotic', no longer seen as a person but as a disturbed mental state.

John Clare speaks for many users of mental health services who feel that they have seen the doctor, but doubt whether the doctor has seen them: 'I AM – yet what I am, none cares or knows' – the feeling of being seen, yet not seen, only serving to intensify their suffering and confusion. Further, if the psychiatrist acts merely on the basis of social norms, he or she risks making value judgements that cannot do justice to each unique human soul, never more so than when dealing with eccentric, creative and unusual people. Engaging only at the psychological level of mind will not help Clare to feel his soul's needs have been understood; a soul-to-soul connection is required to pave the way for his return to the human world.

The first step is to enter into Clare's inner world without imposing one's own value system and to identify the point of contact where Clare would feel that both his anguish and his yearning had been recognised. More than that, it requires being genuinely open to Clare's experience of being held in the arms of God.

To be asked 'How do you feel?', or 'What do you need?', addresses the concerns of the embodied ego. There is a place for this, of course, for the psychiatrist has a duty to see whether Clare's mental state is impoverished, for example, by a serious depression, which could be helped by medication (i.e. needs of the body). Further, the psychiatrist would be attempting to understand Clare's psychological defences against pain and loss, especially since Clare is evidently disengaging from the world of human relationships (i.e. needs of the mind).

However, when the psychiatrist feels free to listen to his or her own heart, revealing their own humanity to Clare and venturing to speak from their own soul to ask Clare 'What might your soul need?', Clare is likely to feel touched in his inmost being, for soul speaks directly to soul.

From this 'holy ground', like ripples widening in a pond, the enquiry can gently extend to what led Clare to the extreme place where he must 'long for scenes where man hath never trod/A place where woman never smiled or wept'. This can be the start of a return journey to the world of minds, bodies and human relationships.

Freud re-visited

Let us compare this approach with how Sigmund Freud may have formulated the problem. Freud set great store by what he called the reality principle (1911). He also made clear his belief that psychological maturity demands that we dispense with the childish illusion that the universe is the creation of a loving God (Freud, 1927). Faced with Clare's longing to return to an Eden-like relationship with God, and his fantasy of sleeping, childlike, in the fused embrace of mother earth and father sky, Freud would have assumed that he was dealing with an infantile regression (Freud, 1926: p. 127f). The spiritual content of Clare's fantasy would have been of little interest to him beyond the fact that it pointed to a catastrophic failure in some developmental task.

Within the framework of the analytic relationship, which may have provided Clare with less exalted but more stable containment than 'the grass below – above the vaulted sky', Freud would have offered the possibility of a process through which Clare's psychotic regression might sufficiently recover for understanding to take the place of incoherence, and mourning for the lost object to replace the denial of loss (Freud, 1917). This would have to take place through the analysis of the transference – the fluctuations in the emotional relationship between patient and analyst as it becomes the theatre in which past emotional entanglements are re-enacted (Racker, 1968).

Jung re-visited

Carl Jung would also have noted the regressive nature of Clare's fantasy, but believing as he did that conscious and unconscious processes function in a compensatory relationship, would have seen this fantasy as an attempt by Clare's psyche to engender self-healing (Jung, 1967). Specifically, Clare's ego had taken refuge in an archetype of divine nurture – suggested by the transpersonal imagery of the third stanza of the poem – where it had found an emergency holding ground.

In health, this archetype finds expression in the unfolding infant–mother relationship and in the ever-widening circle of relationships that develop through childhood (Neumann, 1976). In Clare's case, however, there would seem to have been a breakdown in his object relations and the only comfort he can now find is in the fantasy of sleeping in the arms of God.

Clare's ringing words 'I am and live' could simply be asserting that he is still alive and clinging to his identity. But Jung, familiar with psychotic states of mind, would doubtless have heard an echo with the Hebrew name for God – YHWH, I AM THAT I AM, suggesting that Clare is hovering on the brink of a catastrophic inflation of the ego in which he has identified himself with God (Jung, 1958).

How might Jung have worked with Clare's fragile ego? One possibility would have been to explore whether the fantasy of sleeping sweetly like a child, the grass below and the sky above, could become the beginning of a process of 'active imagination' (Samuels et al, 1986) in which the psyche itself might furnish the ingredients needed for Clare's healing. This would be delicate work.

If it turned out that Clare adhered concretely to his fantasy, indicating that symbolic function was lost, this would suggest that a cognitive behavioural rather than an analytical approach should be attempted. If the attempt to engage the fantasy in active imagination led to a marked rise in Clare's anxiety or excitement, increasing the risk of psychotic fragmentation, psychotherapy with medication as an adjunct might be possible. On the other hand, if Clare proved able to engage with his fantasy in such a way that a story began to unfold, this would suggest that a Jungian approach was suitable for him. Crucial, here, would be the psychiatrist's ability to reflect on the accumulating material in a symbolic way, not directly challenging or disputing Clare's more literal spiritual imagery but gently making connections between the emerging myth and the outward circumstances of his life and developmental history, in so far as this was known.

Freud and Jung had many theoretical and technical differences, but each, in his own way, was devoted to his patients, and would have made enormous efforts to create a relationship with Clare, the one thing he so conspicuously lacked. Who can say to what extent such devotion would not have been the most powerful therapeutic factor?

Converging pathways

In describing the Jungian way of working, we have ventured into the transpersonal field, being concerned with experiences in which the psyche expands beyond the confines of the personal self and connects with a larger, more meaningful reality.

Historically, this vision of the greater whole can be traced to one of the great pioneers of psychology, William James (1842–1910). His humane and pragmatic approach to psychology and, most of all, his lectures on the varieties of religious experience (James, 1960) set the 'gold standard' for the psychological study of religion for the next hundred years. The breadth of his vision is evident in the following passage:

> Our normal waking consciousness, rational consciousness as we call it, is but one special type of consciousness, while all about it, parted from it by the filmiest of screens, there lie potential forms of consciousness entirely different. We may go through life without suspecting their existence; but apply the requisite stimulus, and at a touch they are there in all their completeness [James, 1960: p. 374].

Such shifts in consciousness, in which the ego is transcended, are often accompanied by profound religious or spiritual awakening. The focus, however, can be secular, as in the expression of a compassionate concern for humankind, all life, nature and the planet.

James maintained a down-to-earth approach to the value of religious beliefs, sympathetically evaluating a wide range of first-hand reports of religious experiences and always ready to subject his own beliefs to scrutiny. He remained agnostic about the ultimate source of spiritual experience, yet he was convinced that our lives are in some way continuous with a higher power which, when experienced as benign, has a demonstrably beneficial effect on our lives. (Thus, he anticipated by some 70 years the research that would later show the positive effects of spirituality on health, both physical and mental.) James concluded that for practical purposes, belief in the chance of salvation was enough, because 'the existence of the chance makes the difference ... between a life of which the keynote is resignation and a life of which the keynote is hope' (1960: p. 500).

James reminds us that whatever our own personal beliefs may be, we should never underestimate the importance of our patients being allowed to come to their own meaningful experience of subjective reality and of the healing properties of religious experience. In John Clare's words, 'There to abide with my Creator, God, and sleep as I in childhood sweetly slept', the soul that has not been able to withstand life's anguish seeks replenishment and healing. In our further discussion of soul-centred therapy, we shall be suggesting how the patient's spiritual reality can be directly engaged as a powerful therapeutic tool.

We next turn to Viktor Frankl (1905–1997), a Jewish psychiatrist and psychotherapist who survived four Nazi concentration camps in which his mother, father, brother, and wife perished, included here because, although coming from the mainstream of psychiatry, his ideas form a bridge with more specifically transpersonal interventions.

Frankl's experiences formed the basis for an existential psychotherapy he called 'logotherapy', founded on spirituality in the sense of humankind's 'will to find meaning' (1973: p. 10). Three major insights inform Frankl's work: first, that we can detach from the oppression in which we may find ourselves; second, that in doing so, no matter what the outward circumstance, we are free to choose and uphold the values by which we live and die; and third, that living or dying with dignity requires a framework of meaning that can embrace suffering as well as health. Frankl quotes Nietzsche, 'He who knows a "why" for living, will surmount almost every "how"', and goes on to say, while the concern of most people was summed up by the question, 'Will we survive the [concentration] camp?' – for if not, then this suffering has no sense – the question which in contrast beset me was, 'Has this whole suffering, this dying, a meaning?' – for if not, then ultimately there is no sense to surviving. For a life whose meaning stands or falls upon whether one survives or not, a life, that is, whose meaning depends upon such a happenstance, such a life would not really be worth living at all [Frankl, 1967: p. 102].

Reading John Clare's poem in the light of Frankl's experience, we would seek to discover what part the loss of meaning played in Clare's illness. Was the loss of meaning consequent upon his breakdown or did he break down because he was no longer able to make sense of his existence? Either way, loss of meaning leads to loss of control, for when we cease to understand our experience we lose the ability to take meaningful action in relation to it.

More recently, Frankl's work has influenced the development of spiritually augmented cognitive–behavioural therapy (D'Souza & Rodrigo, 2004). But here we want to highlight Frankl's emphasis on the meaning both of living and dying. A life that only holds meaning in relation to personal survival will always be profoundly threatened by the prospect of loss, whether this is of health or relationships or ultimately death.

The larger, transpersonal perspective is one that bestows on each life an enduring value that transcends death. For those who have children, there is the hope that the love shown to them will bear fruit in the fullness of their lives, and for generations thereafter. For some, it is the value of service to the community and friendships, while for others there is the hope that one's professional work will make a contribution, however small, to the progress of humankind. All these would be expressions of humanistic spirituality.

Frankl tried to help his patients, many of whom were also Holocaust survivors, find value and meaning for continuing to live now. In addition, most religions also hold that this life prepares us for the next one. Regardless of which view psychiatrists and other mental health professionals privately may take, empathically relating to the patient's personal framework of meaning and purpose is crucial when making the diagnosis of a mental disorder.[2]

---

2 This is not easy, for as psychiatrists, we are obliged to make judgements about what is supposed to be normal and abnormal. A delusion is defined as pathological because the fixed idea is held contrary to other people's beliefs; indeed, the diagnosis of illness is sometimes made on these grounds alone. Further, because the suffering that a person with a mental illness inflicts may be more evident on the lives of others than on self (attributed to lack of insight), neither is personal suffering required for the diagnosis of mental illness.

Transpersonal psychology

We will now attempt to demonstrate how a broad understanding of the relationship of spirituality to psychotherapy may be given more specific therapeutic focus by outlining developments within the burgeoning field of transpersonal psychology.

Set against the broad perspectives offered by William James, Carl Jung and Viktor Frankl, transpersonal psychology has evolved as a body of theory and practice along a number of avenues. From within the psychotherapeutic tradition there is the pioneering work of Robert Assagioli (1888–1974), who first formulated psychosynthesis in 1910. Assagioli's metapsychology (Assagioli, 1965) incorporates Jung's collective unconscious but specifically locates a 'central self' positioned midway between the unconscious and what Assagioli calls the 'superconscious'. The central self engages with the attributes of personality listed by Assagioli (thought, intuition, imagination, emotion-feeling, sensation, and impulse-desire), but is not to be confused with these attributes, for it is composed purely of consciousness and will. (The similarity with Buddhism is evident here – meditation enables the self to dis-identify with desires and attachments, since its essence is not the substance of those emotions.)

In psychosynthesis, there are two sequential therapeutic tasks. First, there is the secure integration of personality around the central self, not so different from the aim of much psychotherapy and essential for healthy 'grounding'. The second task is transpersonal, focusing on a point of universal consciousness and will, conceptualised within the superconscious realm and known as the 'transpersonal self'. The therapeutic aim is to find alignment with, and to express, the energies of the transpersonal self. In doing so, we are led to recognise that ultimately we are all one, and with that understanding there arises a global perspective characterised by social cooperation, altruistic love, and a transpersonal vision of spiritual evolution.

Another pathway comes from the religious and mystical tradition. Pierre Teilhard de Chardin (1881–1955) was a visionary French Jesuit, palaeontologist and philosopher who sought to integrate Christian theology with natural science and evolutionary theory. He suggested that the Earth, in its evolutionary unfolding, is growing from the biosphere towards a new organ of consciousness, called the noosphere, analogous on the planetary level with the evolution of the cerebral cortex in the human species. Teilhard saw this emerging global information network as heralding a massive convergence of minds, resulting in what he called the 'Omega Point' (Teilhard de Chardin, 1959). Such a global information flow has been compared to the growth of the internet, but Teilhard's vision is anticipating the spiritual evolution of humankind, characterised by a profound ethic and expressed through universal love.

Teilhard's Western evolutionary spirituality can be compared with that of Sri Aurobindo (1872–1950), a scholar, mystic, yogi and evolutionary philosopher. Educated in England, Aurobindo later returned to India, where he became involved in extreme nationalist politics. He was sent to prison, where he turned to the Bhagavad-Gita. On his release he began a life of intensive meditation, establishing an ashram at Pondicherry and teaching 'integral yoga', which aims to advance global consciousness to the divine level. Sri Aurobindo (1939) linked the ancient tradition of Vedantic thought with spiritual evolution through the generative power of what he called 'supermind'. He envisioned the eventual spiritual destiny of humankind as coming about through the effort of individuals to transform their level of consciousness (cf. the aphorism: 'if you want to change the world, first change yourself'), leading collectively to a divine state of consciousness in which the Absolute is experienced as 'infinite existence, infinite consciousness and infinite delight'.

A further contribution to the transpersonal field comes from the study of entheogens, popularly known as psychedelics. There is a long tradition of the ritual use of entheogens in the shamanic rituals of indigenous cultures worldwide, which has been studied participatively by anthropologists such as Narby (1998).

In the West, there was much interest in Aldous Huxley's book *The Doors of Perception* (1954), in which he gave a detailed account of his experimentation with mescaline. He suggested that ordinary consciousness was the result of the brain filtering out the awareness of information that would otherwise be overwhelming. Certainly the effect of entheogens like lysergic acid diethylamide (LSD), which first became popular as a recreational drug in the 1960s, is to open the mind to a transcendental reality which can be terrifying or ecstatic, according to the susceptibilities of the individual.

At about the same time, the psychiatrist Stanislav Grof began systematically researching non-ordinary states of consciousness using LSD under laboratory conditions. When the drug was proscribed, even for research purposes, Grof developed a breathing/sensory input programme (Holotropic Breathwork™) to induce a comparable altered state of consciousness (Grof, 1993). Grof highlights the role of the birth experience in shaping the emotional disposition of later years and has closely studied the relationship of psychotic breakdown to 'spiritual emergency' (see chapter 11, pp. 227–230, for further details). Grof's clinical findings have been buttressed by the theoretical writings of Ken Wilber (1996) and linked to the Vedic concept of the chakras by the psychiatrist John Nelson (1994).

Yet another contribution to transpersonal psychology comes from a range of experiences that appear to defy the limits of space–time, according to the conventions of classical physics. They include mediumship (Solomon & Solomon, 2003; Fontana, 2005), paranormal experiments (Radin, 1997), research on life after death (Schwartz & Simon, 2002), the near-death experience (Bailey & Yates, 1996), reincarnation studies (Stevenson, 1966; 1997) and, by means of working hypnotherapeutically, past-life regression

(Woolger, 1999), life-between-life therapy (Newton, 1998; 2002) and spirit release therapy (Baldwin, 1992; Powell, 2006). There is heated debate about the scientific status of these areas of work, for they profoundly challenge the world view of material realism. Yet the evidence base for paranormal phenomena is strong and even hardened sceptics need to be aware of the research that is taking place. Simply asserting that such things are 'impossible', which once was a legitimate scientific position to take, now betrays ignorance and prejudice; the case against, if it is to be argued, deserves to be reasoned as carefully as the case for. As for practitioners working with altered states of consciousness, they will generally answer by saying that it is more important for them to be able to help the patient get better than to worry about exactly how it happened.

Soul-centred therapy

How might psychiatrists who find themselves broadly in sympathy with the ideas presented in this chapter offer soul-centred interventions in clinical practice? The Humanistic and Integrative Psychotherapy Section of the UK Council for Psychotherapy accredits a number of relevant trainings but relatively few psychiatrists will wish to undertake such a specialisation. Yet much can be offered by way of simple, compassionate interventions that help the patient to feel deeply supported, acknowledged and encouraged in times of crisis. Therefore, we shall conclude with vignettes which illustrate the kind of situation where an intuitively soul-centred approach can be helpful (case studies 6.1–6.4).

Life and death situations most commonly put us in touch with Soul, yet our intuitive response to loss is not given credence in our society (Powell, 2007). For instance, it is well known that the bereaved may see or hear their loved one in the wake of loss (case study 6.1). However, many psychiatrists dismiss this as an emotionally driven misperception and the patient will probably be simply reassured that to imagine such things is normal.

There is an alternative – to work there and then with a person's intuitive faculties. When we are told, for instance, that the patient saw the deceased standing at the foot of the bed on the night of the funeral, an opportunity arises to treat it not as a statistical happenstance but as communication from Soul and to enquire, 'How did he/she look? Did he/she say anything? How did you feel? What importance has this for you?' Some patients are afraid they may be thought mad; others are apprehensive for religious reasons – for instance, the Bible prohibits contact with 'familiar spirits' (Leviticus 19:31, 20:6; Deuteronomy 18:11). However, when reassured, the patient will frequently report having felt comforted by the visitation. Such experiences are far from rare, if we include sensing as well as seeing; either way, an important connection has been explored.

A problem for secular Western society is that when someone dies, it seems that nothing else remains to be done except helplessly grieving the absence of the loved one. However, where the soul is recognised as continuing on its journey, there is an important role for the bereaved to fulfil in the form of prayers and blessings, specifically to support the departed soul in moving on to its spiritual destination. This is an act of continuing love and concern, the parting being, so to speak, a comma rather than a full stop. Further, the emotions of loss can be usefully harnessed rather than repressed, as can happen when overwhelming defences against loss are activated.

Another difficulty is that prayers and blessings may be felt to be the province of priest and Church, so that the bereaved feel their own personal contribution is less important. Yet transpersonal research suggests that those bereaved are exactly the ones to be actively involved and that nothing is of greater help to a departed soul than being lovingly supported in 'moving on', rather than detained by the anguish of the loved ones left behind.

It is therefore always important respectfully to ask about the patient's religious and spiritual beliefs (Culliford, 2007). If no definitive view is given, it can then be helpful to enquire whether a person believes that life exists only from birth to death. The majority of patients confide that they have wondered whether life continues after death but are liable to add 'you probably think it's silly of me' or words to that effect. Again, with further reassurance, it may be possible to enquire 'If it is so, how do you imagine it might be?' This can open the door to working psychotherapeutically with the patient's intuitive faculty (case study 6.1 and 6.2) (Powell, 1998).

Case study 6.1

Joan presented with depression after the death of her husband Ted, having nursed him through a long and debilitating illness. They had been together some 40 years and her loss had left her stricken with grief. Each new day was a living nightmare. She continually felt Ted's presence around the house but it only brought her pain. Yes, it was possible that life after death continued on in some way, but how could that help her now? So Joan was asked whether she would like to try to make contact with Ted in a way that might help bring her peace of mind.

At the psychiatrist's suggestion Joan shut her eyes, relaxed and was encouraged to see if she could 'find' Ted wherever he might be. After a couple of minutes, a faint smile played on her lips. The psychiatrist asked Joan what she saw. She replied that she could see Ted in his cricket whites playing cricket and looking very fit and happy. The psychiatrist remarked that Ted seemed to be enjoying a game of celestial cricket! Joan's smile widened and she added that cricket had been Ted's great passion. Then a look of deep sadness passed across her face. Asked whether she would like to speak with Ted, she nodded. So the psychiatrist suggested she 'walk up to him' and see what might happen. After a moment, Joan said that she was now standing next to him and he had put his arm around her. What was he saying? He was saying 'Don't worry; everything is going to be all right.' Joan was asked to look around her. Was there anyone else present? Then she could see her deceased sister and parents smiling and waving to her.

Joan's vivid experience (case study 6.1) can be interpreted at the psychological level of object loss or the transpersonal level of connecting with Spirit, or both. It is often best left undefined, simply as an experience that the patient can return to, feel reassured by and as a way of finding healing according to the need.

Case study 6.2

Christine attended with a history of chronic depression that had not responded to antidepressants. Her personal background had been a childhood of severe deprivation. She grew up lonely, wanting to make relationships but unable to access her own capacity to love, or to feel worthy of love.

Christine was asked if she felt able to 'look' into the black cave, which is how she described her depression, and with the help of the psychiatrist to see whether any answers lay within.

Christine's first response to going into this dark place was that it was cold and empty. After a few minutes she reported finding a pair of steel handcuffs on the stone floor. Then she found a rope and soon after, an iron chain. It is not hard to imagine what these objects said about her bleak and lonely inner world. Christine was now getting into something of a panic. She was pressed to go on looking. Then, after what seemed an eternity, her expression changed to one of concern. The psychiatrist asked her 'What now?' She had found a little puppy in a dark corner. He suggested she pick it up and hold it to her. With her eyes still closed, she cradled the puppy. What could she feel? She replied that she could feel the puppy's love for her. She was urged to let her own love flow to the puppy at the same time. She began to cry. After a pause, the psychiatrist asked her to find an image for the emotion that flowed within her and she chose a heart made of gold. Then she was invited to picture a sunbeam falling on this golden heart so she could see it in all its beauty.

In case study 6.2, at the psychological level, the puppy symbolises the child Christine. She loves and nurtures this child-self, which she had thought was lost forever and in doing so discovers that she still has the capacity for love. In terms of spiritual object relations, we can see the experience as helping Christine retrieve her soul that had got buried in the wasteland of her childhood.

From the spiritual perspective, deprivation and abuse in childhood is a double blow. The damage sustained on the psychological level to the child's internal object world would be bad enough. However, the child's 'spiritual object relations' have also been denied. From the transpersonal perspective, this is our pre-existing soul connection with the Divine, which inspires our original sense of goodness and which forms the template on which human object relations are laid. Not surprisingly, reconnecting with Soul is an invaluable asset when seeking integration and healing of the traumatised self, as shown in case study 6.3 and 6.4 (Powell, 2003).

Case study 6.3

Carol's story had been one of terrible abuse and hardship and for many years she had taken refuge in alcohol. During the first interview, she was encouraged to look inside herself and describe what she found there. What Carol saw was 'her heart beating so hard it could burst'. What did she want to do with it? She put it to rest in a silk lined coffin, saying 'only death will bring it peace'. But then after a moment the heart transformed into a little whirligig of energy. It would not be trapped but flew about the room. So she released it and watched it fly away.

Images of the soul are incapable of death, being our personal quotient of eternal and infinite consciousness. But Carol was not ready or able to harness her soul for her own benefit. She did not take up the offer of therapy, which would have meant abstaining from alcohol.

Nearly 4 years later Carol came to see the psychiatrist again, in the meantime having faced up to her drinking. This time, she went inside herself, into a dark cave, where she found a treasure chest. The psychiatrist asked if she could pick up the treasure chest and see if there was any way out. She put it under her arm and soon found an archway and went through. Now she found herself in a sandy desert, by a pool of water and some trees. She sat by the water, resting peacefully and said with a sigh 'This is for me!' (All her life she has rushed around trying to please others). Did she want a drink? She drank deeply of the cool fresh water. Now where did she need to go? She immediately found herself back home, still holding the treasure chest, studded with jewels and very beautiful. She placed it on the floor in the middle of the room. Following this session, therapy was offered and accepted.

Sometimes, when the heart has been sorely wounded, there is a need to find healing (case study 6.4).

Case study 6.4

A young man, Roger, who had suffered great distress as a teenager, sought help. At the time, he had been encouraged to seek guidance from a priest, with disastrous results. The priest was untrained in psychotherapy but took it on himself to convince Roger that his problems all stemmed from the fact that his parents had never loved him. This wasn't true – the priest was massively projecting his own problem onto Roger – but the young man was vulnerable and started to believe his mentor. Soon he became deeply alienated from his parents, which only worsened his isolation and depression.

After a period of psychotherapy, the effects of the abuse by the priest had largely been overcome. However, at follow-up a year later, Roger reported that he could still feel something wrong, for there was a persisting sensation of physical discomfort. He explained, 'it's as if a big splint has entered the right side of my neck and gone down through my chest'.

Case study 6.4 *(contd)*

Roger was asked what this splint, if it could speak, would say. The answer came straight back. 'Anger!' The psychiatrist speculated that Roger's anger with the priest may have acted like a splint to keep him functioning, but rather than trying to interpret this, he asked Roger what should be done about it. Roger replied despairingly 'I don't know – it's part of me.' The psychiatrist suggested he try closing his eyes and allow himself to float upwards and away from his body, then simply to observe himself down there sitting in the chair with his problem. The question was repeated and this time without a second's hesitation Roger said emphatically 'I need to pull it out!' With encouragement, this is what he visualised himself doing, drawing it out inch-by-inch. It left a raw wound in its track. How was he going to dispose of it? Roger answered 'I want to put it in the garden, and let it weather away naturally, like wood'. The session was concluded by spending time envisaging cleansing and anointing the wound until Roger was satisfied with the result.

When we are able to dis-identify with the problem, there is the chance for ego to make way for Soul, which in its wisdom guides us to find the right response, in this case the healing of an old wound.

Conclusion

In this chapter we have set out a unitive way of thinking about the relationship between spirituality, psychiatry and psychotherapy. We have expanded on John Clare's poem *I AM*, because it powerfully articulates the distress of many mental health patients. After a survey of psychotherapeutic approaches including the transpersonal, we have described how soul-centred interventions can engage with the spiritual reality of the patient.

We acknowledge the value of more traditional and lengthy psychotherapeutic approaches but we are well aware of the constraints on time and opportunity when working in the acute clinical services. This is where the brief soul-centred approach can be particularly helpful. Our patients come to us distressed and frequently staring into the abyss, seeking the warmth of genuine human contact, yet often afraid to ask. We know from discussions within the Spirituality and Psychiatry Special Interest Group of the Royal College of Psychiatrists that many mental health professionals have the sincere wish to respond soul-to-soul, a desire echoed by patients' representatives on the National Spirituality and Mental Health Forum; yet, this very human dimension of our work has not received much attention within the profession to date.

We can take heart from our roots. The etymology of psychiatry is *psyche*, soul, and *iatros*, doctor; and for psychotherapy, it is *therapeuein*, to take care of, to heal. Albert Einstein remarked, 'the intuitive mind is a sacred gift and the rational mind is a faithful servant' (1931). When soul leads and science follows, we can be assured of the best of both worlds.

References

Abrams, N. & Primack, J. (2000) Einstein's view of God. In *God for the 21st Century* (ed. R. Stannard). Templeton Foundation Press.

Assagioli, R. (1965) *Psychosynthesis: a Manual of Principles and Techniques*. Psychosynthesis Research Foundation.

Aziz, R. (1990) *C. G. Jung's Psychology of Religion and Synchronicity*. State University of New York Press.

Bailey, L.W. & Yates, J. (1996) *The Near Death Experience: a Reader*. Routledge.

Baldwin, W. (1992) *Spirit Releasement Therapy*. Headline Books.

Bate, J. (2003) *John Clare: a Biography*. Picador.

Bate, J. (2004) *John Clare: Selected Poems*. Faber and Faber.

Black, D. M. (2006) *Psychoanalysis and Religion in the 21st Century: Competitors or Collaborators?* Routledge.

Bomford, R. (1999) *The Symmetry of God*. Free Association Books.

Casement, A. & Tacey, D. (2006) *The Idea of the Numinous, Contemporary Jungian and Psychoanalytic Perspectives*. Routledge.

Culliford, L. (2007) Taking a spiritual history. *Advances in Psychiatric Treatment*, **13**, 212–219.

Dixon, M. & Sweeney, K. (2000) *The Human Effect in Medicine, Theory, Research and Practice*. Radcliffe Medical Press.

D'Souza, R. F. & Rodrigo, A. (2004) Spiritually augmented cognitive–behavioural therapy. *Australasian Psychiatry*, **12**, 148–152.

Einstein, A. (1931) *Cosmic Religion* (1st edn). Covici-Freide.

Emerson. R. W. (1841) The Over-Soul, in *Essays*, first series. In *Nature and Selected Essays* (2003) (ed. E. L. Ziff), p. 207. Penguin Classics.

Field, N., Harvey, T. & Sharp, B. (eds) *(2005) Ten Lectures on Psychotherapy and Spirituality*. Karnac.

Fontana, D. (2005) *Is there an Afterlife?* O Books.

Frankl, V. (1967) *Psychotherapy and Existentialism*. Simon & Schuster.

Frankl, V. (1973) *The Doctor and the Soul, from Psychotherapy to Logotherapy*. Pelican Books.

Freud, S. (1911) Formulations on the two principles of mental functioning. Reprinted (1966) in *The Standard Edition of the Complete Psychological Works of Sigmund Freud, Vol. 12* (trans. & ed. J. Strachey). Hogarth Press.

Freud, S. (1917) Mourning and melancholia. Reprinted (1966) in *The Standard Edition of the Complete Psychological Works of Sigmund Freud, Vol. 14* (trans. & ed. J. Strachey). Hogarth Press.

Freud, S. (1926) Inhibitions, symptoms and anxiety. Reprinted (1966) in *The Standard Edition of the Complete Psychological Works of Sigmund Freud, Vol. 20* (trans. & ed. J. Strachey). Hogarth Press.

Freud, S. (1927) The future of an illusion. Reprinted (1966) in *The Standard Edition of the Complete Psychological Works of Sigmund Freud, Vol. 21* (trans. & ed. J. Strachey). Hogarth Press.

Grof, S. (1993) *The Holotropic Mind*. Harper.

Huxley, A. (1954) *The Doors of Perception and Heaven and Hell*. Chatto & Windus.

James, W. (1960) *The Varieties of Religious Experience: a Study in Human Nature*. Collins Fontana Library.

Jung, C. G. (1958) Schizophrenia. Reprinted (1977) in *C. G. Jung: The Collected Works, Vol. III* (eds H. Read, M. Fordham & G. Adler). Routledge & Kegan Paul.

Jung, C. G. (1967) Symbols of transformation. Reprinted (1956) in *C. G. Jung: The Collected Works, Vol. V* (2nd edn) (eds H. Read, M. Fordham & G. Adler). Routledge & Kegan Paul.

Kabat-Zinn, J. (1995) *Wherever You Go There You Are: Mindfulness Meditation in Everyday Life*. Hyperion.

Kabat-Zinn, J., Massion, A. O., Kristeller, J., *et al* (1992) Effectiveness of a meditation-based stress reduction programme in the treatment of anxiety disorders. *American Journal of Psychiatry*, **149**, 936–943.

King, M. & Dein, S. (1998) The spiritual variable in psychiatric research. *Psychological Medicine*, **28**, 1259–1262.

Klein, J. (2003) *Jacob's Ladder: Essays on Experiences of the Ineffable in the Context of Contemporary Psychotherapy*. Karnac.

Koenig, H. G. & Cohen, H. J. (2002) *The Link between Religion and Health: Psychoneuroimmunology and the Faith Factor*. Oxford University Press.

Koenig, H. K., McCullough, M. E. & Larson, D. B. (2001) *Handbook of Religion and Health*. Oxford University Press.

Lambert, K. (1981) *Analysis, Repair and Individuation*. Academic Press.

Larson, D. B. & Larson, S. S. (2001) *Patient Spirituality and Mental Health: An Expanding Focus in Clinical Care and Research, Parts 1 and 2*. Royal College of Psychiatrists (http://www.rcpsych.ac.uk/pdf/larson1.pdf) (http://www.rcpsych.ac.uk/pdf/larson2.pdf).

Larson, D. B., Larson, S. S. & Koenig, H. G. (2001) The patient's spiritual/religious dimension: a forgotten factor in mental health. *Directions in Psychiatry*, **21**, lesson 21, Nov 2001 (http://www.rcpsych.ac.uk/pdf/larson3.pdf).

MacKenna, C. (2000) Jung and Christianity: Wrestling with God. In *Jungian Thought in the Modern World* (ed. E. Christopher & H. M. Solomon). Free Association Books.

MacKenna, C. (2002) Self-images and God images. *British Journal of Psychotherapy*, **18**, 325–338.

MacKenna, C. (2004) Conscious change and changing consciousness, some thoughts on the psychology of meditation. *British Journal of Psychotherapy*, **21**, 103–118.

MacKenna, C. (2005*a*) A personal journey through psychotherapy and religion. In *Ten Lectures on Psychotherapy and Spirituality* (ed. N. Field, T. Harvey & B. Sharp). Karnac.

MacKenna, C. (2005*b*) Faith in the therapeutic process. *Journal of the British Association of Psychotherapists*, **43**, 108–123.

MacKenna, C. (2006) The last farthing. *British Journal of Psychotherapy*, **23**, 11–26.

MacKenna, C. (2007) The dream of perfection. *British Journal of Psychotherapy*, **23**, 247–267.

Meissner, W. W. (1984) *Psychoanalysis and Religious Experience*. Yale University Press.

Narby, J. (1998) *The Cosmic Serpent, DNA and the Origins of Knowledge*. Gollancz.

Nelson, J. (1994) *Healing the Split*. State University of New York Press.

Neumann, E. (1976) *The Child*. Harper and Row.

Newton, J. (1998) *Journey of Souls: Case Studies of Life between Lives*. Llewellyn Publications.

Newton, J. (2002) *Destiny of Soul*. Llewellyn Publications.

Powell, A. (1998) Soul consciousness and human suffering: psychotherapeutic approaches to healing. *Journal of Alternative and Complementary Medicine*, **4**, 101–108.

Powell, A. (2002) Quantum psychiatry – where science meets spirit. *Nexus*, **9**, 51–55.

Powell, A. (2003) *Love and the Near Life Experience*. Royal College of Psychiatrists (http://www.rcpsych.ac.uk/pdf/Andrew%20Powell%20Love%20and%20the%20Near%20Life%20Experience.x.pdf).

Powell, A. (2004*a*) Consciousness that transcends spacetime: its significance for the therapeutic process. *New Therapist*, **29**, 12–20.

Powell, A. (2004*b*) *Death and Soul Consciousness*. Royal College of Psychiatrists (http://www.rcpsych.ac.uk/pdf/AndrewPowellDeathandSoulConsciousness.pdf).

Powell, A (2006) The contribution of spirit release therapy to mental health. *Light*, **126**, 10–16.

Powell, A. (2007) *Why Must We Suffer? A Psychiatrist Reflects*. Royal College of Psychiatrists (http://www.rcpsych.ac.uk/pdf/ATT01042.pdf).

Racker, H. (1968) *Transference and Counter-Transference*. International Universities Press.

Radin, D. (1997) *The Conscious Universe*. HarperCollins.

Radin. D. (2006) *Entangled Minds*. Paraview Pocket Books.

Rogers, C. R. (1965) *Client-Centered Therapy*. Houghton Mifflin.

Samuels, A., Shorter, B. & Plaut, F. (1986) *A Critical Dictionary of Jungian Analysis*. Routledge & Kegan Paul.

Schreurs, A. (2002) *Psychotherapy and Spirituality: Integrating the Spiritual Dimension into Therapeutic Practice*. Jessica Kingsley.

Schwartz, G. E. & Simon, W. L. (2002) *The Afterlife Experiments*. Atria Books.

Shoenberg, P. (2007) *Psychosomatics*. Palgrave Macmillan.

Singer, J. (1995) *Boundaries of the Soul: the Practice of Jung's Psychology*. Prism.

Solomon, G. & Solomon J. (2003) *The Scole Experiment*. Piatkus.

Sri Aurobindo (1939) *The Life Divine*. Reprinted in 1977 (10th edn). Sri Aurobindo Ashram Trust.

Stein, S. M. (1999) *Beyond Belief, Psychotherapy and Religion*. Karnac.

Stevenson, I. (1966) *Twenty Cases Suggestive of Reincarnation*. Reprinted in 1974. Press of Virginia.

Stevenson, I. (1997) *Reincarnation and Biology. Vol. 1: Birthmarks, Vol. 2: Birth Defects and Other Anomalies*. Praegar.

Symington, N. (1994) *Emotion and Spirit, Questioning the Claims of Psychoanalysis and Religion*. Cassell.

Teilhard de Chardin, P. (1959) *The Phenomenon of Man*. Collins.

Truax, C. B. & Carkhuff, R. R. (1967) *Towards Effective Counselling and Psychotherapy Training and Practice*. Aldine Press.

Wilber, K. (1996) *The Atman Project: a Transpersonal View of Human Development*. Theosophical Publishing House.

Woolger, R. (1999) *Other Lives, Other Selves*. Bantam Books.

World Health Organization (1992) *The ICD–10 Classification of Mental and Behavioural Disorders*. World Health Organization.

Andrew Powell's publications on spirituality and health are available from http://www.rcpsych.ac.uk/college/specialinterestgroups/spirituality/publications.aspx

CHAPTER 7

Intellectual disability

Oyepeju Raji

Spirituality is a deeply personal experience that does not depend on being religious or belonging to a faith group. The spirit is the essence of life. This book considers that spirituality is a universal dimension of human experience, being of fundamental or ultimate importance (Cook, 2004). Spirituality is about wholeness and wholesomeness, interconnection and validation; it shows that all lives have purpose and are positively influencing other lives. Each human life matters – there are no exceptions and there is no hierarchy.

Swinton (1999) defines spirituality as that aspect of human existence that gives it its 'humanness'. To deny that people with intellectual disabilities are spiritual is devaluing their human dignity, for every human being has need to find a sense of meaning of life, a purpose and to feel he or she belongs. 'The desire for wholeness of being is not an intellectual attainment, for it is no less present in people with learning disability, but lies in the essence of what it means to be human' (Royal College of Psychiatrists, 2006: pp. 2–3). Hebrew Scripture declares that 'all are fearfully and wonderfully made' (Psalm 139, verse 14). Thus, every human life is uniquely valuable, independent of another's perception of their 'fitness for purpose'. Each person possesses unique gifts and talents that were meant to be shared; however, it first has to be recognised that all people possess such gifts.

Beliefs about disability across cultures and ages

All human societies hold beliefs, practices and rituals for the expression of spirituality. Different spiritual belief systems ascribe different meanings to disability. Some cultures hold that people with disability are of 'lesser value', considered 'undesirable' or even feared and different cultures deal with these attitudes and feelings in various ways. Some give spiritual explanations for disability that allow control to rest with a superior being, whereas others attempt to find a human understanding of the lives of people with a disability. Some would argue that scriptural bases of religious beliefs form the foundation for the age-old practice of exclusion that people with intellectual disabilities experience in many facets of life. Such attitudes towards disability can result in people internalising negative messages about spirituality and its usefulness. Beliefs about the relationship of disability to sin, adequacy of faith and miraculous healing can be challenging concepts; people wonder what they have done wrong to be 'punished' in this way, with profound psychological consequences (Treloar, 2002). The vulnerability of people with intellectual disabilities and their dependence on carers can lead to spiritual manipulation. People without disability may look patronisingly on those with disabilities as objects of their benevolence. Others, however, appreciate that all human beings are interdependent, for no one can survive on their own, without leaning on other people at some stage in life.

Medieval Christianity explained mental disorder as a manifestation of the devil. A mixture of the magical and the natural was employed in making sense of concepts concerning 'simple-mindedness' and 'madness'. Mental illness was considered both sacred and profane and was dealt with by isolating those afflicted. It was believed that a person with a mental disorder was possessed by the devil and to rid the body of it, the person was subjected to severe physical punishment or even death. Demons were exorcised as treatment for insanity and affected people were thrust out of society (Stockholder, 1994).

In indigenous peoples of sub-Saharan Africa, there is still the tendency to believe in metaphysical/spiritual explanations of disability. In parts of Nigeria, for example, physical and intellectual disabilities and mental illness are held by some to be caused by negative spiritual influences (evil forces) direct from the gods, or invoked by one's enemies, and for which affected people may be subjected to spiritual cleansing and healing. Christian and Islamic influences have modified the practice to some extent, but cultural traditions largely remain in place, giving rise to interweaving influences of spirituality, culture and science. Similar traditions are maintained in Zimbabwe, where the role of traditional and spiritual healers in the care of people with disabilities is formally recognised (Mpofu & Harley, 2002).

In many developing countries, where the science of disability is not understood at the local level, efforts at 'purification' persist, along with segregation from 'normal society'. Yet it must be conceded that segregation can arise no less in highly intellectual and materialistic societies, where the value of a person is closely linked to their intellectual functioning and consequent economic worth.

In 17th-century England, the 'Poor Law' was introduced by an Act of Parliament, requiring all parishes to establish workhouses to provide places where paupers, degenerates, people with mental illness and the 'mentally handicapped', could live. The responsibility was ascribed to parishes on the basis that those who were 'mentally defective' were seen as morally impoverished and in need of salvation. They were also thought to be in need of education and treatment, with the first asylums being founded in the 19th century. This institutionalisation of people with intellectual disabilities and people with mental illness continued to increase during the first half of the 20th century, creating almost impenetrable barriers between them and open society. This process laid the foundation for the organised care of people with learning disabilities in many parts of the world. Positive attitude to disability has been growing since; however, it has been slow and patchy.

Distinguishing between mental illness and intellectual disability

The development of science in the 17th and 18th centuries saw increased interest in the capabilities of the human mind, arriving at a distinction between the psychological processes of people with intellectual disabilities and those who have mental illness. John Locke (quoted in Race, 2002: pp. 23–52) described that whereas the 'lunatic' had lost his mind, the 'idiot' never had one. A lost mind might be restored to sanity in some way, but what had never existed could not be artificially created and the 'idiot' was thus irredeemable. This was the beginning of distinguishing between the concept of intellectual disability and mental illness. Locke indicated that people with intellectual disabilities differed from people who had mental illness in the way they process information. He proposed that a person's mind starts empty and develops on the basis of the senses' interpretation of experiences and the mind's reflection on those experiences. He argued that whereas people with mental illness showed normal intensity of perception but combined ideas abnormally, people with intellectual disabilities did not experience events fully. This was considered to be scientific reasoning at the time, compared to earlier 'superstitious beliefs'.

Locke's idea that people with intellectual disabilities do not experience events fully can still be seen today in the provision of services. Dykens (2006) argues that people with intellectual disabilities have continued to be defined by their pervasive deficits and that workers in the field of intellectual disability have traditionally focused on basic external life conditions (in relation to providing for basic needs and skills acquisition) rather than recognising strengths and positive internal states that include happiness, contentment, hope and engagement. Consequently, the experience of people with disability varies according to the social construct of disability in the culture in which they are living.

Intellectual disability starts before adulthood and has a lasting effect on development, presenting with varying levels of support needs. People with intellectual disabilities have problems with language, reading and writing. They can have major difficulties in communicating their ideas and preferences, struggle with abstract concepts and need help to understand complex ideas.

Do people with intellectual disabilities have a deeper spiritual life?

Spirituality is not dependent on intellectual functioning and neither is the measure of spirituality dependent on eloquence or how it is expressed.

Spirituality is beyond words and may be present even in people who are in vegetative states. Swinton (1997), writing on the belief that a meaningful spiritual life cannot be achieved in the absence of intellectual ability, argues that faith and spirituality are not intellectual concepts but relational realities and that a person's spiritual life should not be evaluated according to intellectual criteria. Finally, faith traditions believe that spirit extends beyond the physical and that spiritual consciousness transcends the finite reality of this world.

It can be argued that freedom from intellectual preoccupation removes a barrier and allows a person to be more in touch with the spiritual. This is the case in meditation, which encourages an awareness that transcends mind and body, going beyond intellectual functioning. The more profound the intellectual disability, the less a person may be hindered by considerations of the here and now. Sulmasy (1997) reported that faith workers found that spirituality was profoundly felt with people with intellectual disabilities who were unhindered by everyday awareness, allowing the beauty of the spirit to be felt in its (pure) form.

The social model

Medical research in Western culture has concentrated on trying to identify causes of intellectual disability in a bid to eliminate or prevent it (according to the 'medical model'). However, the white paper *Valuing People* (Department of Health, 2001) initiated a person-centred approach to the delivery of holistic care for people with intellectual disabilities, with a focus on ordinary living (the social model), that sees the person rather than the disorder. Importantly, spirituality is now being recognised as an important but often overlooked dimension of the lives of people with intellectual disabilities (Swinton, 2001a). In the last quarter of the 20th century, the concept of normalisation (Wolfensberger, 1972) has brought people with intellectual disabilities more into mainstream society, with the aim of achieving social inclusion and with opportunities to build meaningful bonds within the community as fully accepted participants in everyday life. The focus, however, has been largely on meeting the basic material needs of the service users (Sinson, 1996) and the reality is that for some exclusion continues to be a significant aspect of their lives.

Culture

Within some cultures, negative theories about the origin of intellectual disability cause stigma, and affected relatives are kept hidden to avoid embarrassment. People with intellectual disabilities are not fully accepted and have no defined roles, and in this context are excluded from the category of social beings. They are not included in social occasions, ceremonies and celebrations (Raji & Hollins, 2000).

Families of people with intellectual disabilities often find that their own faith, beliefs and practices play an important role in coping with their relative's impairment while dealing with social stigma and indifference. However, progress through the stages of grief does not always result in acceptance, as the family wrestles with the question of whether a supernatural cause or other explanation such as some penalty for their own past actions, e.g. 'karma', or sin, is responsible for their predicament.

Religion

Although a person does not have to be religious to be spiritual, organised religion remains the most common way of understanding and expressing spirituality. Hatton *et al* (2004) found a number of reasons for some confusion as regards religious expression and needs of people with intellectual disabilities among paid and family carers. Scriptural interpretations concerning disability are not consistent. An example can be found in Christian scripture on the relationship of sin to disability. Jesus on the one hand forgives sin as the means to healing a disability (Mark 2:1–12) and on the other challenges the popularly held assumption that another disability was the result of sin (John 9:1–3). In Hebrew scripture, Moses commanded that extra care should be taken of the disabled (the blind) (Deuteronomy 27:18). In Islam, society is obliged to assist and respect people with intellectual disabilities (Qur'an, surah 51:19). In Hinduism, disability may be understood as the outcome of karma. A more inclusive view of disability can be found in Buddhism, where it is considered that those who are 'disabled' are not so much those with physical or intellectual impairment as those who are unable to attain spiritual enlightenment; intellectual disability itself is no hindrance to following this path. Similarly, Sikh scriptures stipulate that disability refers less to any physical or mental impairment than it does to disability of the soul, which hinders people from achieving their purpose in life.

Evidently, theology need not discourage those with intellectual disability from joining in faith practices and it is nothing but prejudice to suppose that people with functional impairments are disadvantaged when it comes to spiritual practice. Indeed, religious leaders and philosophers have been influential in developing a more positive view of how society should respond to people with a disability. One such example is found in the Jewish way of life, which is strongly community-oriented. Bunning & Steel (2006) report models of inclusion where Jewish organisations provide culturally appropriate services to Jewish parents and children with special needs in specifically Jewish ways, to enable group identity and harness a positive sense of self.

Religion attends to spiritual need by providing shared rituals, narratives, symbols and guidance through scriptures, prayer and modes of social support, furthering a sense of belonging that sustains the 'self' in the construction of both personal and group identity. Yet people who cannot (verbally) communicate their 'inner world', with its hopes, dreams and needs can miss out on this important human experience, if such needs are not recognised. Studies have found that even though spirituality plays a significant role in the lives of many people with intellectual disabilities, carers and support workers are often unaware of this and consequently fail to address it (Swinton, 2001b).

Although the practice of religion is to an extent bound by culture, a person's ethnic or cultural background does not necessarily predict their religious or spiritual needs. Some services for people with intellectual disabilities only considered people's religious needs in line with their culture, their religion in effect being denoted by their country of origin (Hatton et al, 2004). Ignoring spiritual needs contravenes Article 13 of the Human Rights Act 1998, which stipulates that religious expression is a fundamental human right.

Persons with physical or mental disabilities, and their families, often turn to religious institutions for comfort and belonging. However, they are not always made welcome. Lack of knowledge and understanding leads to insensitivity, and congregations can be too focused on the disability rather than relating to the person. Indeed, religious institutions sometimes fail to create the necessary accommodation for people with disabilities and even show covert signs of hostility towards them. Possible reasons for this exclusion stem from the most ancient of beliefs about the nature of disability. Such beliefs have contributed in Western society to the establishment of a medical model that views disability as pathology.

Assessing spiritual needs of people with intellectual disiabilities

There is still very little research into the significance of spirituality for people with intellectual disabilities, be it theistic, non-theistic or any combination thereof. Many accounts of spiritual experience are in single case/experiential reports. Coulter (2002) considers whether it is possible 'scientifically' to study spirituality when the objective purpose and methods of science do not seem well suited to such a study. He argues that it is possible to study the objective correlates of spirituality such as health or behaviour. However, it is important not to confuse these objective correlates with the subjective essence of spirituality. Swinton (2004a) found that people with intellectual disabilities recognise the importance of the spiritual dimension to include love, care, acceptance and connectedness with God and others and these are not easily measured.

In modern cultures, the concept of spirituality has widened beyond the confines of traditional religion to embrace what might be termed 'secular spirituality', relating to the aspect of a person that links the deeply personal to the universal, providing an understanding of one's interrelationship with nature as well as people. It includes joining with others in an appreciation

127

of beauty, music and the creative arts and engenders a sense of harmony. It connects all the different pieces into a meaningful whole, with a sense of one's own place in it. Yet the continuing perception that spirituality equates with institutional religion was demonstrated in a recent audit survey of local residential homes for adults with intellectual disabilities conducted by the author.[1] Staff were asked about the spiritual needs of the residents under their management and the most common responses equated spirituality with organised religious practices; there was no reference made to secular spirituality. A person's spiritual need was usually written into the care plan by a group of formal and informal carers on behalf of the client, whose acquiescence was taken as participation. The belief among caregivers that spirituality is synonymous with religious practice may mean that those who do not express signs of spiritual needs in religious terms are likely to be overlooked (McSherry, 2000). Further, holding different religious beliefs or no religious belief can make staff feel unable to support the spiritual needs of those they care for. The audit found that staff are more likely to address the spiritual needs of residents if they identify themselves as spiritual.

How do we assess the spiritual needs and experience of people with intellectual disabilities? This area is often explored by using abstract rather than concrete representations, yet most people with intellectual disabilities have communication difficulties and struggle with abstract concepts. There is no standard 'language' of spirituality for people with intellectual disability. Rather, spirituality is the sum total of all the life experiences that have helped to create meaning, and which can be further explored through studies, teachings, meetings and discussion. Avenues for learning and development may not be easily accessed by people with intellectual disabilities. Nevertheless, the experience of meaning does not require explicit verbal expression. The danger is in operating with a verbal mindset where needs, if not expressed, are deemed absent (Raji *et al*, 2003). Gardner (1999) has argued that people who happen to be intellectually disadvantaged may nonetheless have a rich spiritual life.

Indeed, it is clear that people with intellectual disabilities do have spiritual experiences. Swinton (2004*b*) ran focus groups in which such people were able to talk about spirituality and what gives meaning to their lives. His research found that support workers are generally not equipped to recognise and respond to people's spiritual needs. The report recommends ways for carers and faith communities to enable people with intellectual disabilities to express their spiritual needs. Exploration of the spiritual needs of people with intellectual disabilities calls for sensitive handling; person-centred planning puts the person at the centre of the exploration, creating an understanding of their internal world and not just resulting in another ticked box on the care plan.

---

[1]   O. Raji, R. Lawrence & B. Cramer (2007) 'Meeting the spiritual needs of people with learning disabilities living in residential homes. An audit survey carried out in south London' (details available from O.R. on request).

Coping with disability

Many factors affect coping with disability, including the cause, nature and timing of the disability. Spiritual strategies used in coping with disability have been shown to bring positive outcome (Larson *et al*, 1993). Spirituality has been described as that which enables a person to survive bad times, to be strong and to overcome difficulties. Although there is a growing body of evidence on the positive effect of spirituality on health and coping (Treloar, 2002), there is little recognition or understanding of how people with intellectual disabilities might benefit from spiritual support. Yet the questions they often asked include 'Why me?' (Bicknell, 1983) or 'How can a good God allow this to occur?' (Baldacchino & Draper, 2001). The effect of spirituality on the lives of caregivers is attracting more attention (Singer & Irvin, 1989). They turn to clergy for support (Miltiades & Pruchno, 2002), are more likely to use prayer as a coping strategy and thus have a positive relationship with the care recipient (Wood & Parham, 1990).

Parents have traditionally been the primary providers and caretakers of children with intellectual disabilities. High levels of cohesion and harmony in families positively affect the social and cognitive development of children with disabilities (Trute & Hauch, 1988). A reciprocal benefit was described by Stainton & Besser (1998), who found that families reported the positive impact of having children with intellectual disabilities. They described increased sense of purpose and priorities, with expanded personal and social networks and community involvement, and finding their children to be a source of joy and happiness.

Religion can play a critical role in sustaining human relationships that are strained by the everyday realities and necessities of providing and receiving care. Kaufman *et al* (1990) considered that the social or spiritual aspect of religious participation had a buffering effect on parents' stress levels. On the other hand, even though religious beliefs can help family values and provide 'meaning for life' experiences (Taylor & Chatters, 1986), parents of people with disabilities do not always have positive experiences of faith communities, feeling rejected and excluded when their children are not welcome. Children and adults with intellectual disabilities may not be included in faith communities because of their behaviour. This can lead to segregation and isolation.

Bereavement and grief

All too often, it is assumed that people with intellectual disabilities are not affected by the death of a loved one and their grief is not acknowledged. Yet, losing a loved one is an important spiritual experience. The greater the level of disability, the more the person's communication depends on observer interpretation. It is probably for this reason that the reaction of people with intellectual disabilities to bereavement has received relatively little attention (Raji *et al*, 2003).

Normal grief has been extensively described (Bowlby, 1961; Parkes, 1972), suggesting a progression through several non-discrete stages, with some overlap or return to earlier stages but resolving over time. Yet continuing, unresolved grief is a spiritual experience that is part of the lives of many people with intellectual disabilities. Swinton (2004*b*) found grief, loss and a sense of disconnectedness were common phenomena among people with intellectual disabilities. Some factors that contribute to poor adjustment to loss include inhibition of the experience and expression of grief (Parkes, 1972; Oswin, 1991). Grief, if denied expression, is potentially pathological, and people with intellectual disabilities may present to services with severe emotional problems following an experience of disenfranchised grief (Hollins & Esterhuyzen, 1997). Such people may grieve in ways that are not understood and which may therefore be ignored, or discounted as challenging behaviour.

Funerary rituals reinforce group ties, provide cultural identity and form a source of valuable social support, which can be important in both practical and emotional terms. The exclusion of people with intellectual disabilities from these mourning customs excludes them from valuable emotional support. Sometimes people with intellectual disabilities are not told about a death, even of a close relative. They will be sensitive to the changes around them but are not helped to make sense of them by sharing fully in the experience. They are left bewildered and unable to play a useful part in the rituals of loss and grieving.

It is known that predictors of depression following bereavement include insecure attachment patterns in childhood (Marris, 1991) and having to adjust to a new life over which one has little control, while not understanding why things have changed. These factors are prevalent in people with intellectual disabilities. Narayanasamy *et al* (2002) described a counselling approach to spiritual support during crisis for people with intellectual disability. This included giving time and space to build trusting relationships with a sense of security, showing love and compassion, and helping staff and other residents achieve a sense of meaning and purpose.

Psychiatry of learning disability

Psychiatrists are increasingly becoming interested in spirituality because of its potential benefits to mental health. Mental well-being can be described as a state of harmony within the individual and between the individual and the environment. Traditionally, psychiatrists have had responsibility for the medical care of people with intellectual disabilities. Normalisation is now having a significant effect on the way services for people with intellectual disabilities are structured throughout the UK and in other parts of the world. The UK has a highly specialised psychiatric service specifically for people with intellectual disabilities, steered by the Faculty of Psychiatry of Learning Disability in the Royal College of Psychiatrists. This includes developments to map the spiritual needs of people with intellectual disabilities within the context of their mental health and well-being. It is becoming increasingly clear that science alone is not enough to provide a basis for understanding and caring for another human being.

Many people with intellectual disabilities have psychiatric, behavioural and emotional problems. Assessing the presence of mental health problems in people with intellectual disabilities is a complex process, which raises distinct theoretical questions and methodological dilemmas. Most categories of mental illness have been reported in people with intellectual disabilities (Eaton & Menolascino, 1982; Sovner & Hurley, 1983). Opinion varies about how the severity of intellectual disability affects a person's vulnerability to developing different psychiatric disorders (Corbett, 1979; Gostason, 1985; Iverson & Fox, 1989; Doody et al 1998). There is currently also limited evidence regarding factors predicting the presence of mental health problems in individuals with intellectual disabilities. However, there is general agreement that the rate of psychopathology in people with intellectual disabilities is substantially raised when compared with the general population, with increased vulnerability over the whole spectrum of psychopathology and especially with certain diagnostic groups such as the autism–spectrum disorders. Reported rates of psychopathology vary significantly, from 10 to 40% (Borthwick-Duffy, 1994; Cooper et al, 2007). Psychiatric illnesses can be difficult to detect in this population, because of problems with communication and atypical presentations. If a person with intellectual disability is brought to the attention of a psychiatrist, the clinician lacking training and experience in the field may inaccurately ascribe any problem identified as being purely due to the intellectual disability itself, so-called 'diagnostic overshadowing'. Most assessment techniques rely on verbal accounts and utilise parallel interviewing of both the patient and a key informant. The greater the level of disability, the more reliant the assessor on third-party involvement. Information about how the individual with intellectual disabilities regards his or her current experience is limited and often totally absent.

The same standards for everyone?

People with learning disabilities form a heterogeneous group and decisions about presence and type of mental illness are based on diagnostic criteria standardised for the general population. Costello & Bouras (2006) have argued that the application of measurement techniques developed for the general population may be inappropriate in people with intellectual disabilities. However, in the absence of other evidence, these generic assessments have been extrapolated to form the basis of understanding of this group of service users' needs.

Mental health assessments should include issues of spirituality. However, this is not generally addressed during evaluation and the planning of care and support (Berlin & Miller, 1992). The available literature considers either the spiritual or mental health needs of people with intellectual disabilities but rarely a combination of the two. An exception is found in the publications of the L'Arche International Faith Community (www.larche.org), which has a Christian focus.

Lack of time, uncertainty about spirituality and how to incorporate spiritual care into the role of the professional, lack of education in the spiritual dimension of people's experiences and fear of imposing values on people have all been reported as barriers to the implementation of spiritual care for people with intellectual disabilities (Swinton, 2004b). There is a tendency simply to translate a person's spiritual experiences into the language of psychology or psychiatry, since distress may be interpreted more easily within the boundaries of a familiar, psychological framework than by engaging with a spiritual paradigm (Swinton, 2001b). Last, the attitude of carers who equate spirituality with religion may mean that for people with intellectual disabilities issues of secular spirituality may be missed (Gilbert & Watts, 2006).

Treatment approaches in people with intellectual disabilities

Several treatment approaches have been demonstrated to be effective for persons with mental health disorders and intellectual disabilities. Although psychopharmacology is widely used, a number of studies have shown that psychotherapy is often effective in improving coping abilities or relieving symptoms of psychopathology (Fletcher, 1993). The basis of psychotherapy is similar to that for the general population (Rubin, 1982; Levitas & Gilson, 1989; Fletcher & Duffy, 1993), but techniques must be adapted to the developmental skills of the individual being treated (Szymanski, 1980; Blotzer & Ruth, 1995). Psychotherapy provides a tool for finding the self and 'healing the soul', through a relationship between therapist and patient that requires a connection with another human being, highlighting shared characteristics that help to find meaning in life. Group therapy provides a shared connection with others in similar circumstances, which fosters group cohesion and peer support. This can help reduce feelings of isolation (Fletcher, 1984), leading to a sense of unity with the wider world.

Behaviour management programmes are widely used to modify inappropriate behaviour and teach adaptive skills. In a different approach, McGee (1993) described a combined psychotherapeutic and behaviour modification programme called 'Gentle Teaching', involving the building of a therapeutic relationship between therapist and individual that McGee refers to as 'bonding'. This technique attempts to redirect maladaptive behaviour towards meaningful human engagement.

Empirical indicators of spiritual well-being for people with intellectual disabilities are not readily available. Studies show that spiritual support is delivered in a variety of ways using different approaches and that there is better recognition of religious than spiritual needs (Narayanasamy & Owen, 2001; Narayanasamy *et al*, 2002). Nevertheless, evidence suggests that responding to the spirituality of people with intellectual disabilities can be rewarding for clients, their families and professional carers. Research has shown that although staff experienced initial difficulty in identifying with their role and doubted their own abilities to deliver, they discovered a sense of achievement and satisfaction when meeting clients' spiritual needs. It also gave staff a greater sense of cohesiveness and improved morale (Montgomery, 1991; Benson & Stark 1996; McNair & Leguit 2000; Narayanasamy *et al*, 2002).

Patient spiritual care and staff spirituality

Spirituality can enrich the working life of staff and help to find meaningfulness in the workplace (Gilbert & Watts, 2006). Spiritual care requires provision of time that is increasingly lacking in healthcare and a degree of closeness that may even be considered unprofessional. One viewpoint is that closeness limits objectivity in decision-making. Coulter (2002) and Royce-Davis (2000) recommend that practitioners should be given the opportunity for personal exploration of spiritual issues. The absence of any training in spiritual skills (Ingersoll, 1994) may explain why many service professionals do not emphasise spiritual needs to the same degree as other issues in mental health assessment. To provide optimal care, professionals need to understand their clients' spirituality, focusing on the person, without foisting their own spiritual or religious beliefs on vulnerable people (Royce Davis, 2000).

People with intellectual disabilities are increasingly becoming valued members of society. However, they still rely heavily on 'services' to enable them make the most of life and its meaning; therefore, in concentrating on providing efficient and effective services, it is possible to lose sight of their ordinariness and their humanity (Hart & Pettingell, 2005). Progress has been patchy and *ad hoc*, driven by organisational and professional goals rather than having the person with intellectual disabilities at the centre of change. People with intellectual disabilities must have opportunities to achieve all that life has to offer, including experiences that help to make sense of who they are and the purpose of their life here on earth.

Spiritual care of people with intellectual disabilities

Issues of spirituality and faith remain a big challenge in caring for people with intellectual disabilities, especially at times of transition and during major life events. Such people require ways of communicating that get around their cognitive and linguistic difficulties. These include using simple language, visual cues and making abstract concepts as concrete as possible.

Religious communities in Europe and North America are increasingly coming to the realisation that traditional worship and rituals are inappropriate to the needs of many people with intellectual disabilities and are finding alternative approaches that enable more meaningful participation (see L'Arche (www.larche.org), SPRED (Special Religious Development; www. spred.org.uk) and Causeway Prospects (www.prospects.org.uk)). They are taking into consideration the special ways in which people with intellectual disabilities grow in faith, concluding that strongly relational, intuitive experiences are more fruitful than explanations, and that silence can be more profound than words.

In the UK and the USA, people with intellectual disabilities face tremendous obstacles in gaining access to appropriate, quality healthcare and inadequate physician training is partly the cause (Hogg, 2001; Voelker, 2002). There is a need to educate generic mental health professionals on intellectual disabilities early on in their training and through continuing professional development. Seidel (2003) reported that the European Association for Mental Health in Mental Retardation stated at its annual conference that all persons with intellectual disabilities have a right to the best mental healthcare available to the health and social care system of any country. Training is required to enable those supporting people with intellectual disabilities to recognise and respond to their spiritual needs (Swinton, 2004a). In the past, the lifestyles of persons with mental health problems and intellectual disabilities were governed by programme models developed for them, but without their input. However, the trend today is toward a service system that is individualised and based on personal choice and satisfaction. The aim must be to supply whatever support may be necessary to enable affected individuals to improve functioning, and to help them find personal success and satisfaction in the environment of their choice.

Conclusion

People with intellectual disabilities are marginalised in society, with limited opportunity to find meaning in their lives. Their spiritual needs should be incorporated into person-centred care plans, enabling them to experience and explore their spirituality in its widest meaning. Staff need to bear in mind that spirituality is not dependent on consciousness or the ability to communicate easily and that it transcends the bounds of ability and disability. Spirituality may not be apparent in some people because of their disability and it is important for caregivers to find a way of understanding a person's spiritual experience. Further, care staff should be open and receptive to the spiritual experiences that people with intellectual disabilities may have, without imposing their own spiritual or religious views.

Spirituality is now recognised to have a positive link to health and well-being in both preventative and restorative capacities. In developing ways of helping people with intellectual disabilities to define their own spirituality, it is necessary to move away from a verbal mindset and from the measurement of externally perceived needs, in favour of an understanding of the internal state.

Research on the spiritual needs and experiences of people with intellectual disabilities who additionally have mental health needs is seriously lacking and more is needed on both scientific and naturalistic fronts. The emphasis should change from doing things 'to' or 'for' to doing them 'with' the person with intellectual disabilities.

Beliefs inherent within the major faith traditions can act as barriers to those with disabilities. What is urgently required is an inclusiveness that welcomes people with intellectual disabilities into both religious and secular life. There are developments to address these; faith communities can and should be powerful sources of friendship and support, research showing that membership of a supportive and inclusive religious community benefits a person's mental health (Larson *et al*, 1997). In the field of mental healthcare, spirituality extends far beyond the ambit of faith traditions (Swinton, 2004*b*). Available in equal measure to those with intellectual disabilities and their personal and professional carers, its inclusion in the care process can only enhance, dignify and enrich the life of persons with intellectual disabilities. As human beings, to this they are fully entitled.

References

Baldacchino, D. & Draper, P. (2001) Spiritual coping strategies: a review of the nursing research literature. *Journal of Advanced Nursing*, **34**, 833–841.

Benson, L. A. & Stark, M. (1996) *Timeless Healing: Power and Biology of Belief*. Simon & Schuster.

Berlin, S. & Miller, P. (1992) Practitioner's personal and professional attitudes and behaviours toward religion and spirituality: issues for education and practice. *Journal of Social Work Education*, **28**, 190–203.

Bicknell, D. J. (1983) The psychopathology of handicap. *British Journal of Medical Psychology*, **56**, 167–178.

Blotzer, M. A. & Ruth, R. (1995) *Sometimes you just want to feel like a human being: case studies of empowering psychotherapy with people with disabilities*. Brookes.

Borthwick-Duffy, S. (1994) Epidemiology and prevalence of psychopathology in people with mental retardation. *Journal of Consulting and Clinical Psychology*, **62**, 17–27.

Bowlby, J. (1961) Process of mourning. *International Journal of Psychoanalysis*, **42**, 317–340.

Bunning, K. & Steel, G. (2006) Self-concept in young adults with a learning disability from the Jewish community. *British Journal of Learning Disabilities*, **35**, 43–49.

Cook, C. C. H. (2004) Addiction and spirituality. *Addiction*, **99**, 539–551.

Cooper, S.-A., Smiley, E., Morrison, J., *et al* (2007) Mental ill-health in adults with intellectual disabilities: prevalence and associated factors. *British Journal of Psychiatry*, **190**, 27–35.

Corbett, J. A. (1979) Psychiatric morbidity and mental retardation. In *Psychiatric Illness and Mental Handicap* (ed. F. E. James & R. P. Snaith), pp. 11–25. Gaskell.

Costello, H. & Bouras, N. (2006) Assessment of mental health problems in people with intellectual disabilities. *The Israel Journal of Psychiatry and Related Sciences*, **43**, 241–251.

Coulter, D. (2002) Recognition of spirituality in healthcare: personal and universal implications. In *Spirituality and Intellectual Disability: International Perspectives on the Effect of Culture and Religion on Healing Mind, Body and Soul* (International Association for the Scientific Study of Intellectual Disabilities Congress, eds W. Gaventa (Jnr), W. Gaventa & D. Coulter). Haworth Press.

Department of Health (2001) *Valuing People: A New Strategy for Learning Disabilities for the 21st Century*. TSO (The Stationery Office).

Doody, G. A., Johnstone, E. C., Sanderson, T. L., *et al* (1998) 'Pfropfchizophrenie' revisited: Schizophrenia in people with mild learning disability. *British Journal of Psychiatry*, **173**, 145–153.

Dykens, E. M. (2006) Toward a positive psychology of mental retardation. *American Journal of Orthopsychiatry*, **76**, 185–193.

Eaton, L. F. & Menolascino, F. J. (1982) Psychiatric disorders in the mentally retarded: types, problems and challenges. *American Journal of Psychiatry*, **139**, 1297–1303.

Fletcher, R. J. (1984) A model day service for the mentally retarded-mentally ill population. In *Handbook of Mental Illness in the Mentally Retarded* (eds F. Menolascino & J. Stark). Plenum Press.

Fletcher, R. J. (1993) Mental illness-mental retardation in the United States: policy and treatment challenges. *Journal of Intellectual Disability Research*, **37** (suppl.1), 25–33.

Fletcher, R. J. & Duffy, T. (1993) Group therapy with mentally retarded persons. In *Mental Health Aspects of Mental Retardation: Progress in Assessment and Treatment* (eds R. J. Fletcher & A. Dosen). Lexington Books.

Gardner, H. (1999) *Intelligence Reframed*. Basic Books.

Gilbert, P. & Watts, N. (2006) Don't mention God. *A Life in the Day*, **10**, 20–25.

Gostason, R. (1985) Psychiatric illness among the mentally retarded: a Swedish population study. *Acta Psychiatrica Scandinavica*, **318**, 111–117.

Hatton, C., Turner, S., Shah, R., *et al* (2004) *Religious Expression, a Fundamental Human Right: the Report of an Action Research Project on Meeting the Religious Needs of People with Learning Disabilities*. Foundation for People with Learning Disabilities.

Hart, S. & Pettingell, J. (2005) Valuing people with learning disabilities. *Journal for the Royal Society for the Promotion of Health*, **125**, 16–17.

Hogg, J. (2001) Essential healthcare for people with learning disabilities: barriers and opportunities. *Journal of the Royal Society of Medicine*, **94**, 333–336.

Hollins, S. & Esterhuyzen, A. (1997) Bereavement and grief in adults with learning disabilities. *British Journal of Psychiatry*, **170**, 497–501.

Ingersoll, R. E. (1994) Spirituality, religion and counselling: dimensions and relationships. *Counselling and Values*, **38**, 98–111.

Iverson, J. C. & Fox, R. A. (1989) Prevalence of psychopathology among mentally retarded adults. *Research in Developmental Disability*, **10**, 77–83.

Kaufman, A. V., Campbell, V. A. & Adams, J. P. (1990) A lifetime of caring: older parents who care for adult children with mental retardation. *International Journal of Family Care*, **2**, 39–54.

Larson, D., Wood, G. & Larson, S. (1993) A paradigm shift in medicine toward spirituality. *Journal of Mind-Body Health*, **9**, 39–49.

Larson, D., Sawyers, J. & McCullough, M. (1997) *Scientific Research on Spirituality and Health: a Consensus Report*. National Institute for Healthcare Research.

Levitas, A. & Gilson, S. (1989) Psychodynamic psychotherapy with mildly and moderately retarded patients. In *Mental Retardation and Mental Illness: Assessment, Treatment and Services for The Dually Diagnosed* (eds R. Fletcher & F. Menolascino). Lexington Books.

Marris, P. (1991) The social construction of uncertainty. In *Attachment across the Life Cycle* (by C. M. Parkes). Routledge.

McGee, J. (1993) Gentle teaching for persons with mental retardation: the expression of a psychology of interdependence. In *Mental Health Aspects of Mental Retardation: Progress in Assessment and Treatment* (eds R. J. Fletcher & A. Dosen). Lexington Books.

McNair, J. & Leguit, G. (2000) The local church as an agent of natural support to individuals with developmental disabilities. *Issues in Transition*, **2**, 11–16.

McSherry, W. (2000) *Making Sense of Spirituality in Nursing Practice*. Churchill Livingstone.

Miltiades, H. B. & Pruchno, R. (2002) The effect of religious coping on caregiving: appraisals of mothers of adults with developmental disabilities. *Gerontology*, **42**, 82–91.

Montgomery, C. (1991) The caregiving relationships: paradoxical and transcendent aspects. *Journal of Transpersonal Psychology*, **23**, 91–105.

Mpofu, E. & Harley, D. (2002) Disability and rehabilitation in Zimbabwe: lessons and implications for rehabilitation practice in the US. *Journal of Rehabilitation*, **68**, 26–40.

Narayanasamy, A. & Owen, J. (2001) A critical incident study of nurses' responses to the spiritual needs of learning disabilities clients. *Journal of Advanced Nursing*, **33**, 446–455.

Narayanasamy, A., Gates, B. & Swinton, J. (2002) Spirituality and learning disabilities: a qualitative study. *British Journal of Nursing*, **11**, 948–957.

Oswin, M. (1991). *Am I Allowed to Cry? A Study of Bereavement Among People Who Have Learning Difficulties*. Human Horizons.

Parkes, C. M. (1972) *Bereavement: Studies of Grief in Adult Life*. Tavistock.

Race, D. G. (2002) *Learning Disability: a Social Approach*. Routledge.

Raji, O. & Hollins, S. (2000) Exclusion from funerary rituals and mourning: implications for social and individual identity. In *Madness, Disability and Social Exclusion: the Archaeology and Anthropology of 'Difference'* (ed. J. Hubert). Routledge.

Raji, O., Hollins, S. & Drinnan, A. (2003) How far are people with learning disabilities involved in funeral rites? *British Journal of Learning Disabilities*, **31**, 42–45.

Royal College of Psychiatrists (2006) *Help is at Hand: Spirituality and Mental Health* (leaflet). Royal College of Psychiatrists.

Royce-Davis, J. (2000) The influence of spirituality on community participation and belonging: Christina's story. *Counselling and Values*, **44**, 135–142.

Rubin, R. L. (1982) Bridging the gap through individual counselling and psychotherapy with mentally retarded people. In *Bridging the Gap* (eds F. J. Menolascino & B. McCann). University Park Press.

Seidel, M. (2003) The Declaration of Rome 2003 with regard to the promotion of interest and services for people with intellectual disabilities with mental health needs. *Journal of Policy and Practice in Intellectual Disability*, **1**, 101–103

Singer, G. H. & Irvin, L. K. (1989) Family care giving, stress and support. In *Support for Caregiving Families: Enabling Positive Adaptation To Disability*, pp. 3–25. Paul H. Brooke.

Sinson, J. (1996) Normalisation and community integration of adults with severe mental handicaps relocated to group homes. *Journal of Developmental and Physical Disabilities*, **6**, 255–270.

Sovner, R. & Hurley, D. A. (1983) Do the mentally retarded suffer from affective illness? *Archive of General Psychiatry*, **49**, 61–67.

Stainton, T. & Besser, H. (1998) The positive impact of children with an intellectual disability on the family. *Journal of Intellectual and Developmental Disability*, **23**, 57–70.

Stockholder, J. E. (1994) Naming and renaming persons with intellectual disabilities. In *Disability is not Measles: New Research Paradigms in Disability* (eds M. H. Rioux & M. Bach), pp. 153–179. L'institut Roeher Institute.

Sulmasy, D. P. (1997) *The Healer's Calling: Spirituality for Physicians and Other Healthcare Professionals*. Paulist Press.

Swinton, J. (1997) Restoring the image: spirituality, faith and cognitive disability. *Journal of Religion and Health*, **36**, 21–28.

Swinton, J. (1999) Reclaiming the soul: a spiritual perspective on forensic nursing. In *Forensic Nursing and the Multidisciplinary Care of the Mentally Disordered Offender* (eds A. Kettles & D. Robinson). Jessica Kingsley.

Swinton, J. (2001a) *A Space to Listen: Meeting the Spiritual Needs of People with Learning Disabilities*. Mental Health Foundation.

Swinton, J. (2001*b*) *Spirituality in Mental Healthcare: Rediscovering a Forgotten Dimension.* Jessica Kingsley.

Swinton, J. (2004*a*) *Why are We Here? Spirituality and the Lives of People with Learning Disabilities.* Mental Health Foundation.

Swinton, J. (2004b) *No Box to Tick. A Booklet for Carers and Support Workers on Meeting the Spiritual Needs of People with Learning Disabilities.* Mental Health Foundation.

Szymanski, L. S. (1980) Individual psychotherapies with retarded persons. In *Emotional Disorders of Mentally Retarded Persons* (eds L. Szymanski & P. Tanquay). University Park Press.

Taylor, R. J. & Chatters, L. N. (1986) Church-based informal support among elderly Blacks. *The Gerontologist*, **26**, 637–642.

Treloar, L. L. (2002) Disability, spiritual beliefs and the Church: the experiences of adults with disabilities and family members. *Journal of Advanced Nursing*, **40**, 594–603.

Trute, B. & Hauch, C. (1988) Building on family strength: a study of families with positive adjustment to the birth of a developmentally disabled child. *Journal of Marital and Family Therapy*, **14**, 185–193.

Voelker, R. (2002) Improved care for neglected population must be 'rule rather than exception'. *Journal of American Medical Association*, **288**, 299–301.

Wood, J. B. & Parham, I. A. (1990) Coping with perceived burden: ethnic and cultural issues in Alzheimer's family caregiving. *Journal of Applied Gerontology*, **9**, 325–339.

Wolfensberger, W. (1972) *The Concept of Normalization in Human Services*. National Institute on Mental Retardation. Canada.

CHAPTER 8

Substance misuse

Christopher C. H. Cook

Substance misuse psychiatry is concerned with what happens when people use psychoactive substances in such a way that they cause harm to themselves and others. It is, therefore, a field of clinical practice and scientific enquiry that is concerned with people's relationships with themselves and others and the wider order of things, but especially with the object of their 'addiction'. Necessarily, this engages it with spiritual concerns and in fact the field has a history of engaging with spiritual as well as medical ways of thinking. The definition of spirituality offered in chapter 1 (p. 4) emerged from a study of the addictions literature.

Much has been said about exactly how behavioural patterns of substance misuse should be defined. Such definitions are largely beyond the scope of this chapter, but of central importance to the field today is the concept of the dependence syndrome, which has influenced both ICD–10 (World Health Organization, 1992) and DSM–IV (American Psychiatric Association, 1994) classifications of substance use disorders. This has largely replaced, or else has come to define, the concept of addiction in clinical practice and scientific research. It is a bio-psychosocial understanding of addiction that has now withstood the test of several decades of research. It has the benefit of clarifying what addictive behaviour is about so as to enable us to see both what the spiritual issues entailed in that behaviour might be, and also what the bio-psychosocial correlates of spirituality are.

For example, the element of subjective compulsion, defined within the dependence syndrome in such a way as to include both craving and impaired control over substance-related behaviour, touches on important concerns of both Buddhist and Christian spirituality (Groves & Farmer, 1994; Groves, 1998; Cook, 2006). Because these traditions each have something important to say about the spiritual nature of addiction, it is not surprising that Christian, Buddhist and other faith-based treatment programmes have been founded as a response to the suffering with which addiction is associated. On the other hand, the model of the dependence syndrome reminds us that there is a bio-psychosocial dimension to spiritual problems. This is true not only within the field of substance misuse but in all areas of human experience. Spiritual problems are inextricably linked to the business of being human and are generally not well understood, if completely divorced from this physical, psychological and social reality.

The substance misuse field also has another important lesson to offer about the relationship between spirituality and psychiatry in general. Although dependence is a particularly important complication of substance use, it is not best understood in isolation. Rather, it is a problem that emerges when, of a group of people who engage in psychoactive substance use, only some become dependent. It is therefore a problem of appetitive behaviour, an aspect of human experience in which we are all involved. (Plato considered the appetitive or desiring faculty to be one of two 'irrational' aspects of the human soul, alongside a third, rational, faculty (Lee, 2003: pp. 139–149).) The spirituality of substance misuse is therefore not only a concern of patients or addicts; neither is it only a concern of those who consider themselves to be in some way 'religious', for it is a matter that concerns us all.

Historical perspective

Whatever the conceptual relationship between spirituality and addiction, history helps to illuminate why spirituality has become a particular concern of substance misuse psychiatry. In the Western world, at least up until the end of the 18th century, problems such as drunkenness were not particularly distinguished from other social and moral concerns, for example theft, adultery or gluttony. For some, the failure to distinguish between such problems is understood as being the basis of the now discredited 'moral model' of addiction. But it is doubtful that this model ever properly existed in quite the way that some people seem to imagine. Rather, drunkenness was something that people were responsible for, in the same way that they were responsible for other social and personal vices. A few people were, perhaps, relative saints, but most people in society were sinners, of one kind or another.

In 17th-century Europe, thought and belief about almost all aspects of human life began to be influenced by the intellectual movement now known as the Enlightenment. The Enlightenment emphasised reason and science as the basis for understanding human problems, thus excluding the authority of religious traditions and scriptures (see, for example, Honderich, 1995: pp. 236–237). From the late 18th century onwards, this movement appears to have begun to influence thinking about drunkenness. In 1785, Benjamin Rush published *An Inquiry into the Effects of Ardent Spirits upon the Human Body and Mind with an Account of the Means of Preventing and of the Remedies for Curing Them* (Rush, 1785) and in 1804 Thomas Trotter published *An Essay, Medical, Philosophical and Chemical, on Drunkenness and Its Effects on the Human Body* (Trotter, 1804). Addiction (or 'chronic inebriety') became a medical concern in addition to being a religious concern. In this context, a disease model of addiction became popular, although it was rarely completely divorced from the moral model. This disease was understood, in one form or another, as a disease of the will, caused by alcohol.

The disease model, in a modified form, was adopted in the 20th century by Alcoholics Anonymous (AA), and it was this organisation that has had particular influence over the perception of addiction as a spiritual problem in North America and Europe. Founded in Akron, Ohio, by two alcoholics in 1935, AA drew on both religious and medical sources for its understanding of alcoholism. The former came mainly from the Oxford Group, an evangelical Christian movement of the time. The latter came from, among other places, Dr William Silkworth, the physician who treated one of the founders of AA and who later contributed a medical foreword to the 'Big Book' of AA (Alcoholics Anonymous, 1976: pp. xxiii–xxx). It is estimated that Silkworth treated more than 50 000 alcoholics during the course of his lifetime (Kurtz, 1991: pp. 21–22). Although he adopted a specific physical disease model of alcoholism that did not stand the test of time (he understood alcoholism as being a form of physical allergy to alcohol), he also saw very little hope for recovery, unless the alcoholic experienced a 'psychic change'. For this change to come about, he saw the need for 'something more than human power' (Alcoholics Anonymous, 1976: p. xxvii).

The founders of AA were also influenced by the work of William James, who wrote a seminal book on the psychology of religion, *The Varieties of Religious Experience* (1985). Within the pages of this volume may be found many psychological accounts of religious experience, which include reference to those who struggled with chronic drunkenness or, as we would say, alcohol dependence. The case of S. H. Hadley is recounted by James at some length (ibid., pp. 201–203). Hadley saw himself as a hopeless case, a 'homeless, friendless, dying drunkard', who had delirium tremens (ibid., p. 210). Having found himself praying in a prison cell, he went on his release to a meeting at a Mission Hall at which Jerry M'Auley, a man known for his work among drunkards, was preaching. Responding to the call at the end of the meeting, Hadley describes how, with a breaking heart, he prayed to Jesus to help him. At this, a profound affective change came about: 'indescribable gloom' was replaced with 'glorious brightness'. Hadley concludes his account:

> From that moment till now I have never wanted a drink of whiskey, and I have never seen money enough to make me take one. I promised God that night that if he would take away the appetite for strong drink, I would work for him all my life. He has done his part, and I have been trying to do mine [James, 1985: p. 203].

The Varieties of Religious Experience left its mark on AA. Although initially a Christian movement, it acquired a wariness of established religion that bears much of the character of James' own suspicion of doctrinal formulation and religious belief. It saw, nonetheless, a key need for spiritual transformation in recovery from alcoholism and it offers a 'spiritual but not religious' way of finding this, which is accessible to people of all faiths or none. It is, essentially, a secular form of spirituality (Kurtz, 1996).

From the story of two alcoholics seeking to help one another in America in the 1930s, AA has become a worldwide organisation of more than 2 million members in over 100 000 groups operating in more than 150 countries (www.alcoholics-anonymous.org.uk). The philosophy of AA was also adopted by various sister organisations seeking to help people with different addictions, including Narcotics Anonymous (NA), Cocaine Anonymous (CA) and Gamblers Anonymous (GA), and also those seeking to help families and children of those who are addicted, including AlAnon (for spouses and partners of alcoholics), Alateen (for teenage children of alcoholics) and Families Anonymous (FA, for families of members of NA). Furthermore, although firmly rooted as a mutual help movement, the philosophy of AA has also influenced professionally-led treatment and has been adopted by both residential and community-based programmes (Cook 1988a,b). In general, all mutual help groups based upon the philosophy of AA, as expressed in its '12 steps', are referred to as '12-step groups'. Treatment programmes based upon this philosophy are often referred to as '12-step treatment programmes' or, more popularly, the 'Minnesota Model', reflecting the early development of programmes of this sort in Minnesota in the 1940s and 1950s.

Whereas AA and its sister organisations offer a non-religious, non-denominational approach to spirituality as a pathway to recovery from addiction, various religious or faith-based organisations continue to offer different forms of spirituality anchored within their own faith traditions. Thus, Christian (National Institute on Drug Abuse, 1977; Moos *et al*, 1978), Buddhist (Barrett, 1997), Islamic (Abdel-Mawgoud *et al*, 1995), Native American (Garrett & Carroll, 2000) and other programmes have been described, each offering their own distinctive approach to spirituality either as a response in itself, or else in combination with various secular and scientific interventions.

At the same time, mainstream healthcare provision and scientific research within the addictions field in the Western world have tended to focus on physical, social and psychological interventions that do not require, or even allude to, the need for any spiritual change. Other mutual help groups have been established that do not require the assent to spirituality, even in a secular form, that is so central to AA (Humphreys, 2004: pp. 33–93). The field of substance misuse treatment today is thus heterogeneous. However, the worldwide impact of the spirituality of AA and the significant non-statutory provision of faith-based organisations have ensured that spirituality is a subject for discussion among lay people and professionals, those with their own experience of addiction and those who study the addictive behaviour of others, within treatment communities and faith communities. Spirituality has become a feature of the addictions treatment landscape.

Spirituality as a protective factor

Before moving on to the treatment studies, it would be worth considering briefly the field of research suggesting that spirituality is a protective factor against substance misuse. Various measures of religious behaviour, religious affiliation or 'religiosity' are inversely correlated with substance use and misuse (Chamberlain & Hall, 2000: pp. 189–197; Koenig *et al*, 2001: pp. 169–172; Koenig, 2005: pp. 109–112). There is debate about how this effect may operate. For example, affiliation with a faith community may instil moral values which guard against substance use – especially illicit substance use – or substance misuse. However, religion is also associated with various measures of mental well-being (Chamberlain & Hall, 2000: pp. 118–137; Koenig, 2005: pp. 43–81) and may reduce substance misuse by improving coping skills or reducing perceived stress. On the other hand, the effect may simply be a function of conforming to the norms of a social group in which substance use or misuse is less acceptable. Church-affiliated young people are clearly offered drugs at a rate not very different to that of other young people and so, whatever the mechanism of the protective effect may be, it is not simply a case of their being hidden away from drug-using peers (Cook *et al*, 1997).

Measures of religiosity are clearly related to spirituality and it would appear that spirituality is also protective against substance misuse (Zimmerman & Maton, 1992; Stewart, 2001; Leigh *et al*, 2005). Spirituality appears to exert a protective effect in both high- and low-risk groups (Ritt-Olson *et al*, 2004).

It may be helpful to consider an example of this kind of research. In a study of 7661 church-affiliated young people (age 12 to 30 years), agreement with statements reflecting church attendance, Christian belief and spiritual practices (prayer and Bible reading) were generally found to be associated with lesser likelihood of them having smoked cigarettes, drunk alcohol or used illicit drugs (Hope & Cook, 2001). However, church attendance appeared to be more important for the 12- to 16-year-olds, whereas belief and Bible reading appeared to be more important for the 17- to 30-year-olds. Perhaps for younger people, socialisation within a faith community provides protection against substance misuse, but for older people it is the internalisation of faith and its expression in personal spirituality that provides protection.

Spirituality in substance misuse treatment programmes

Spirituality may be variously understood and spiritual issues differently addressed in different kinds of treatment programmes. Broadly speaking, they can be considered in three groups: 12-step spirituality, spirituality rooted in the faith traditions of faith-based organisations, and non-specific explorations of spirituality that might take place in any other treatment programme.

12-step spirituality

The principles adopted by 12-step groups and 12-step programmes are summarised in the so-called '12 steps' as written down by the original founders of AA, adapted with only minor modifications by AA's sister groups. They are expressed in the first person, reflecting their origins in the personal experiences of the founders:

1   We admitted we were powerless over alcohol – that our lives had become unmanageable.

2   Came to believe that a Power greater than ourselves could restore us to sanity.

3   Made a decision to turn our will and our lives over to the care of God *as we understood Him.*

4   Made a searching and fearless moral inventory of ourselves.

5   Admitted to God, to ourselves and to another human being the exact nature of our wrongs.

6   Were entirely ready to have God remove all these defects of character.

7   Humbly asked Him to remove our shortcomings.

8   Made a list of all persons we had harmed, and became willing to make amends to them all.

9   Made direct amends to such people wherever possible, except when to do so would injure them or others.

10 Continued to take personal inventory, and when we were wrong, promptly admitted it.

11 Sought through prayer and meditation to improve our conscious contact with God *as we understood Him* praying only for knowledge of His will for us and the power to carry that out.

12 Having had a spiritual awakening as the result of these steps we tried to carry this message to alcoholics and to practise these principles in all our affairs.

(Alcoholics Anonymous, 1977; original emphases preserved)

The influence of the Oxford Group's spirituality is visible here, with its emphasis on personal confession and repentance of sin. However, the influence of *The Varieties of Religious Experience* (James, 1985) may also be discerned – in the lack of religious doctrinal language and emphasis upon God (or a 'Higher Power') as understood and experienced by the individual members of AA.

The first three steps relate to relationship, especially that with the object of addiction (in this case alcohol) over which the individual finds him- or herself powerless, and relationship with a transcendent power towards which the individual must turn for help. This transcendent or 'Higher Power' provides a subject for much debate. The explicit reference to 'God' in steps 3, 5, 6 and 11 undoubtedly provides the reason for many a person attending AA only once or twice and then declaring that it is 'too religious'. However, in practice, all 12-step groups and programmes are open to people from all faiths and none. God is understood by the individual according to their own faith tradition, folk religion or a personal notion of the Divine which is unique to that individual. Alternatively, a 'Higher Power' is construed in some even less religious way as 'the group', or the 12-step programme itself. What is important is that a power outside of oneself is identified – a power greater than self which is not self. It is not so much that the member of AA has to believe in God (although many do) as that they must believe that they are 'not God'.

Steps 4 to 10 are concerned with confession and repentance, to use Christian terminology, but are referred to here as the taking of a moral inventory and making amends. The concern with relationship between self and a transcendent order is anchored here in relationships with others – especially those who have been harmed by the addict in the course of the history of their addictive behaviour. It is sometimes said that the disease model offers a way of avoiding personal responsibility but, in contrast, members of AA, at least those who work through the steps in a serious way, are engaged deeply with personal responsibility, both for what they have done and for working at their own recovery.

Finally, steps 11 and 12 are concerned with ongoing spiritual practice and sharing with others what has been learnt. It is clear that this ongoing spirituality is founded in the personal spiritual experience of the individual. It is not a theoretical programme, but one that can only be based upon a personal spiritual 'awakening' or conversion. Such an experience might be sudden, as in the case of S. H. Hadley, or it might be gradual, but it is in such an experience that hope is to be found.

What does all this mean in practice? Attendance at meetings of AA and/or its sister fellowships (as they are called) is considered to be vital to the process. The steps are 'worked' by individual members with the assistance and guidance of a 'sponsor', a more experienced member who acts as mentor and guide. In general, asking whether or not a member of AA or other 12-step fellowship has a sponsor provides a good indication of whether they are actually taking the programme seriously. There is also an extensive literature supportive of 12-step spirituality and recovery. A key place within this literature is held by the 'Big Book' (Alcoholics Anonymous, 1976), which outlines the nature of the problem, the approach taken by AA in response and provides accounts of the experiences of some of the early members. The 'Big Book' of AA is paralleled by comparable works in each of the other 12-step fellowships (e.g. Narcotics Anonymous, 1986).

Spirituality in the programmes of faith-based organisations

It is not possible to review here the spiritual traditions of all the world's religions. Chapter 12 explores the general relationship between spirituality and religion in further detail. However, some examples can be given of the various connections made between the spiritualities of particular religions and the spiritual condition of addiction. It is also important to consider what takes place in practice in addiction treatment programmes provided by faith-based organisations.

For Christianity, the problem is less in making connections between spirituality and addiction than in choosing between various possible theological understandings of what addiction is all about. At some level, there appears to be a general consensus that it is connected with 'sin' or rebellion against God, but this can mean very different things to different people. For some it implies that 'addiction is (a) sin', for others that 'sin is addiction'. Even these two, apparently similar, models can result in very different approaches to helping people caught in the web of addiction. The one appears very much like the moral model in religious clothing. The other reduces addiction to being merely an expression of the human condition, a condition of which we are all a part, and risks losing any distinctive understanding of what it is to be addicted. There are, of course, many nuances and subtleties that distinguish the ways in which these models might be expressed, such as that put succinctly by Linda Mercadante in the title of her book *Victims and Sinners* (Mercadante, 1996).

Elsewhere (Cook, 2006), I have explored some of the common ground that is mapped out both by scientific studies of addiction and some foundational Christian texts. Like Mercadante, I conclude that for Christian theology, grace rather than sin is central and it is grace that (in non-theological language) the 12-step programmes have also identified as vital to recovery from addiction. Grace, in Christian terms, is concerned with the relationship between God and human beings, a relationship within which God is always generously self-giving despite, and even because of, human powerlessness and self-imprisonment. Christian spirituality, like 12-step spirituality, is more concerned with the human need to look beyond ourselves than it is to focus on our own faults and failings – the solution is to be found in relationship with the Divine reality that is both deeply within us and also outside and beyond us.

Buddhism also finds resonance with the language of addiction. For Buddhism, concepts such as 'dependence' and 'craving' are associated with the very problems that are at the root of all human suffering. Thus, for example, Paramabandhu Groves defines craving as: 'the urge or desire to obtain an experience other than the one we are experiencing at present' (Groves, 1998). Such urges and desires can express themselves in subtle and varied ways, but they are not alien to any of us. As with Christian spirituality, we find here a reminder that the phenomenon of addiction is something that affects us all and is a part of the human condition. However, the focus is more on recognising why craving is unhelpful and how we may better deal with it. The answer to the latter is to be found in the development of 'skilfulness' – a quality that includes elements of wisdom, attentiveness and compassion – which enables us to view our actions and motives differently and to break away from the unhealthy motivation that is inherent within craving. In contrast to Christianity, Buddhism does not require a focus on relationship with God, but it shares a recognition that unhealthy attachments to things that are 'not God' are at the root of human suffering.

Even these two brief examples will immediately draw attention to the different ways in which faith traditions might suggest remedies for the addictive state. Thus, within the revealed monotheistic faiths, Judaism, Christianity and Islam, spirituality in the programmes offered by their associated faith-based organisations is most likely to take the form of prayer, worship and study of scripture. For Buddhist groups, spirituality might look much more like cognitive therapy (Avants & Margolin, 2004) coupled with meditation rather than prayer. However, nor will all Christian programmes look alike. In some, visible reliance is placed upon secular psychological and medical techniques, with spirituality providing more of a motivating factor or rationale (see, for example, Judge, 1971). In others, exactly the opposite is true, with the emphasis entirely upon prayer, Bible study and Christian faith, and with secular therapies almost or completely absent (see, for example, Gruner, 1979).

Spirituality in secular treatment programmes

Treatment programmes that follow neither a 12-step design nor the spiritual tradition of a faith-based organisation might be considered 'non-spiritual'. Although a chaplain or a chaplaincy team is usually available within NHS trusts in the UK, it is very much up to the individual patient whether or not he or she takes the opportunity to talk to a chaplain about the spiritual aspects of their problem. It seems that patients in substance misuse services in the UK rarely take this opportunity. However, various surveys show that such patients (at least in the USA) do consider spirituality to be important (McDowell *et al*, 1996; Carroll *et al*, 2000; Arnold *et al*, 2002; Dermatis *et al*, 2004).

There are implicit and explicit ways in which spirituality may be addressed, even within secular and medical substance misuse treatment programmes, that do not follow the traditions of a faith-based organisation or a 12-step programme. It seems almost impossible to discuss problems of substance misuse without a spiritual dimension to the conversation, even if the word 'spirituality' is not actually used. For example, the definition of spirituality used in chapter 1 (p. 4) was derived from a review of the body of research on addiction and spirituality (Cook, 2004). This analysis of some 263 publications revealed 13 conceptual components the authors had used to define spirituality:
1 Relatedness
2 Transcendence
3 Humanity
4 Core/force/soul
5 Meaning/purpose

6   Authenticity/truth
7   Values
8   Non-materiality
9   (non)Religiousness
10 Wholeness
11 Self-knowledge
12 Creativity
13 Consciousness.

Of these, the first two, relatedness and transcendence, are the most commonly cited (34 and 41% respectively of papers studied, but included in 62 and 53% respectively of questionnaires used to measure spirituality in addictions research). Inevitably, interventions for substance misuse involve considerations of relatedness, for it is the relationship with the object of addiction that is at the heart of the problem, and relationships with self and others almost inevitably suffer as a result. Transcendence, if understood in the narrower sense of the Divine or a 'Higher Power', is not integral to secular treatments for substance misuse. However, if understood in a broader sense of recognising the inadequacy of personal resources, failed previous attempts to address the problem, or of the need to accept help from others, transcendence may be considered a key premise to engaging in any helping relationship – including that offered by a substance misuse treatment service.

This very brief analysis of spirituality within secular substance misuse treatment must obviously be balanced by the recognition that there are particular dynamics, including biological as well as psychological and social disturbances, which are unique to the dependence syndrome and are not experienced by all human beings. However, the extent to which spirituality and addiction touch on universal aspects of the human condition – in particular our relationships with ourselves, others and the world around us – is important. It is this which creates a point of contact between therapist and service user, and it is this which offers an antidote to the stigma associated with the moral model.

There are explicit ways in which spirituality may be addressed within secular treatment programmes. For example, where relapse prevention programmes address the need for lifestyle balance, spiritual as well as biological, psychological and social aspects of human lifestyle can constructively be addressed (Moss *et al*, 2007). Even where plurality of faith tradition makes it difficult to address spirituality through any common understanding of religion, many NHS and other substance misuse treatment programmes allow some educational input from 12-step group members, or else allow such groups to meet on their premises. This is not to suggest that such treatment programmes adopt 12-step spirituality, but at least patients are afforded the opportunity to be acquainted with what these groups have to offer and to discuss concerns they may have. Similarly, techniques of mindfulness and skilfulness, although associated with the Buddhist tradition, find parallels within cognitive–behavioural psychology and may be accessible to people who would not ordinarily think of themselves as interested in Buddhism.

It is also possible to introduce discussion of spirituality in a neutral way, without favouring any particular spiritual tradition, and doing so in a non-threatening and non-judgemental way can be helpful (Jackson & Cook, 2005). There is evidence that in the UK staff attitudes may not make this easy to do in practice (Day *et al*, 2005), but in the USA they appear to be more positive (McDowell *et al*, 1996; Forman *et al*, 2001). Staff personal awareness of their own spirituality, and the preferences and prejudices associated with this, is undoubtedly important as a first step to ensuring that service users are given the opportunity to discuss spirituality during the course of their treatment.

Treatment outcome research

Only three relevant outcome studies of addiction treatment programmes with good methodology (longitudinal design, comparison groups, high follow-up rates and reliable/valid measures) have been published to date (Humphreys & Gifford, 2006). Two of these studies are of 12-step programmes and one is of a Christian programme.

1   Rudolf Moos and his colleagues (Moos *et al*, 1978) studied 97 men in a residential Salvation Army treatment programme for the treatment of 'skid row' alcoholics. The spiritual components of the Salvation Army programme included attendance at AA meetings as well as more specifically Christian counselling and worship. The programme also included therapy groups and community meetings, educational input, vocational rehabilitation and opportunity for recreation. Residents improved significantly on seven out of nine outcome measures, and those who participated more actively did significantly better on four of these measures in comparison with those who participated less actively. Comparisons with half-way house and hospital-based programmes were favourable.

2   Project MATCH compared the efficacy of 12-step facilitation with cognitive–behavioural and motivational enhancement therapy (Project MATCH Research Group, 1997) over a 12-week period, using manual-based treatments for alcoholism. Twelve-step facilitation aimed to encourage involvement in AA and a beginning of working the 12 steps. As many as 952 patients were randomised between interventions in the out-patient arm of the study, and 774 in an aftercare arm of the study that followed in-patient or day-patient treatment. Outcomes between groups were comparable, with 12-step facilitation clients faring as well as those in other groups, and with benefits maintained at 3-year follow-up (Project MATCH Research Group, 1998). In fact, 12-step facilitation, if anything, showed slight advantages.

3   Humphreys & Moos (2001) studied 1774 substance-dependent veterans treated either in a 12-step orientated in-patient programme

or in a cognitive–behaviourally orientated in-patient programme. The 12-step programme patients spent on average 39% of their time in programme-related activities, as compared with only 4% for patients in the cognitive–behavioural programme. Patients in the 12-step group showed higher rates of abstinence at follow-up 1 year after treatment (46% v. 36%) and they also had significantly lower treatment costs.

A larger number of studies have been published where various measures of outcome and spirituality have been related, although they do not meet all of the criteria specified by Humphreys & Gifford (2006). Table 8.1 (pp. 153–157) provides details of 13 studies in which abstinence and spirituality have been related. The relationship is almost invariably positive (i.e. spirituality is associated with abstinence), with the main exception being the study of clergy alcoholics published by Fichter in 1982 in which spirituality appeared to be unrelated to abstinence. The study by Fiorentine & Hillhouse (2000) is perhaps also an exception, and will be discussed here further (p. 151).

In Table 8.2 (pp. 158–160) details are provided of six studies in which length of sobriety and abstinence have been related. Here again there appears to be a positive relationship, with spirituality usually predicting longer sobriety, although again there are two studies, by Brown & Peterson (1991) and by Rush (2000), in which no significant relationship of this kind was found.

The limitations of this evidence base are apparent. All of the studies in Table 8.2 and all but one of the studies in Table 8.1 were conducted in the USA, which may limit applicability of the findings to Europe or other parts of the world. Similarly, the studies in both tables are concerned primarily with 12-step spirituality. Exceptions to this include one study in which attendance at religious services predicted abstinence as a treatment outcome (Brown et al, 2004) and another in which the focus of interest was traditional spiritual practices of Native Americans (Stone et al, 2006). In many studies, the faith tradition of participants was not specified, and where it was, the bias was almost always towards Christianity (except Stone et al, 2006). The instruments used to measure spirituality as a variable and the underlying conception of spirituality that they reflect were diverse.

Despite the various limitations of these studies, on the basis of the evidence to date it would appear that treatment in programmes that incorporate spirituality is at least as effective as other forms of treatment. Further, there is reason to believe that spirituality is positively associated with abstinence and/or length of abstinence as an outcome measure following treatment of various kinds and/or involvement in 12-step mutual help groups.

Treatment process research

Spirituality may be conceived of as either an independent or a dependent variable in treatment research. If spirituality is a universal attribute, measurable in a similar way to personality, it may prove to reflect receptiveness to treatment or to certain kinds of treatment, or it may function as a prognostic indicator. It may mediate other outcomes such as abstinence or reduced substance use, or it may simply be understood as reflecting a better quality of outcome or a better quality of life. In addition to this, spirituality might be considered a function of treatment environment and the spirituality of therapists (in relation to the spirituality of patients/clients) might be an important influence in treatment. These possibilities suggest complex and various ways in which spirituality could influence treatment process, and multivariate studies of high-quality methodology will be required to unravel them.

Table 8.3 (pp. 161–164) summarises ten studies in which spirituality has been examined in relation to the process of treatment of, and/or recovery from, substance misuse. Again, it will be seen that there is a universally positive relationship between spirituality and the treatment process, with spirituality tending to increase during treatment/recovery and/or being perceived by treatment recipients as an important part of the treatment/recovery process. However, in one study (Borman & Dixon, 1998) spirituality increased during treatment in both 12-step and other types of treatment programmes. This perhaps provides a reminder that spirituality is an aspect of the treatment process that may be implicit as well as explicit, and that it deserves attention not only in explicitly spiritual approaches to treatment, but in all forms of treatment for substance misuse.

Two further studies are worthy of further comment. The study by Chen (2006) arguably qualifies for Humphreys' and Gifford's criteria of longitudinal design, comparison groups, high follow-up rates and reliable/valid measures (Humphrey & Gifford, 2006). Attrition rates were low (28% among those attending NA and participating in a 12-step course, and 26% in a group attending NA only) and valid/reliable measures were used. The study was of prison inmates, but it remains to be seen how they fare when they are released from prison. However, those participating in a 12-step 'course' (a total of 480 hours over 6 months, providing comprehensive explanations of the 12 steps) in addition to NA attendance demonstrated a higher sense of coherence and meaning in life, and reduced anxiety, depression and hostility over the 12-month course of the study, as compared with those who did not participate in such a course.

The study by Fiorentine & Hillhouse (2000; see also Table 8.1) is also of interest in terms of the light that it sheds on treatment process. This was also a prospective longitudinal study of good design, although without a comparison group. Measures of spirituality were concerned here with embracement of 12-step ideology and it is again disappointing that other, more generally relevant measures were not employed. Although acceptance of 12-step ideology was found to predict attendance at 12-step meetings, it was also found that acceptance of the ideology predicted abstinence independently of this. In particular, the aspects of ideology that were found to be important for attendance were recognition of the need for lifelong attendance at 12-step meetings and the need to surrender to a 'Higher Power'. The aspect of ideology predicting abstinence, however, was the idea that a return to controlled or non-problematic use would never be possible. The authors comment that their 'findings suggest that the spiritual emphasis of 12-step programmes does not assist in the process of recovery' (p. 385). This is argued on the basis that the spiritual emphasis of the programme (which they understand only in relation to the aspects of ideology relating directly to a 'Higher Power') must exclude some potential members. Although this may be the case, their overall conclusion regarding spirituality is highly debatable. Clearly there is a complex relationship between the component beliefs of 12-step ideology, some of which might appear more immediately 'spiritual' than others, but all of which are interrelated as comprising a whole package.

The qualitative studies summarised in Table 8.3 show that individuals recovering from substance misuse believe that spirituality is an important part of the process of their recovery and that this may take different forms, according to faith tradition, involvement with a 12-step programme and other factors. Taken together, the studies quoted in this table, both quantitative and qualitative, reveal varying understandings of what spirituality is, among both researchers and participants. These understandings generally reflect different selections, emphases upon, and combinations of the 13 component concepts of spirituality discussed earlier (also described in more detail in Cook, 2004). Future research needs to more clearly identify them and examine their interrelationships and interdependence.

Conclusion

Spirituality and substance misuse are intimately related. This relationship is partly a product of history, especially the history of religious concern with the morality of substance misuse and the history of the 12-step movement and its spiritual response to addiction. There also appears to be a more fundamental relationship which touches upon the very core of what it means to be a human being: the experience of being related to self, others and a wider, 'transcendent' reality, and the experiences of personal freedom and choice which are so severely compromised in the addictive state. These relationships are borne out by qualitative and quantitative research, which shows that there is an evidence base both for a protective effect of spirituality against the development of substance misuse and also for spirituality as an important variable for study in substance misuse treatment research.

Yet, if spirituality is reduced merely to a variable of objective importance for evidence-based medicine, its true significance will have been missed. It is concerned both with the objective and subjective aspects of the practice of substance misuse psychiatry and with the subjectivity of what it is to be human. This is something which should draw together therapist and patient in a way that both respects and transcends the social boundaries that are defined by professional relationships.

Table 8.1 Studies of spirituality and abstinence in recovery from substance misuse

Study	Study design	Substance	Participant characteristics Male n	Female n	Age years	Religion	Ethnicity	Selection criteria	Measure of spirituality	Findings
The rehabilitation of clergy alcoholics: ardent spirits subdued (Fichter, 1982)	Cross-sectional	Alcohol	677	0	n/s	Christian	n/s	Clergy treated for alcoholism	Clergy Lifestyle Project; tape-recorded interviews	Level of spirituality unrelated to abstinence but is related to AA involvement
The role of spirituality in recovery from chemical dependency (Johnsen, 1993)	Cross-sectional (6 months after discharge from treatment)	Various	40	10	mean 36.8	n/s	n/s	Random sample of in-patients from a California 12-step treatment programme	Spiritual Practices Questionnaire	Use of prayer/meditation significantly associated with abstinence at 6 months' follow-up
Measurement of materialism and spiritualism in substance abuse research (Mathew et al, 1995)	Cross-sectional comparison of groups, plus test–retest reliability (7 days' interval)	Various	79	64	mean 43/38/33[a]	Christian 82%, agnostic/other 18%	n/s	Three groups: 1 Individuals recovering from substance use disorder, for >6months 2 Clergy controls 3 General population controls	Mathew Materialism–Spiritualism Scale (MMSI)	Michigan Alcohol Screening Test positive controls lower than recovering group for G, M & C subscales of MMSI
AA through the eyes of its older members (Washburn, 1996)	Qualitative	Alcohol	3	3	60–82	n/s	n/s	Older AA members	Ethnographic interview	Spirituality perceived as a key theme by older abstinent AA members

Table continues

153

Table 8.1 Continued

Study	Study design	Substance	Participant characteristics					Selection criteria	Measure of spirituality	Findings
			Male n	Female n	Age years	Religion	Ethnicity			
The effects of spiritual practices on recovery from substance abuse (Carter, 1998)	Cross-sectional comparison of two groups	Various	39	22[b]	n/s	n/s	n/s	Two groups: 1 Addicts in recovery 2 Addicts with history of multiple relapses	Brown–Peterson Recovery Progress Inventory	Alcoholics/addicts with fewer relapses and long-term recovery indicated increased spiritual practices
Factors influencing recovery from different addictions (Koski-Jännes & Turner, 1999)	Cross-sectional	Various	38	38	25–76	n/s	Finnish	Recovered addicts (abstinent for 3 years) responding to newspaper advertisements	Questionnaires and interviews	Spirituality (and 12-step groups) important in maintaining change in recovery following 12-step treatment for alcohol/drug addictions
Exploring the additive effects of drug misuse treatment and twelve-step involvement: does twelve-step ideology matter? (Fiorentine & Hillhouse, 2000)	Prospective longitudinal, 8-month follow-up	Various	121	235	18–55	n/s	White 30%, African American 43%, Mexican/Central American 23%, other 4%	Out-patients in substance misuse treatment programmes in Los Angeles	Embracement of 12-Step Ideology Scale (modified)	Acceptance of 12-step ideology predicts attendance at 12-step meetings; acceptance of ideology predicts abstinence independently of attendance

Study	Design	Substance			Age			Sample	Measures	Findings
Spirituality and addiction: Relationship to recovery and relapse (Jarusiewicz, 2000)	Cross-sectional comparison of two groups	Various	24	16	31–72	n/s	n/s	Recovering (n=20) and relapsing (n=20) patients at addiction treatment facility in New Jersey	Spiritual Beliefs Scale; Faith Development Interview Guide	Recovering individuals have greater faith and spirituality than those relapsing
Spirituality, religious problem-solving and sobriety in Alcoholics Anonymous (Oakes et al, 2000)	Cross-sectional with retrospective report	Alcohol	41	37	23–71	Mostly Christian	White 85%, African American 8%, Native American 6%, other 1%	AA members drawn from groups in six US states	AA Involvement Scale; Religious Problem Solving Scale; Spiritual Experience Index; Religious Background and Behaviour Questionnaire; Purpose in Life Questionnaire	AA involvement is single most important predictor of abstinence and sobriety; religious problem solving/ coping style possible mediator of relationship between spirituality and sobriety; difficulties of definition of spirituality acknowledged
Spiritual and religious support in recovery from addiction among HIV-positive injection drug users (Avants et al, 2001)	6-month longitudinal design	Drugs	30	13	mean 40	n/s	White 40%, African American 49%, Hispanic 12%	HIV-positive drug users in methadone maintenance programme	Spiritual Support (one item only)	Perceived spiritual comfort and support at entry to treatment with methadone maintenance was an independent predictor of abstinence from drug use by HIV-positive injection drug users

Table continues

Table 8.1 *Continued*

Study	Study design	Substance	Male n	Female n	Age years	Ethnicity	Religion	Selection criteria of spirituality	Measure	Findings
Alcoholics Anonymous and church involvement as predictors of sobriety among three ethnic treatment populations (Roland & Kaskutas, 2002)	Longitudinal, 12-month follow-up	Alcohol	506	345	more than half aged 30–44	n/s	White 63%, African American 30%, Hispanic 7%	Enrolled in alcohol treatment programme in north California	Religious Background and Behaviour Questionnaire	African American participants more religious than White/Hispanic participants; high AA attendance associated with higher rate of sobriety in all groups
Factors associated with treatment outcomes in an aftercare population (Brown et al, 2004)	Longitudinal, 6-month follow-up	Various	145	49	mean 35	n/s	African American 96%	Probationers and parolees in drug-free out-patient programmes in Baltimore	Religious service attendance; Beck Hopelessness Scale	Optimism/ pessimism and religious observance significant predictors of substance use in follow-up

Participant characteristics

| Traditional practices, traditional spirituality, and alcohol cessation among American Indians (Stone et al, 2006) | Cross-sectional but part of an ongoing longitudinal study | Alcohol | 696 | 284 | 17–77 | Native American | Native American | Parents of children age 10–12 years on four Native American reservations involved in 3-year ongoing study | Measure of Traditional (Native American) Spirituality (4-item) | $n=133$ 'non-alcohol users'; of the remaining: 37% had stopped using alcohol, 34% had one or more alcohol/drug treatments; 68% of total sample had a lifetime history of alcohol abuse; participation in traditional activities and traditional spirituality associated with positive effect on alcohol cessation |

n/s, not specified; AA, Alcoholics Anonymous

a. mean age of each of the three study groups

b. gender not specified, $n=2$

Table 8.2 Studies of spirituality and length of sobriety in recovery from substance misuse

Study	Study design	Participant characteristics[a]					Selection criteria	Measure of spirituality	Findings
		Substance	Male n	Female n	Age years	Ethnicity			
Assessing spirituality in addiction treatment and follow-up: development of the Brown–Peterson Recovery Progress Inventory (B-PRPI) (Brown & Peterson, 1991)	Cross-sectional (but with pre- and post-treatment measures in sample 3)	Various	55	53	17–63	n/s	Three samples: 1 Members of AA groups in north-central Mississippi (n=35) 2 Members of 12-step groups in central and south-west Mississippi (n=58) 3 12-step out-patient treatment (n=15)	Brown–Peterson Recovery Progress Inventory	No correlation between spirituality and length of sobriety
Spirituality and purpose in life in alcoholism recovery (Carroll, 1993)	Cross-sectional	Alcohol	100	0	26–81	Majority White	Members of AA groups in north California	Step Questionnaire; Purpose in Life Questionnaire (PIL)	AA attendance and practice of step 11 both correlated with PIL and length of sobriety
The spiritual experience in recovery: a closer look (Sandoz, 1999a)	Cross-sectional	Alcohol	26	30	Mean 45	White 90%	Members of AA groups in south New Jersey	AA Practices and Spiritual Experience	Claimed spiritual experience associated with: older age, longer sobriety, heard more 5th steps, made more 12th-step calls

Study	Design	Substance		N	Age	Ethnicity	Sample	Measure	Findings
Power, spirituality, and time from a feminist perspective: correlates of sobriety in a study of sober female participants in Alcoholics Anonymous (Rush, 2000)	Cross-sectional	Alcohol	0	125	Mean 47	White 94%, other 6%	Snowball sample of female AA members	Spiritual Orientation Inventory	Number of AA meetings attended weekly contributed significantly to spirituality; spirituality higher for those involved in their religion; no correlation between spirituality and length of sobriety
Spirituality, contentment, and stress in recovering alcoholics (Poage et al, 2004)	Cross-sectional	Alcohol	35	18	24–77	White 89%, Hispanic 6%, African American 4%, Native American 2%	Members of AA groups in west Texas	Spirituality Assessment Scale (composite from other scales)	Length of sobriety significantly associated with spirituality; spirituality and contentment positively related; spirituality correlated with lower stress in women but not men

Table continues

Table 8.2 *Continued*

Study	Study design	Substance	Participant characteristics				Selection criteria	Measure of spirituality	Findings
			Male n	Female n	Age years	Ethnicity			
Helping, spirituality and Alcoholics Anonymous in recovery (Zemore & Kaskutas, 2004)	Cross-sectional	Alcohol	118	80	21–82	White 83%, African American 7%, Latino 7%, Asian–Pacific Islanders 2%, Native American 1%, other 1%	Convenience sample of recovering alcoholics	Daily Spiritual Experiences Scale	Longer sobriety predicted higher theism, self-transcendence and AA achievement

n/s, not specified; AA, Alcoholics Anonymous

a. In none of the studies was the participants' religion specified.

Table 8.3 Studies of spirituality as part of the substance misuse treatment/recovery process

Study	Study design	Substance	Participant characteristics					Selection criteria	Measure of spirituality	Findings
			Male n	Female n	Age years	Religion	Ethnicity			
A retrospective study of the concept of spirituality as understood by recovering individuals (Mathew et al, 1996)	Retrospective comparison pre/post-recovery	Poly	65	58	Mean 43/33[a]	n/s	n/s	Recovering addicts in the USA with min. 6 months' abstinence (n=62); normal controls (n=61)	Mathew Materialism and Spiritualism Scale (MMSS); Cognitive Pattern Questionnaire	Increase in spirituality in recovery
Spirituality and the 12 steps of substance abuse recovery (Borman & Dixon, 1998)	Retrospective comparison pre/post-treatment	Various	n/s[a]	n/s	n/s	n/s	n/s	Out-patients in 12-step (n=28) and non-12-step (n=14) treatment programmes in central Indiana	Spiritual Well-Being Scale (SWBS)	Spirituality increased during treatment in both 12-step and non-12-step groups
Exploring the spiritual experience of the Twelve Steps of Alcoholics Anonymous (Sandoz, 1999b)	Cross-sectional	Alcohol	27	30	45	Protestant 26%, Catholic 64%, other 11%	White 93%, African American 4%, mixed 4%	AA members, recruited from groups in south New Jersey	AA Practices and Spiritual Experiences	82% AA members claimed to have had a spiritual experience (72% slow, 22% slow and sudden, 6% sudden); spiritual experience significantly associated with completion of steps 4, 5, 8 and 9.

Table continues

Table 8.3 *Continued*

Study	Study design	Substance	Participant characteristics					Selection criteria	Measure of spirituality	Findings
			Male n	Female n	Age years	Religion	Ethnicity			
The relationship among substance abuse counselors' spiritual well-being, values, and self-actualizing characteristics and the impact on clients' well-being (Brooks & Matthews, 2000)	Pre and post-treatment measurement of SWBS	Poly	14	31[b]	n/s	n/s	n/s	Three samples from Virginia: 1 random sample of in-patient counsellors (n=11); 2 convenience sample of out-patient counsellors (n=34); 3 convenience sample of in-patient treatment programme patients (n=94)	Rokeach Value Survey; SWBS; Personal Orientation Inventory	Half variance of SWBS accounted for by self-acceptance (POI), loving and wisdom (RVS); wisdom negatively correlated with SWB; patients' SWB increased during in-patient treatment
The role of religion and spirituality in recovery from drink problems: A qualitative study of Alcoholics Anonymous members and south Asian men (Morjaria & Orford, 2002)	Qualitative	Alcohol	10	0	36–57	Catholic 50%, Hindu 30%, Sikh 20%	South Asian 50%, White 50%	Two UK samples: 1 White AA members (n=5) 2 South Asian in NHS/non-statutory treatment for alcohol problems (n=5)	Taped semi-structured interview	AA members experienced conversion (cf. 'Big Book' of AA); South Asian men underwent re-affirmation of existing religious beliefs

A focus group analysis of relapse prevention strategies for persons with substance use and mental disorders (Davis & O'Neill, 2005)	Qualitative	Various	15	12	Mean 44	n/s	African American 77%, European–American 22%	People in later stages of substance abuse treatment at a Chicago rehabilitation centre	Focus groups	Engaging in prayer or relying on a 'Higher Power', participating in a meaningful activity and thinking differently about life are important strategies in sustaining abstinence
Qualitative interviews on substance abuse relapse and prevention among female trauma survivors (Harris, Fallot & Berley, 2005)	Qualitative	Various	0	27	Mean 42	n/s	African American 81%, White 19%	Women with history of physical or sexual abuse and mental health and substance abuse disorders at an urban US mental health agency	Semi-structured interview	Connection, self-awareness, sense of purpose and meaning and spirituality all considered by participants to be supportive of recovery; individual relapse prevention skills alone appeared insufficient to sustain abstinence
Correlates of therapeutic involvement among adolescents in residential drug treatment (Hawke, Hennen & Gallione, 2005)	Cross-sectional	Drugs	142	38	13–18	n/s	Hispanic 20%, African American 36%, White 46%	Adolescents in five residential drug treatment programmes in New Jersey	Spirituality items from Personal Experience Inventory	Self-esteem and spirituality strongly correlated with therapeutic involvement

Table continues

Table 8.3 *Continued*

Study	Study design	Substance	Participant characteristics						Selection criteria	Measure of spirituality	Findings
			Male *n*	Female *n*	Age years	Religion	Ethnicity				
Social support, spiritual program, and addiction recovery (Chen, 2006)	Longitudinal – 1 year study period	Drugs	93	0	Mean 36	n/s	Jewish 71%, Arab 29%		Inmates of 3 Israeli prisons: 1 NA & 12-step programme (*n*=43) 2 NA attendance only (*n*=50)	Meaningfulness subscale of Antonovsky's Sense of Coherence Scale	12-step programme participants had higher sense of coherence and meaning in life and reduction of negative emotions
Religious and spiritual elements of change in Sikh men with alcohol problems: a qualitative exploration (Morjaria-Keval, 2006)	Qualitative	Alcohol	15	0	0	Sikh	South Asian		Sikh men living in UK Midlands showing successful change of drinking behaviour for at least 4 months	Taped, semi-structured interview	Transition from 'amli' (drunk) to 'amritdhari' (baptised) associated with critical transformation process involving religious adherence, purification and seeking redemption.

n/s, not specified; AA, Alcoholics Anonymous; NA, Narcotics Anonymous; SWBS, Spiritual Well-Being Scale; SWB, spiritual well-being; NHS, National Health Service

a. 42 study participants, gender not specified; b. gender not specified in 94 participants.

References

Abdel-Mawgoud, M., Fateem, L. & Al-Sharif, A. I. (1995) Development of a comprehensive treatment program for chemical dependency at Al Amal Hospital, Damman. *Journal of Substance Abuse Treatment*, **12**, 369–376.

Alcoholics Anonymous (1976) *Alcoholics Anonymous* (3rd edn). AA World Services.

Alcoholics Anonymous (1977) *Twelve Steps and Twelve Traditions*. AA World Services.

American Psychiatric Association (1994) *Diagnostic and Statistical Manual of Mental Disorders: DSM–IV* (4th edn). APA.

Arnold, R., Avants, S. K., Margolin, A., *et al* (2002) Patient attitudes concerning the inclusion of spirituality into addiction treatment. *Journal of Substance Abuse Treatment*, **23**, 319–326.

Avants, S. K. & Margolin, A. (2004) Development of Spiritual Self-Schema (3-S) therapy for the treatment of addictive and HIV risk behavior: a convergence of cognitive and Buddhist psychology. *Journal of Psychotherapy Integration*, **14**, 253–289.

Avants, S. K., Warburton, L. A. & Margolin, A. (2001) Spiritual and religious support in recovery from addiction among HIV-positive injection drug users. *Journal of Psychoactive Drugs*, **33**, 39–45.

Barrett, M. E. (1997) Wat Thamkrabok: a Buddhist drug rehabilitation program in Thailand. *Substance Use and Misuse*, **32**, 435–459.

Borman, P. D. & Dixon, D. N. (1998) Spirituality and the 12 steps of substance abuse recovery. *Journal of Psychology and Theology*, **26**, 287–291.

Brooks, C. W. & Matthews, C. O. (2000) The relationship among substance abuse counselors' spiritual well-being, values, and self-actualizing characteristics and the impact on clients' well-being. *Journal of Addictions and Offender Counseling*, **21**, 23–33.

Brown, B. S., O'Grady, K., Battjes, R. J., *et al* (2004) Factors associated with treatment outcomes in an aftercare population. *American Journal on Addictions*, **13**, 447–460.

Brown, H. P. & Peterson, J. H. (1991) Assessing spirituality in addiction treatment and follow-up: development of the Brown–Peterson Recovery Progress Inventory (B–PRPI). *Alcoholism Treatment Quarterly*, **8**, 21–50.

Carroll, J. F. X., McGinley, J. J. & Mack, S. E. (2000) Exploring the expressed spiritual needs and concerns of drug dependent males in modified therapeutic community treatment. *Alcoholism Treatment Quarterly*, **18**, 79–92.

Carroll, S. (1993) Spirituality and purpose in life in alcoholism recovery. *Journal of Studies on Alcohol*, **54**, 297–301.

Carter, T. M. (1998) The effects of spiritual practices on recovery from substance abuse. *Journal of Psychiatric and Mental Health Nursing*, **5**, 409–413.

Chamberlain, T. J. & Hall, C. A. (2000) *Realized Religion*. Templeton Foundation Press.

Chen, G. (2006) Social support, spiritual program, and addiction recovery. *International Journal of Offender Therapy and Comparative Criminology*, **50**, 306–323.

Cook, C. C. H. (1988a) The Minnesota model in the management of drug and alcohol dependency: miracle method or myth? Part I: The philosophy and the programme. *British Journal of Addiction*, **83**, 625–634.

Cook, C. C. H. (1988b) The Minnesota model in the management of drug and alcohol dependency: miracle method or myth? Part II: Evidence and conclusions. *British Journal of Addiction*, **83**, 735–748.

Cook, C. C. H. (2004) Addiction and spirituality. *Addiction*, **99**, 539–551 (see also corrigendum: *Addiction* (2006), **101**, 761).

Cook, C. C. H. (2006) *Alcohol, Addiction and Christian Ethics*. Cambridge University Press.

Cook, C. C. H., Goddard, D. & Westall, R. (1997) Knowledge and experience of drug use among church affiliated young people. *Drug and Alcohol Dependence*, **46**, 9–17.

Davis, K. E. & O'Neill, S. J. (2005) A focus group analysis of relapse prevention strategies for persons with substance use and mental disorders. *Psychiatric Services*, **56**, 1288–1291.

Day, E., Gaston, R. L., Furlong, E., *et al* (2005) United Kingdom substance misuse treatment workers' attitudes toward 12-step self-help groups. *Journal of Substance Abuse Treatment*, **29**, 321–327.

Dermatis, H., Guschwan, M. T., Galanter, M., *et al* (2004) Orientation toward spirituality and self-help approaches in the therapeutic community. *Journal of Addictive Diseases*, **23**, 39–54.

Fichter, J. H. (1982) *The Rehabilitation of Clergy Alcoholics: Ardent Spirits Subdued*. Human Sciences Press.

Fiorentine, R. & Hillhouse, M. P. (2000) Exploring the additive effects of drug misuse treatment and twelve-step involvement: does twelve-step ideology matter? *Substance Use and Misuse*, **35**, 367–397.

Forman, R. F., Bovasso, G. & Woody, G. (2001) Staff beliefs about addiction treatment. *Journal of Substance Abuse Treatment*, **21**, 1–9.

Garrett, M. T. & Carroll, J. J. (2000) Mending the broken circle: treatment of substance dependence among Native Americans. *Journal of Counseling and Development*, **78**, 379–388.

Groves, P. (1998) Doing and being: a Buddhist perspective on craving and addiction. In *Psychiatric Nursing: Ethical Strife* (eds P. Barker & B. Davidson), pp. 202–210. Edward Arnold.

Groves, P. & Farmer, R. (1994) Buddhism and addictions. *Addiction Research*, **2**, 183–194.

Gruner, L. R. (1979) Comparative analysis of therapeutic models of using the Teen Challenge paradigm. *Cornell Journal of Social Relations*, **14**, 191–211.

Harris, M., Fallot, R. D. & Berley, R. W. (2005) Qualitative interviews on substance abuse relapse and prevention among female trauma survivors. *Psychiatric Services*, **56**, 1292–1296.

Hawke, J. M., Hennen, J. & Gallione, P. (2005) Correlates of therapeutic involvement among adolescents in residential drug treatment. *American Journal of Drug and Alcohol Abuse*, **31**, 163–177.

Honderich, T. (ed.) (1995) *The Oxford Companion to Philosophy*. Oxford University Press.

Hope, L. C. & Cook, C. C. H. (2001) The role of Christian commitment in predicting drug use among church affiliated young people. *Mental Health, Religion and Culture*, **4**, 109–117.

Humphreys, K. (2004) *Circles of Recovery: Self-Help Organizations for Addictions*. Cambridge University Press.

Humphreys, K. & Gifford, E. (2006) Religion, spirituality and the troublesome use of substances. In *Rethinking Substance Abuse: What the Science Shows and What We Should Do About It* (eds W. R. Miller & K. Carroll), pp. 257–274. Guilford.

Humphreys, K. & Moos, R. (2001) Can encouraging substance abuse patients to participate in self-help groups reduce demand for healthcare? A quasi-experimental study. *Alcoholism, Clinical and Experimental Research*, **25**, 711–716.

Jackson, P. & Cook, C. C. H. (2005) Introduction of a spirituality group in a community service for people with drinking problems. *Journal of Substance Use*, **10**, 375–383.

James, W. (1985) *The Varieties of Religious Experience*. Penguin.

Jarusiewicz, B. (2000) Spirituality and addiction: relationship to recovery and relapse. *Alcoholism Treatment Quarterly*, **18**, 99–109.

Johnsen, E. (1993) The role of spirituality in recovery from chemical dependency. *Journal of Addictions and Offender Counseling*, **13**, 58–61.

Judge, J. J. (1971) Alcoholism treatment at the Salvation Army: a new men's social service center program. *Quarterly Journal of Studies on Alcohol*, **32**, 462–467.

Koenig, H. G. (2005) *Faith and Mental Health*. Templeton Foundation Press.

Koenig, H. G., McCullough, M. E. & Larson, D. B. (2001) *Handbook of Religion and Health*. Oxford University Press.

Koski-Jännes, A. & Turner, N. (1999) Factors influencing recovery from different addictions. *Addiction Research*, **7**, 469–492.

Kurtz, E. (1991) *Not-God: A History of Alcoholics Anonymous.* Hazelden.

Kurtz, E. (1996) Twelve step programs. In *Spirituality and the Secular Quest* (ed. P. H. van Ness), pp. 277–302. SCM.

Lee, D. (ed.) (2003) *Plato: The Republic* (2nd edn). Penguin.

Leigh, J., Bowen, S. & Marlatt, G.A. (2005) Spirituality, mindfulness and substance abuse. *Addictive Behaviors,* **30,** 1335–1341.

Mathew, R. J., Mathew, V. G., Wilson, W. H., *et al* (1995) Measurement of materialism and spiritualism in substance abuse research. *Journal of Studies on Alcohol,* **56,** 470–475.

Mathew, R. J., Georgi, J., Wilson, W. H., *et al* (1996) A retrospective study of the concept of spirituality as understood by recovering individuals. *Journal of Substance Abuse Treatment,* **13,** 67–73.

McDowell, D., Galanter, M., Goldfarb, L., *et al* (1996) Spirituality and the treatment of the dually diagnosed: an investigation of patient and staff attitudes. *Journal of Addictive Diseases,* **15,** 55–68.

Mercadante, L. A. (1996) *Victims and Sinners.* Westminster John Knox Press.

Moos, R. H., Mehren, B. & Moos, B. (1978) Evaluation of a Salvation Army alcoholism treatment program. *Journal of Studies on Alcohol,* **39,** 1267–1275.

Morjaria, A. & Orford, J. (2002) The role of religion and spirituality in recovery from drink problems: a qualitative study of Alcoholics Anonymous members and South Asian men. *Addiction Research and Theory,* **10,** 225–256.

Morjaria-Keval, A. (2006) Religious and spiritual elements of change in Sikh men with alcohol problems: a qualitative exploration. *Journal of Ethnicity in Substance Abuse,* **5,** 91–118.

Moss, R., Cook, C. C. H. & Sandoz, J. (2007) Maintenance and relapse prevention. In *Foundations of Addictions Counseling* (eds D. Capuzzi & M. D. Stauffer), pp. 268–282. Pearson.

Narcotics Anonymous (1986) *Narcotics Anonymous* (3rd edn). World Service Office.

National Institute on Drug Abuse (1977) *An Evaluation of the Teen Challenge Treatment Program.* National Institute on Drug Abuse.

Oakes, K. E., Allen, J. P. & Ciarrocchi, J. W. (2000) Spirituality, religious problem-solving and sobriety in Alcoholics Anonymous. *Alcoholism Treatment Quarterly,* **18,** 37–50.

Poage, E. D., Ketzenberger, K. E. & Olson, J. (2004) Spirituality, contentment, and stress in recovering alcoholics. *Addictive Behaviors,* **29,** 1857–1862.

Project MATCH Research Group (1997) Matching alcoholism treatments to client heterogeneity: Project MATCH post-treatment drinking outcomes. *Journal of Studies on Alcohol,* **58,** 7–29.

Project MATCH Research Group (1998) Matching alcoholism treatments to client heterogeneity: Project MATCH three-year drinking outcomes. *Alcoholism, Clinical and Experimental Research,* **22,** 1300–1311.

Ritt-Olson, A., Milam, J., Unger, J. B., *et al* (2004) The protective influence of spirituality and 'Health-as-a-Value' against monthly substance use among adolescents varying in risk. *Journal of Adolescent Health,* **34,** 192–199.

Roland, E. J. & Kaskutas, L. A. (2002) Alcoholics Anonymous and church involvement as predictors of sobriety among three ethnic treatment populations. *Alcoholism Treatment Quarterly,* **20,** 61–77.

Rush, B. (1785) An Inquiry into the Effects of Ardent Spirits upon the Human Body and Mind with an Account of the Means of Preventing and of the Remedies for Curing Them. Reprinted 1943 in *Quarterly Journal of Studies on Alcohol,* **4,** 325–341.

Rush, M. M. (2000) Power, spirituality, and time from a feminist perspective: correlates of sobriety in a study of sober female participants in Alcoholics Anonymous. *Journal of the American Psychiatric Nurses Association,* **6,** 196–202.

Sandoz, C. J. (1999a) The spiritual experience in recovery: a closer look. *Journal of Ministry in Addiction and Recovery,* **6,** 53–59.

Sandoz, C. J. (1999b) Exploring the spiritual experience of the Twelve Steps of Alcoholics Anonymous. *Journal of Ministry in Addiction and Recovery,* **6,** 99–107.

Stewart, C. (2001) The influence of spirituality on substance use of college students. *Journal of Drug Education*, **31**, 343–351.

Stone, R. A., Whitbeck, L. B., Chen, X., *et al* (2006) Traditional practices, traditional spirituality, and alcohol cessation among American Indians. *Journal of Studies on Alcohol*, **67**, 236–244.

Trotter, T. (1804) *An Essay, Medical, Philosophical, and Chemical, on Drunkenness and Its Effects on the Human Body*. Reprinted 1988. Routledge.

Washburn, N. (1996) AA through the eyes of its older members. *Journal of Geriatric Psychiatry*, **29**, 185–204.

World Health Organization (1992) *The ICD–10 Classification of Mental and Behavioural Disorders: Clinical Descriptions and Diagnostic Guidelines*. WHO.

Zemore, S. E. & Kaskutas, L. A. (2004) Helping, spirituality and Alcoholics Anonymous in recovery. *Journal of Studies on Alcohol*, **65**, 383–391.

Zimmerman, M. A. & Maton, K. I. (1992) Life-style and substance use among male African-American urban adolescents: a cluster analytic approach. *American Journal of Community Psychology*, **20**, 121–138.

CHAPTER 9

Neuroscience of the spirit

Peter Fenwick

Since the 1980s there has been a growing recognition that organ-based medicine is very limiting when considering the genesis of disease in humans. Mind–body medicine is still a growing area, but it has been shown that psychological experience, emotional states and pathological styles of behaviour can all lead directly to physical illness. This recognition has led to the field of psychoneuroimmunology, which has now developed to the point where mental states can be seen to be linked to heart disease and cancers through specific physiological pathways.

It is in this setting that there has been a re-evaluation, particularly by the medical profession, of spiritual medicine that brought widespread recognition that a spiritual component must be considered in both physical and mental illness. In this chapter I will first consider some of the reductionist mechanisms underlying spiritual medicine. Spiritual medicine may be perceived as the spiritual dimension of healing, in which the highest-order holistic processes of the individual are expressed and their expression leads to healing; for example, the aims and goals of the individual, their interaction within their social systems and their transpersonal beliefs.

I will look at the consequences for reductionist science, if the effects of prayer and distant healing are accepted into the main body of scientific knowledge. I will also touch on miracles, that is spiritual healing where the locus of the healing is not yet understood by reductionist science and so can be attributed to forces outside the materialistic realm and consequently outside our reductionist paradigm.

Science has always been reluctant to approach spiritual matters seriously, but this attitude is changing. There are numerous reasons for this, but the most important for conventional medicine is simply that spiritual medicine has been shown to work (Koenig *et al*, 2001). There is, in addition, an ever-growing demand from students for medical courses that include a spiritual dimension. The percentage of US medical schools teaching courses in spiritual medicine has increased dramatically during the past decade; from 3% in 1995, to 40% in 1998 (Levin *et al*, 1997), to 100% in 2001. In 2001, the Templeton Foundation supported the publication of the *Handbook of*

Religion and Health (Koenig *et al*, 2001), which draws together the numerous scientific studies that underpin this field. It is clear from the book that absence of spiritual values is very important in the genesis of illness as is their presence in the healing of illness. So why has Western science been so resistant to exploring this area?

The nature of Western science

Western science is based on the rationalism of Descartes, Galileo, Locke, Bacon and Newton. Galileo defined a two-dimensional universe, consisting of matter and energy. These 'stuffs', he said, had primary and secondary qualities. Primary qualities were those aspects of nature that could be measured, such as velocity, acceleration, weight and mass. Secondary qualities were the qualities of subjective experience, such as smell, vision, truth, beauty and love. Galileo maintained that the domain of science was the domain of primary qualities; secondary qualities were non-scientific.

> To excite in us tastes, odours and sounds I believe that nothing is required in external bodies except shapes, numbers, and slow or rapid movements. I think that if ears, tongues and noses were removed, shapes and numbers and motions would remain but not odours or tastes or sounds [Morton, 1997: p. 58].

Western primary quality science has been outstandingly successful in examining and quantifying the world around us and in producing our current technology. Some philosophers of science have used the reductionist scheme to attempt an understanding of consciousness. Daniel Dennett (1991), for example, argues that only what we can observe in the physical structure of the brain and its function should be included in our understanding of experience and consciousness. The peep show of the private world of the individual's mind should not be included in our theories. This leads to a very limited view of consciousness and results in Dennett claiming that if we understand neuronal function in its entirety, we will then completely understand conscious experience, a view denied by many scientists.

However, the scientific position with regard to consciousness is still very much the same as that Sir Charles Sherrington (1940) noted nearly 70 years ago: science puts its fingers to its lips and is largely silent when the question of consciousness arises. The reason for this is that consciousness is a secondary quality and thus not the domain of science. This leaves our science very lopsided, as only the physical aspects of any phenomenon – a 'view from nowhere' as it has been described – can be investigated by the scientific method (Nagel, 1974). Yet a moment's thought, as Max Velmans points out in his recent book, shows that all objectively described phenomena, the things 'out there', are essentially psychological entities (Velmans, 2000). It is the way that the evidence is obtained that makes the difference between 'objective' and 'subjective' qualities. Objective qualities are tested by asking many different individuals whether their psychological concepts of 'what is out there' match. For instance, do we all see the same pointer readings when we look at the same meter?

In the West, a science of secondary qualities, which asks whether we all have the same internal psychological state in the same circumstances, is only just beginning. This form of science, used to investigate mind directly, is very much an Eastern perspective. In the East, mindfulness techniques are used to expand consciousness. In many of these, watching the breath and holding the mind focused are the essential features. An excellent example of this very precise observation of the mind while doing a standardised practice is zen sesshin, practised widely in Japan, which involves up to a week of concentrated mindfulness practice with no social interaction taking place between the practitioners. This technique has been finely honed over the years to produce an expansion of consciousness in its practitioners (Austin, 2000, 2006).

There is some evidence that the neuroscience community is slowly changing its view. A paper given at the Royal Society by Schwartz *et al* (2005) on quantum physics in neuroscience and psychology discusses John von Neumann's mathematical treatment of quantum mechanics, in which he infers two processes. Process 2 is equivalent to the old Newtonian theories of reductionist science, whereas Process 1 incorporates consciousness into the mathematical explanation of how particles and systems behave, for von Neumann's mathematics stretches from the very small up to at least brain-sized structures. When discussing how this applies to brain behaviour, the authors say,

> [...] behaviour that appears to be caused by mental effort is actually caused by mental effort: the causal efficacy of mental effort is no illusion. Our wilful choices enter neither as redundant or epiphenomenal effects, but rather as fundamental dynamical elements that have the causal efficacy that the objective data appear to assign to them [Schwartz *et al*, 2005: p. 1325].

Recently, John Searle, an eminent philosopher of consciousness, has argued that mind is separate from brain, although arising from it; it is an emergent property, but nevertheless has it own 'mind' properties. This view allows that the mind may have an effect on brain function through the brain as an independent entity (Searle, 2007).

Spiritual medicine

Let us start with a definition of the spiritual dimensions of healing – a type of healing in which understandable and already verified scientific mechanisms are involved but in which transpersonal concepts are used. For example, in the Dean Ornish programme for heart disease, meditation, group discussions and diet are all combined to produce opening of the coronary arteries and changes in the blood flow (Dean Ornish Research Group; see Pischke *et al*, 2007). Miracles, prayer and distant healing, on the other hand, can be defined as healing for which no known or no accepted scientific mechanism can provide an explanation.

Scientific concepts behind the spiritual dimension of healing

In the past decade, a number of studies have shown the success of spiritual medicine. These studies come from a wide range of fields and deal with many aspects of religious and spiritual practice.

Koenig *et al* (2001) in their *Handbook of Religion and Health* look at the various factors relating to health and show the importance for a person's health of having religious or spiritual beliefs. They have shown that many different factors are involved in susceptibility to disease. A lot of these factors can be influenced by the behaviours that flow from an active religious faith, for example the limitation of self-damaging behaviours such as smoking, drugs and alcohol, the social support network involved in religious belief and attendance at church and church services. A strong faith, positive relationships and positive thinking up-regulate the immune system, reducing the risk of cancer, improving general health and protecting the cardiovascular system.

The field is now so large that it is not possible to review the whole area, but looking in detail at some studies relating to the functioning of the immune system and cardiovascular parameters give a flavour of progress made in this area.

The immune system

Changes in immune system function having been correlated with many factors, among which are social support, cognitive styles of behaviour and thought content. There is a dense network of communication from the higher centres of the brain, some situated in the structures of the frontal lobe, which carry information about the individual's social functioning and mood states and feed into the hypothalamus and thence through the pituitary gland to the immune system. This hypothalamic network centres round the secretion of cortisol, a stress hormone, and the cellular response via the cytokines. The important point is that high levels of cortisol are correlated with depression and anxiety.

With such a dense and widely linked network, it is no surprise to find that what we think, our emotional feelings and our relationships, all interact with the immune system. There have been many studies of the effects of mental and spiritual states on the immune system. A number of these have looked at the development of cancer and correlated its onset with psychosocial stress. Prigerson *et al* (1997) studied 150 individuals after their spouses had died. Those who showed high traumatic grief scores had an increased probability ($P=0.0001$) of developing a new cancer between the 6th and 15th month after their spouse's death. All individuals in the group that developed cancer had high traumatic grief scores. A 6-year follow-up study by Everson *et al* (1996) looked at 2400 middle-aged Finnish men, of whom 174 died, 87 from heart disease and 40 from cancer. The death rate of those with moderate to high levels of hopelessness as scored on a rating scale was two to three times higher than those with low levels of hopelessness. High levels of hopelessness predicted new cases of cancer and heart disease. The groups were matched for blood pressure, cholesterol, smoking, drinking, social class, education and prior depression and social isolation.

Uchino *et al* (1996) reviewed 81 studies, monitoring the effect of social support on the immune system and showed improved immune functioning with higher support. Cardiovascular systems were also improved and more stable and there was an overall reduction in cortisol levels. Interleukin 6 is a cytokine related to inflammation and is a measure of immune system functioning. It is not found in the serum until the age of 65, and then it is a measure of down-regulation of the immune system. High levels of interleukin 6 have been associated with cancer, myocardial infarction, hypertension, Alzheimer's disease, osteoporosis and rheumatoid arthritis. Koenig *et al* (1997) have shown the effect of church attendance on the immune system and on interleukin 6 – over 65-year-olds who went to church at least once a week had lower levels of interleukin 6. In a further study, Koenig *et al* (1999) looked at a sample of nearly 4000 65-year-old people over a 6-year period and was able to show that those who go to church at least once a week are more likely to be alive after 6 years.

As Koenig points out, sceptics of such studies often attribute the mortality effect of religious attendance to confounding by health status (i.e. sick people with impaired mobility are both less likely to attend church and more likely to die (Sloan *et al*, 1999). However, other studies have taken this into account in a very detailed way, and in the Strawbridge *et al*'s study (1997) a number of variables relating to health, social support, habits etc. were all taken into account, with the conclusion that women who attended religious services once a week or more showed a greater than one-third reduction in the likelihood of dying during the 28-year follow-up.

Kiecolt-Glaser *et al* (1993) studied the effects of negative and positive thinking on the immune system, looking at 90 newly-wed couples and rating a 30 min discussion between them. If hostile behaviour was displayed between the couples, there was a significant decrease in non-killer cell activity, a weaker blastogenic response to two mytogens, weaker proliferative response of monoclonal antibodies to the T3 receptor, a large increase in T lymphocytes and helper T lymphocytes, and higher antibody titres to latent Epstein Barr virus, all indicating a down-regulated immune system. There was also a prolonged increase in blood pressure in this group. This study shows the effect on immune system functioning and blood pressure of anger and stress in the marital relationship.

The power of compassion and positive thinking was shown by McClelland & Krishnit (1988). They studied a group of students, 70 of whom watched a film of Mother Teresa healing with compassion, while 62 others, the controls, viewed a film about the Axis powers in the Second World War.

The measure was salivary IgA, an immunoglobulin. The results of the study showed that there was a significant increase ($P=0.025$) in salivary IgA following watching of the film of Mother Teresa compared with the control group. The authors suggested this was due to an up-regulation of the immune system.The study has been used to point out that positive thinking and feelings of compassion can lead to positive bodily changes for the thinker.

The protective value of optimism was well demonstrated in a long-term study by Peterson and Bossio (over a period of 35 years) of 268 men who had taken part in the Harvard study of adult development and had been found to have good physical and psychological health and a high level of academic success. Peterson and Bossio asked the men to write about their war experiences, how successful they had been with their commanders and those serving under them and what their own opinion of themselves was. These essays were then rated so as to extract their score on a scale that ranged from extreme optimism to extreme pessimism. Correlations with the participants' health over the years showed that those who scored optimistically at the beginning of the study were healthier later in life than men who had more pessimistic ratings. This correlation became strongest at the age of 45, two decades after the optimism was assessed (Peterson & Bossio, 1991).

A second study by these authors looked at a group of undergraduates in 1993 (Peterson & Bossio, 1993). Questionnaires estimated their level of optimism and the number of day's illness they had had during the previous month. One year later it was found that the more optimistic students had fewer days of illness and fewer doctor visits than did the more pessimistic students. A study by Kamen-Siegel *et al* (1991) also showed that more optimistic individuals had higher helper:suppressor cell ratios, suggesting that their immune system was better able to combat disease.

In summary, these studies show the close correlation between religious and spiritual practice, as well as positive thinking, and positive changes in a number of stress-related hormonal systems. Social, religious and spiritual beliefs, when practised, can lead to an upgrading of the immune system. A positive rather than a negative attitude may contribute to a healthier life with the possibility of an extended lifespan.

Forgiveness

Forgiveness can be defined as ceasing to feel angry or resentful towards those who have hurt you. It entails an empathetic understanding of the other person, and the ability to judge whether you can forgive them or not. Some innovative work on a neuroscience of forgiveness has been done in Sheffield by a neuroimaging group under the direction of Sean Spence (Farrow *et al*, 2001) who found that there are brain areas which are specifically responsible for making an empathy judgement. The 'theory of mind' area in the left frontal cortex is used in 'mind judgement' – intuiting how other people are thinking – and an area in the middle temporal gyrus is activated when imagining a known person's response. An area deep in the centre of the brain known as the cingulate gyrus, thought to relate to higher social cognitive processing, is involved in making the 'forgivability' judgement – whether, for example, it is easier to forgive someone who steals a pint of milk from a supermarket than someone who steals it from one's doorstep.

It follows that if forgiveness is underpinned by neurological processes, then it should be possible to train people to forgive. Forgiveness therapy has, in fact, been used to great effect in the treatment of post-traumatic stress disorder, which has been shown to resolve more quickly in individuals who show forgiveness (Reed & Enright, 2006). Forgiveness involves a personal strengthening of identity, which leads to a change in mental content, so that the person thinks more positive thoughts and this in itself reduces stress and allows healing. A study by Kretzer et al (2007) used a Hawaiian conflict resolution technique to teach repentance, forgiveness and transmutation of self-image, to reduce blood pressure. After the patients started using this technique, their spirituality scores increased and there was a significant reduction in both systolic and diastolic blood pressure.

Meditation

Spiritual techniques for raising the level of consciousness and increasing attention and focus throughout the day have been practised by most religions. Long-term meditation has two aims. The first is to understand the finest components of mind, and this has been taken to extreme levels in Eastern religions. The second is to enter that part of the mind where experience of love for the Divine is experienced and to work in this area so that union with the Divine may be achieved. A spin-off from these practices is an improvement in health and a strong sense of psychological well-being. A recent study has shown interesting brain changes in long-term meditators, which confirm the effects of practised attention over a number of years. In a functional magnetic resonance imaging (fMRI) study of long-term meditators (Lazar et al, 2005), the authors assess cortical thickness, arguing that this should be changed in the areas used in meditation practice. They found that the brain regions associated with attention, interoception and sensory processing, together with the prefrontal cortex and right anterior insular, were thicker in the meditators than in the controls. These structures are used in attentional processes. But of more interest, the older participants had an increase in prefrontal cortical thickness compared with their matched groups, suggesting that meditation might offset age-related cortical thinning. The authors argued that this was the first time that experience-dependent cortical plasticity had been demonstrated to be associated with meditation practice.

A large number of studies have looked at meditation. Because many different types of meditation have been used in these studies, it is difficult to compare them, especially as most lack a comprehensive description of meditation practice. Some studies use highly experienced meditators who may have spent over 40 years in meditation practice, while others have used meditators with only 2 or 3 years' experience. The number of meditation studies is now so large that in this short review I will only look in detail at four of the more recent ones, selected because they use different sophisticated methods of analysis.

The main changes that occur in meditation are now well recognised. The process of meditation initiates the relaxation response with a decrease in blood cortisol levels and a decrease in pulse rate and blood pressure. There is also some reduction in the galvanic skin response. Concomitant changes in the electroencephalogram (EEG) have also been described, and some of these continue beyond the meditation sessions in individuals who have practised meditation over a number of years.

Newburg et al (2001) published a single-photon emission tomography (SPET) scan study in a group of eight meditators. The participants were doing a form of mantra meditation, but the exact practice is not described. The researchers compared the meditators with nine controls, whose scans were part of the control group in another project. Perfusion in the left frontal lobe was enhanced during the meditation sessions and the authors suggest that this related to a cognitive–attentional component. There was hypoperfusion of the superior parietal lobule, which they argued related to attentional processing and an altered sense of space. They also noted an increase in thalamic activity and pointed out that there was a thalamic asymmetry in the baseline of the meditators, which was different from the controls'. The authors argue that these baseline changes are due to a long-term effect of the meditational practice. They also suggest that the changes in the frontal and parietal cortices during the meditation session are closely related to the positive mental states that are described during meditation.

In a further study, Newburg et al (2003) looked at three Franciscan nuns who had a verbal-based meditation involving the internal repetition of a particular phrase, again using SPET. There was increased blood flow in the pre-frontal cortex (by 7%), inferior parietal lobes (7%) and inferior frontal lobes (9%). There was a strong inverse correlation between the blood flow change in the prefrontal cortex and the ipsilateral and superior parietal lobes. These findings are supportive of strong attentional effects and verbal effects mediated by the frontal lobes, with an alteration in body image produced by the reduction in superior parietal flow. There were only three participants and thus conclusions can only be provisional. It is clear that whatever correlates there are of altered mental states, it is impossible to get an understanding of the very wide changes that may occur in subjective experience.

A further paper looking at Carmelite nuns extended the idea of meditation into transcendent ecstatic states, when the nuns were subjectively in a state of union with God. Before the study, the nuns were asked to practise going into a transcendent state of union with God. They were later asked to reproduce this state in the fMRI scanner. The results suggest a widespread area of activation involving several brain regions and systems. The significant foci of activation were in the right medial orbito-frontal cortex, right middle temporal cortex, right inferior and superior parietal lobules, right caudate, left medial prefrontal cortex, left anterior cingulate cortex, left inferior parietal lobule, left insula, left caudate, and the left brainstem. The authors suggest that the caudate nucleus activation, which has been implicated in previous studies with happiness, romantic love and maternal love, is one of the main structures that is activated in the mystical condition and is related to feelings of joy and unconditional love (Beauregard & Paquette, 2006).

A number of studies have looked at EEG changes during meditation. The most frequently reported changes are an increase in frontal and temporal theta activity, an increase in central beta spindling and an increase in generalised coherence. (Coherence is the frequency correlation coefficient, and thus an increase in coherence suggests an increase in similarity in the frequency domain between different brain areas). All these changes correlate with a level of consciousness that lies between sleeping and waking. This suggests that the door to the wider states of consciousness experienced by the meditator is reached at this level of alertness.

The newer EEG studies, owing to the more sophisticated analysis, have added further information to the above picture. A study by Aftanas & Golocheikine (2001) has examined the EEG during sahaja yoga meditation. The authors measured the EEG during this practice in 11 short-term meditators with half a year's experience and 16 long-term meditators with 3 to 7 years' experience. They describe three phases: the incoming phase, the thoughtless phase when feelings of bliss arise and dominate and which is the deepest stage of meditation (this may last for about an hour), and finally the outcome phase. The authors were particularly interested in the correlation of the electrical activity with feelings of bliss and the difference between long-term and short-term meditators. They found that before meditation, the long-term meditators showed an increase in generalised theta activity. During the meditation session, the long-term meditators showed a high coherence (i.e. frequency correlation) of the left frontal lobe with many other different brain areas. This was not seen in the short-term meditation group. They also noticed a positive correlation between frontal theta power and feelings of bliss and a negative correlation between the appearance of thoughts and frontal theta activity. This study again confirms the EEG changes in long-term meditators and suggests that both the reduction in thoughts and an increase in feelings of bliss are related to frontal theta activity, with the left frontal lobe being very important for the higher and wider subjective mental states. This is a very comprehensive study and shows the way forward for future electrophysiological analysis.

Finally, I would like to mention an interesting positron emission tomography (PET) scan study (Kjaer *et al*, 2002), which to my knowledge is the first study to examine dopamine levels during meditation using the radioactive dopamine ligand C-Ralopride. The meditation practice in this study, yoga nidra, is characterised by a reduced level of desire for action and involves giving up personal goals and loss of executive control while attending to internal sensations and withdrawing from action. The study found that there was an increase in dopamine levels during the meditation sessions, particularly prominent in the ventral striatum, a nuclear complex deep in the brain. The subjective accounts correlated with a decrease in readiness for action and an increase in visual imagery. It was also noted that there was an increase in EEG power in the theta band which correlated with the increase in dopamine. The paper confirms the widespread effects of meditation and suggests that subcortical structures such as the thalamus are significantly involved. This change in dopamine levels in those structures which are related to movement is of particular interest, as there are many subjective reports of an alteration/improvement in movement after meditation (Kjaer *et al*, 2002).

To summarise, the more recent imaging studies show a further indication of the specific brain areas and electrical changes which are involved in meditation. The attention mechanisms of the dorso-lateral prefrontal cortex are prominent, as are parietal lobe changes which relate to the body image in space. Feelings of bliss and emotional changes certainly correlate with frontal theta activity, some of which will be arising from the anterior cingulate gyrus. Frontal theta also links in with specific attentional frontal lobe mechanisms. The idea of a network of areas being involved in meditation has been summarised by Lou *et al* (2005). The studies relating to changes in dopamine are interesting as dopamine is also involved in the reward system (i.e. generates positive feelings). It would be interesting to speculate that some of the dopamine changes may be related to the positive affect that flows from meditation sessions. Finally, the relationship of changes in dopamine levels to motor activity is also important, as there are anecdotal accounts of positive changes in movement in long-term meditators.

Meditation in clinical practice

A recent paper shows the effect on the brain's response to pain in individuals practising transcendental meditation, a mantra method of meditation. Functional MRI outside the meditation period in response to thermally induced pain showed that 40–50% fewer boxels (small analysis areas in the pain centres) were responding to pain in the thalamus and other brain areas than in healthy matched controls. These controls then learnt meditation and practised it for 5 months. When again challenged with the thermal pain stimulus their responses had decreased by 40–50% in the thalamus, prefrontal cortex and, marginally, in the anterior cingulate cortex. What is of interest about this study is that there was no change in the pain intensity for the meditators, but there were major reductions in the effective response to the pain, with a significant reduction in distress (Orme-Johnson et al, 2006).

Meditation has also been found to be generally helpful in those clinical conditions where high arousal and anxiety are part of the pathology. A study by Sudsuang et al (1991) looked at dhammakaya Buddhist meditation. The authors found that consistent meditation was related to a decrease in blood pressure, pulse rate and serum cortisol; these effects were not maintained if the meditation was intermittent. Kabat-Zinn et al (1992) used mindfulness meditation to treat general anxiety or panic disorders in his Massachusetts clinic. He gave an 8-week programme of weekly 2-hour sessions. These comprised a 2-hour structured class on relaxation and stress reduction each week and in the 6th week a 7.5-hour silent meditation retreat. Overall, 20 of the 22 people involved in the study significantly improved at the end of the course, and 18 of the 22 remained so at a 3-year follow-up. This study shows the significant results that may be obtained by linking meditation to group therapy. This programme has been found to be so effective as a way of reducing anxiety that it is now being funded by insurance companies in Massachusetts.

A study by Majundar showed that the technique used by Kabat-Zinn can be successfully transferred to other cultures, and the mindfulness meditation study has been replicated in Germany (Majundar et al, 2002). Mindfulness meditation has also been taken up as a treatment for a number of conditions, such as attention-deficit hyperactivity disorder (Zylowska et al, 2008), intellectual disability (Singh et al, 2007) and rheumatoid arthritis (Pradhane et al, 2007), among others.

A single-blind trial of transcendental meditation in 111 African Americans aged between 55 and 85 years looked at changes in blood pressure, the index group having a mean blood pressure of 179/104 (Schneider et al, 1995). These meditators were paired with a group that was given progressive muscular relaxation and a group who had lifestyle education. After 3 months, those practising transcendental meditation showed a significant reduction in both systolic and diastolic pressure. However, although this method was effective, the mean changes were only 10 mm Hg for systolic and just over 6 mm Hg for the diastolic pressure, which still leaves the participants in the high-risk category. Clearly, further longer-term studies are still required. Transcendental meditation has been practised by some individuals since the time of The Beatles in the 1960s and it should be possible to look at ultra long-term studies of a group of meditators to see whether meditating over a number of years really does increase long-term physical and mental health and life expectancy.

Meditation techniques are associated with a number of unusual phenomena which are reported anecdotally in the esoteric literature but for which there is no scientific explanation. St Teresa of Avila, for example, was said to have been irritated during her meditation sessions by her continual levitation to the roof. St Francis of Assisi was said to have been surrounded by light during his meditation practice. Other accounts suggest that there is some form of mental communication between disciples and masters during meditation. This concept of the linking of meditating minds has not yet been fully tested by science and would be rejected by most scientific grants committees. There are, however, straws in the wind that point in this direction. In an old study, Orme-Johnson *et al* (1982) measured EEG coherence between three meditating individuals on the same site but in different rooms both before and during the time when 2500 students were meditating in a meditation programme over 1000 miles away. After the meditation course was over the experiment was repeated as a control. On the experimental days, EEG coherence between the three individual meditators increased during the experimental period, compared with the 15 min baseline before the distant students started meditating. There was a significant difference on the experimental days compared with the control days. These changes were seen mainly in the alpha and beta frequencies. This was the first good study to be published in a respectable journal that showed the effect of remote meditation on measured individuals carrying out the same form of meditation.

An intriguing new series of experiments have been carried out by Edge *et al* (2003). In this study, the meditating person pressed a button every time their mind came off the meditation process. In a remote room a second person was attempting to help them meditate for a period followed by another period when they were relaxing. The helping and relaxation periods were intermixed and randomised. The experiment showed highly significant results, again suggesting that consciousness is a field and that meditating individuals enhance the field effect.

A more recent study by Wackermann *et al* (2003) has taken this idea of mental linking during emotional connectedness a step further. They allowed the pair of active participants to spend 20 minutes or so together, enhancing their feelings of connectedness, and then put each one into a separate, isolated room. In one room the person received flashes of light, and in the other room the brainwaves of the second person were analysed; it was found that there was a response to the flashes shown to the first person. This experiment suggests a bonding between the two individuals, demonstrated by changes in brainwave activity that can be picked up. Acceptance of these experiments by the scientific community would have a very high cost for science.

In summary, the findings for both the magnetic resonance imaging and the clinical studies show that attentional techniques can alter cortical function, which underpins the many physiological effects that have been found. These changes lead to an enhancement of quality of life and raise the question of whether it may be time for these methods to be valued more in our society and taught and made available on a wider basis.

Spiritual healing

There are numerous studies on the therapeutic effects of spiritual healing. These range from prayer studies of sick people, through miraculous healings, to 'intention to heal' of animals, plants and DNA. Benor reviews this area in his book *Spiritual Healing: Scientific Validation of a Healing Revolution* (2002), where he cites more than 500 such studies. Out of the 191 controlled studies of healing, 124 demonstrate significant effects and of 37 of the most rigorous of these studies, 25 show highly significant effects (Benor, 2002).

A second review book by Benor, *Consciousness, Bioenergy and Healing* (2004), looks at a number of studies in the area of complementary and alternative medical practices and extends this into energy medicine, with assessment of cranio-sacral therapies and other forms of bioenergy therapy. Many of these studies are in the early stages of scientific investigation and validation and so Benor concludes that further scientific work still needs to be done.

A number of interesting recent studies have continued the examination of spiritual healing. Vuckovic and colleagues (2007) looked at shamanic treatment of temporo-mandibular joint disorders. They chose this group of disorders because they are recurrent, chronic, long-standing and non-progressive. They comment that some of these patients are least likely to respond to allopathic treatment if they show 'marked biological responsiveness to external stressors and concomitant emotional and psychosocial difficulties'. They considered that this group was a suitable one for shamanic healing, which they describe as an ancient form of spiritual healing. In their study, 23 women who had temporo-mandibular dysfunction were given five treatments on different visits and were asked to rate their pain on different scales. The study demonstrated a significant reduction in pain with functional improvement. The treatment was so successful that only four women were left with a clinical diagnosis of temporo-mandibular dysfunction at the end of the treatment sessions.

The value and healing power of stories has recently come into prominence. This was highlighted by an article in the *New England Journal of Medicine* by Charon (2004). She described the importance in medicine of the stories patients tell about themselves and their illnesses. This has led to a number of papers in this area and its application to shamanic healing. When patients consult either Western or shamanic healers, they come with a story of their pain and the story of how this fits into their life situation. A recent paper by Watson (2007) looks at this question of stories the patients give and the role of the shaman or the doctor in changing the story and thus stimulating healing. His point is an important one, as it shows the power of storytelling and its value in shamanic practices.

Prayer

Prayer is a widespread practice in the USA. In 2005 a national poll conducted by *Newsweek* found that 64% of Americans prayed every day and a further 10% did so several times a week (http://www.beliefnet.com/News/2005/08/Newsweekbeliefnet-Poll-Results.aspx). One of the early indications of the change in scientific thinking and the recognition that spiritual values could be tested by science was the publication of a paper on prayer by Byrd (1988). Since then, there have been a number of high-quality double-blind randomised controlled trials of intercessory prayer. Not all of these have been positive, but many have produced some supportive evidence that prayer may be effective in healing.

In this scientific era, how are we to conceptualise prayer? Prayer in most theistic traditions is a *novus actus interveniens*, which implies that God interacts directly with his creation and changes physical and mental phenomena. This view of prayer raises many problems for scientists who wish to study whether or not prayer is effective and to find, if possible, a reductionist mechanism. The Cochrane Committee, who keep a database on all medical subjects of reviews of double-blind randomised controlled trials that have been properly carried out, note that proper double-blind prayer trials may be difficult to do if God is involved in the process of prayer, as 'God may not wish to comply with the conditions' of such a trial. They also note that there is a significant background of prayer, as many churches regularly pray for the healing of the sick. Their first conclusion, after reviewing a very small sample of prayer studies (three), was that there was no evidence for the efficacy of prayer, although there was also no evidence against it (Roberts *et al*, 2007).

The first good double-blind randomised controlled trial of prayer is that of Byrd (1988), carried out in a coronary care unit. The names of the active group were sent to a prayer group who were instructed to pray that those named would get better quicker, have fewer complications, etc. The results were promising; in the prayed for group there was a five-fold reduction in the use of antibiotics, a three-fold reduction in the occurrence of pulmonary oedema, fewer individuals required intubation and fewer (though not significantly fewer) died than in the control group. This paper became the model for a number of further studies.

Harris *et al* (1999) looked at 999 consecutive patients attending a coronary care unit. They were randomised to a group who were to be prayed for and a control group. There were no differences in coronary care and length of hospital admission, but when a coronary care unit score, comprising many different variables, was analysed, those in the prayer group had a significantly lower value than those who were not prayed for.

Roberts and colleagues from Westcott House (a Church of England theological college) reviewed (2007) the outcome of prayer studies to that date. They pointed out that there was little difference in death rates and also little change in heart problems with bad or intermediate outcome. However, odds were increased against being readmitted to a coronary care unit for those prayed for. The authors concluded that it was too early to support a definite effect of prayer.

Aviles *et al* (2001) looked at 799 coronary care patients and found that prayer had no significant effect on medical outcome. Abbot (Research Council of Complementary Medicine, 2000) reviewed the scientific studies of prayer. He examined 22 full trials, of which 10 reported significant effects of healing. However, the methods varied. He noted that two well-conducted, large-scale trials using the same method replicated positive effects, but overall the trials were too varied to draw a far-reaching conclusion. He concluded that there was sufficient positive evidence to continue research, but insufficient evidence to accept that prayer was effective in healing. Astin *et al* (2000) from the University of Maryland reviewed 23 trials, noted that they were too heterogeneous for meta-analysis and came to the same conclusion.

A recent large-scale study, which it was hoped would provide definitive evidence on the efficacy of prayer, came from Herbert Benson's analysis of the effects of prayer on 1500 cardiac bypass patients in a multicentre trial. However, although the study had a complex design and gave standardised scripts to those praying, it failed to show any significant effect of prayer. Indeed, it was slightly negative, as those people who knew they were certain to receive intercessory prayer had a higher incidence of complications. This study caused considerable discussion in the scientific community, with a number of people suggesting that its design was likely to produce a negative rather than a positive effect (Benson *et al*, 2006). A study on patients recovering from alcoholism (Walker *et al* 1997) found both positive and negative results. Negative results were found if family members were asked to pray for the recovery, suggesting that the motivation for the family, which may not always be positive, is important to take into account in prayer studies. Clearly, we are going to have to define much more accurately what prayer is and the mental state of those praying.

The whole area of prayer is exciting and contains studies that show both its positive and negative effects. The work on prayer for the next decade is to formalise and quantify methods of prayer. The evidence so far is that intention to heal and the way this intention is used (either as directed prayer, or non-directed heart-centred prayer) is most likely to be the important variable and this will then need to be tested in further research. As current studies have predominantly come from the USA, it would be interesting to see whether European and Asian studies show a similar or different profile.

Testing prayer mechanisms

A good start on the investigation of mechanism underlying the spiritual healing power of prayer has been made by the US Spindrift organisation, which has used prayer in a biological setting to protect either growing yeast or growing seeds against the stress of being retarded by salt solutions. It can be argued that the important variable is the mental state of the person praying rather than the nature of the prayee, and this is equivalent to healing intent. This is a mechanical view of prayer but it certainly helps in trying to distinguish the variables that may be important in prayer studies. There is also the point that *in vitro* experiments are easier to quantify as the healing intent is directed towards physiological changes, whereas in an *in vivo* experiment the person praying may ask for non-specific changes – for example, that the person prayed for 'will have God's peace' or something similar – and this may be difficult to quantify.

In a large number of experiments it has been shown that the plants that were given a healing intent grew more than the controls and that the mechanism of action may be the focused healing intent (The Spindrift Papers, 1993; Sweet, 2003). There will need to be many more such studies before this comes to be accepted by the mainstream scientific community but at least a start has been made.

The limited evidence available suggests that the attitude of the person praying is all important and that prayer for the general well-being of the prayee is more effective than directed prayer. Further, the generally accepted feeling among those who do prayer studies is that there is no evidence that any particular religion or faith makes any difference to the outcome. What is clear is that there are sufficient studies now to suggest that prayer may work, together with mental intent and methods of hands-on healing such as therapeutic touch.

Miracles

The Christian tradition has a long history of healing by miracles, usually associated with special people or special places, such as Lourdes (West, 1957; Dowling, 1984). A miracle is best defined as an act of healing attributed to the intervention of God without a clear physical mechanism to bring the change about. The miracles of St Thomas of Hereford (1218–1282) are such an example (Ross & Jancey, 1987). One miracle attributed to him recounts how a man with a long-term dysphasia and dysphagia who was congenitally without a tongue, slept at the shrine of St Thomas. During the night, St Thomas came to him in a dream, pulling out his tongue. The next morning he had grown a lovely new tongue! Our current era, led as it is by rational science, has been sceptical of such happenings; despite a body of mostly anecdotal evidence to support miraculous healing, miracles are not recognised in mainstream scientific circles.

Gardner (1983) tried to put miracles into a more modern setting. He chose the miracles of St Cuthbert, discussing whether, if St Cuthbert was alive today, he would see the sort of miracles that were commonly seen in his lifetime. A number of modern miracles involving prayer that he had seen in his own medical practice were described. He relates the case of a man in Africa who fell off a church roof and suffered a potentially fatal rupture to his spleen. The group gathered round the dying man to pray for his recovery. With the prayer came a change in the patient's condition and he recovered. Why, asked Gardner, were miracles of this type not more common in our own culture? He quotes the following story:

> When modern missionaries left some Gospel books behind in Ethiopia and returned many years later, they not only found a flourishing Church but a community of believers among whom miracles like those mentioned in the New Testament happened every day – because there had been no missionaries to teach that such things were not to be taken literally [Gardner, 1983: pp. 1927–1933].

This story raises the interesting question of whether we have all been so conditioned by 'scientific missionaries' that we either no longer allow miracles to occur or are blind to those that do.

The need for a wider scientific paradigm

There is, rightly, always resistance to new scientific data that seem to go beyond our current materialistic paradigm. However, physics has shown through quantum mechanics that every particle is linked to every other in the universe and that we no longer live in the clockwork universe of discrete particles suggested by Newton and Galileo. The biological sciences are now carrying out studies whose results also seem to point in this direction. There is the beginning of evidence that mind may be non-local to the brain. There is also some evidence that what the experimenter thinks and expects to find is revealed in the study outcome, suggesting that the experimenter is very much part of the experimental system. It is right that these studies should not be accepted until the evidence is overwhelming, because if they are confirmed, they would indicate a degree of connectivity between individuals and nature which is at the moment unthinkable. Unfortunately, it is difficult to find funding for the types of studies required to continue validating the phenomena that have been described in this chapter. However, the scientific climate is slowly changing and it is to be hoped that funding will become more readily available.

Conclusion

Current work in the field of neuroscience shows very clearly that practising spiritual methods changes brain function. There is also a clear relationship between practising these methods and an improvement in mental and physical health.

Our beliefs, relationships and the way we think all have an influence on our health and should all be taken into account by any treating physician. This chapter shows the close correlation between religious and spiritual practice and positive changes in a number of stress-related hormonal systems. The conclusion for patients is to remember that it is extremely important what we think, as this directly affects our physical health and the physical health of those around us. So far as the doctor is concerned, it is very important to find out what the patient believes, and that he or she understands the protective value of faith, of a committed belief and social structure such as that given by a church group or a positive thinking and supportive social group. Social, religious and spiritual beliefs, when practised, can lead to an upgrading of the immune system, with positive changes in brain function and a positive attitude, all of which may contribute to a healthier life and the possibility of an extended lifespan.

There is also some evidence that our intentions to heal can be effective at a distance, as can our mental state, which may, in a way not yet understood, directly affect the brains/minds of those around us. The non-local effects of mind have been shown in many studies, and it looks as though we may now have to accept that mind may not be limited to the brain. At the moment we cannot offer a scientific explanation for this but, as St Augustine remarked, 'miracles do not happen in contradiction to nature, but only in contradiction to that which is known to us in Nature'.

References

Abbot, N. C. (2000) Healing as a therapy for human disease: a systematic review. *Journal of Alternative Complementary Medicine*, **6**, 159–169.

Aftanas, L. I. & Golocheikine, S. A. (2001) Human anterior and frontal midline theta and lower alpha reflect emotionally positive state and internalised attention: high resolution EEG investigation of meditation. *Neuroscience Letters*, **310**, 57–60.

Astin, J. A., Harkness, E. & Ernst, E. (2000) The efficacy of distant healing: a systematic review of randomized trials. *Annals of Internal Medicine*, **132**, 903–910.

Austin, J. (2000) *Zen and the Brain*. MIT Press.

Austin, J. (2006) *Zen-Brain Reflections*. MIT Press.

Aviles, J. M., Whelan, S. E., Hernke, D. A., *et al* (2001) Intercessory prayer and cardiovascular disease progression in a coronary care unit population: a randomized controlled trial. *Mayo Clinic Proceedings*, **76**, 1192–1198.

Beauregard, M. & Paquette, V. (2006) Neural correlates of mystical experience in Carmelite nuns. *Neuroscience Letters*, **405**, 186–190.

Benor, J. (2002) *Spiritual Healing: Scientific Validation of a Healing Revolution* (eds J. Benor & L. Dossey). Vision Publications.

Benor, J. (2004) *Consciousness, Bioenergy and Healing*. Holistic Healing Publications.

Benson, H., Dusek, J., Sherwood, J., *et al* (2006) Study of the therapeutic effects of intercessory prayer (STEP) in cardiac by-pass patients: a multi-centre randomised trial of uncertainty and certainty of receiving intercessory prayer. *American Heart Journal*, **152**, e25.

Byrd, R. C. (1988) Positive therapeutic effects of intercessory prayer in a coronary care unit population. *Southern Medical Journal*, **81**, 826–829.

Charon, R. (2004) Narrative and Medicine. *New England Journal of Medicine*, **350**, 862–864.

Dennet, D. (1991) *Consciousness Explained*. John Little.

Dowling, St J. (1984) Lourdes cures and their medical assessment. *Journal of the Royal Society of Medicine*, **77**, 634–668.

Edge, H., Suryani, L. K., Tiliopoulos, N., *et al* (2003) A DMILS study in a non-EuroAmerican culture. In *Proceedings of Presented Papers: The Parapsychological Association 46th Annual Convention*, pp. 49–67. Parapsychologial Association.

Everson, S., Goldber, D. E. & Kaplan, G. A. (1996) Hopelessness and risk of mortality and incidence of myocardial infarction and cancer. *Psychosomatic Medicine*, **58**, 113–121.

Farrow, T., Ying Z., Wilkinson, I. D., *et al* (2001) Investigation of the functional anatomy of empathy and forgiveness. *NeuroReport*, **12**, 2433–2438.

Gardner, R. (1983) Miracles of healing in Anglo-Celtic Northumbria as recorded by the Venerable Bede and his contemporaries: a reappraisal in the light of 20th century experience. *BMJ*, **287**, 1927–1933.

Harris, W. S., Gowda, M., Kolb, J., *et al* (1999) A randomised, controlled trial of the effects of remote, intercessory prayer on outcomes in patients admitted to the coronary care unit. *Archives of Internal Medicine*, **159**, 2273–2278.

Kabat-Zinn, J., Massion, A., Kristeller, J., *et al* (1992) Effectiveness of a meditation based stress reduction program in the treatment of anxiety disorders. *American Journal of Psychiatry*, **149**, 936–943.

Kamen-Siegel, L., Radin, J., Seligman, M. E., *et al* (1991) Explanatory style and cell mediated immunity in elderly men and women. *Health Psychology*, **10**, 229–235.

Kiecolt-Glaser, J. K., Malarkey, W. B., Chee, M., *et al* (1993) Negative behaviour during marital conflict is associated with immunological down-regulation. *Psychosomatic Medicine*, **55**, 395–409.

Kjaer, T. W., Bertelsen, C., Piccini, P., *et al* (2002) Increased dopamine tone during meditation-induced changes in consciousness. *Brain Research: Cognitive Brain Research*, **13**, 255–259.

Koenig, H. G., Cohen, J. J., George, L. K., *et al* (1997) Attendance at religious services, interleukin-6 and other biological indicators of immune function in older adults. *International Journal of Psychiatry in Medicine*, **27**, 233–250.

Koenig, H. G., Hays, J. C., George, L. K., *et al* (1999) Does religious attendance prolong survival? A six year follow-up study of 3968 older adults. *Journal of Gerontology: Medical Sciences*, **54A**, M370–377.

Koenig, H. G., McCullough, M. E. & Larson, D. B. (eds) (2001) *Handbook of Religion and Health*. Oxford University Press.

Kretzer, K., Davis, J., Easa, D., *et al* (2007) Self-identity through ho'oponopono as adjunctive therapy for hypertension management. *Ethnicity and Disease*, **17**, 624–628.

Lazar, S., Kerr, C., Wasserman, R., *et al* (2005) Meditation experience is associated with increased cortical thickness. *NeuroReport*, **16**, 1893–1897.

Levin, J. S., Larson, D. B. & Puchalski, C. M. (1997) Religion and spirituality in medicine: research and education. *Journal of the American Medical Association*, **178**, 792–793.

Lou, H. C., Nowak, M. & Kjaer, T. W. (2005) The mental self. *Progress in Brain Research*, **150**, 197–204.

Majundar, M., Grossman, P., Dietz-Waschkowski, B., *et al* (2002) Does mindfulness meditation contribute to health? Outcome and evaluation. *Journal of Alternative and Complementary Medicine*, **8**, 719–730.

McClelland, D. C. & Krishnit, C. (1988) The effect of motivational arousal through films on salivary immunoglobulin. *Psychology and Health*, **2**, 31–52.

Morton, P. A. (1997) *A Historical Introduction to the Philosophy of Mind: Readings with Commentary, p. 58.* Broadview Press.

Nagel, T. (1974) 'What is it like to be a bat?' *Philosophical Review*, **83**, 435–450.

Newburg, A., Alavi, A., Baime, M., *et al* (2001) The measurement of regional cerebral blood flow during the complex cognitive task of mediation: a preliminary SPECT study. *Psychiatry Research: Neuroimaging*, **106**, 113–122.

187

Newburg, A., Pourdehnad, M., Alavi, A., *et al* (2003) Cerebral blood flow during meditative prayer: preliminary findings and methodological issues. *Perceptual and Motor Skills*, **97**, 625–630.

Orme-Johnson, D., Dillbeck, M. C., Wallace, R. K., *et al* (1982) Intersubject EEG coherence. Is consciousness a field? *International Journal of Neuroscience*, **16**, 203–209.

Orme-Johnson, D., Schneider, R., Young, D., *et al* (2006) Neuroimaging of meditation's effect on brain reaction to pain. *Cognitive Neuroscience and Neuropsychology*, **17**, 1359–1363.

Peterson, C. & Bossio, L. M. (1991) *Health and Optimism*. Free Press.

Peterson, C. & Bossio, L. M. (1993) Health attitudes: optimism, hope and control. In *Mind/Body Medicine: How to Use Your Mind for Better Health* (eds D. Goleman & J. Gurin), pp. 351–366. Consumer Reports Books.

Pischke, C. R., Weidner, G., Elliott-Eller, M., *et al* (2007) Lifestyle changes and clinical profile in coronary heart disease patients with an ejection fraction of ≤40% or >40% in the Multicenter Lifestyle Demonstration Project. *European Journal of Heart Failure*, **9**, 928–934.

Pradhane, E., Baumgarten, M., Langenberg, P., *et al* (2007) Effect of mindfulness-based stress reduction in rheumatoid arthritis patients. *Arthritis and Rheumatism*, **57**, 1134–1142.

Prigerson, H. G., Bierhals, A. J., Kasl, S. V., *et al* (1997) Traumatic grief as a risk factor for mental and physical morbidity. *American Journal of Psychiatry*, **154**, 616–623.

Reed, G. L. & Enright, R. D. (2006) The effects of forgiveness therapy on depression, anxiety and post traumatic stress for women after spousal emotional abuse. *Journal of Consulting and Clinical Psychology*, **74**, 920–929.

Roberts, L., Ahmed, I. & Hall, S. (2007) Intercessory prayer for the alleviation of ill health. *Cochrane Database of Systematic Reviews*, **Issue 1**, CD000368, doi: 10.1002/14651858. CD000368.pub2.

Ross, J. H. & Jancey, M. (1987) The Miracles of St Thomas of Hereford. *BMJ*, **295**, 1590–1594.

Schneider, R. H., Staggers, F., Alexander, C., *et al* (1995) A randomised controlled trial of stress reduction for hypertension in older African Americans. *Journal of Hypertension*, **26**, 820–829.

Searle, J. R. (2007) Dualism revisited. *Journal of Physiology (Paris)*, **101**, 169–178.

Sherrington, C. S. (1940) *Man on his Nature*. Cambridge University Press.

Schwartz, J. M., Stapp, H. P. & Beauregard, M. (2005) Quantum physics in neuroscience and psychology: a neurophysical model of mind–brain interaction. *Philosophical Transactions of the Royal Society B*, **360**, 1309–1327.

Singh, N., Lancioni, G., Winton, A., *et al* (2007) Mindfulness training assists individuals with moderate mental retardation to maintain their community placements. *Behaviour Modification*, **31**, 800–814.

Sloan, R. P., Baglella, E. & Powell, T. (1999) Religions, spirituality and medicine. *Lancet*, **353**, 664–667.

The Spindrift Papers (1993) *Exploring Prayer and Healing Through the Experimental Test*. Spindrift.

Strawbridge, W. J., Cohen, R. D., Shema, S. J., *et al* (1997) Frequent attendance at religious services and mortality over 28 years. *American Journal of Public Health*, **87**, 957–961.

Sudsuang, R., Chentanez, V. & Veluvan K. (1991) Effect of Buddhist meditation on serum cortisol and total protein levels, blood pressure, pulse rate, lung volume and reaction time. *Physiology and Behaviour*, **50**, 543–548.

Sweet, B. (2003) *A Journey into Prayer*. Xlibris.

Uchino, B. N., Cacioppo, J. R. & Kiecolt-Glaser, J. K. (1996) The relationship between social support and physiological processes: a review with emphasis on underlying mechanisms and implications for health. *Psychological Bulletin*, **119**, 488–531.

Velmans, M. (2000) *Investigating Phenomenal Consciousness: New Methodologies and Maps*. John Benjamins.

Vuckovic, N. H., Gullion, C. M., Williams, L. A., *et al* (2007) Feasibility and short-term outcomes of a Shamanic treatment for tempero-mandibular joint disorders. *Alternative Therapies in Health and Medicine*, **13**, 18–29.

Wackermann, J., Seiter, C., Keibel, H., *et al* (2003) Correlations between brain electrical activities of two spatially separated human subjects. *Neuroscience Letters*, **336**, 63–64.

Walker, S. R., Tonigan, J. S., Miller, R. W., *et al* (1997) Intercessory prayer in the treatment of alcohol abuse independence: a pilot investigation. *Alternative Therapies in Health and Medicine*, **3**, 79–86.

Watson, S. (2007) An extraordinary moment: the healing power of stories. *Canadian Family Physician*, **53**, 1283–1287.

West, D. J. (1957) *Eleven Lourdes Miracles*. Helix.

Zylowska, L., Ackerman, D., Yang, M., *et al* (2008) Mindfulness meditation training in adults and adolescents with ADHD: a feasibility study. *Journal of Attention Disorders*, **11**, 737–746.

CHAPTER 10

Spiritual care in the NHS

Sarah Eagger, Peter Richmond and Peter Gilbert

Meeting the varied spiritual needs of patients, staff and visitors is fundamental to the care the NHS provides [Department of Health, 2003a: p. 5]

Spirituality has been a part of the professional code of practice for physicians and other healthcare professionals in the UK since the inception of the National Health Service (NHS) in 1947. At that time, legislation was passed to ensure that the religious and faith needs of patients were met in the healthcare system (Speck, 2005). This was reinforced by *The Patient's Charter* (Department of Health, 1991) and in a subsequent health service guidance letter, *The Provision of Spiritual Care to Staff, Patients and Relatives* (Department of Health, 1992). This guidance was replaced in 2003 to reflect new organisational relationships and to provide better support for the multi-faith needs of patients (Department of Health, 2003a).

One could, however, be forgiven for not having a clear picture of how spiritual care is provided within today's NHS. The issues around delivering such care are indeed complex. Orchard (2001: p. 17) notes that 'the NHS is an organism that demands of its services an ability to think through its considerable complexities and to respect its need for a degree of discipline in the way care is developed and delivered'. However, this does not appear to be the case with services for spiritual care and Orchard calls for those services to be 'effective, equitable and better able to respond to those who call on them'. There is a lack of published material on the provision of formal spiritual care services within the health sector. It certainly appears to be a hotchpotch of policies and influences. It would seem that in the reforms that saw mental health trusts splitting off from acute and community trusts, many pastoral care departments were left behind. With no specific service level agreements or funding streams, this area of care was, and still is, often ignored.

What is spiritual care?

It is not only chaplains who provide spiritual care to patients. In chapter 2, 'Assessing spiritual needs', the authors call for collaboration between professionals in this area of patient care. The notion of what spiritual care actually entails requires consideration. Murray *et al* (2004), in a study of patients with life-threatening illnesses, defined spiritual needs as 'the needs and expectations which humans have to find meaning, purpose and value in their life. Such needs can be specifically religious but even people who have no religious faith or are not members of an organised religion have belief systems that give their lives meaning and purpose' (pp. 40–41). They went on to state that 'spiritual care is about helping people whose sense of meaning and worth is challenged by illness'. Cobb & Robshaw (1998) further elaborate that spiritual care is a response to the spiritual needs of a person, understood through exploring life events, beliefs, values and meaning. It is a means of therapeutic support to enable a person challenged by illness, trauma or bereavement to find meaning in their experiences of vulnerability, loss or dislocation. This is certainly relevant to psychiatry and describes what most members of the multidisciplinary team would see as their day-to-day work.

Bloch & Green (2006) resonate with these ideas in their formulation of a modern ethical framework for psychiatry. They describe ethics of care as a contemporary variant of virtue theory that also draws on feminism and psychological constructs, particularly the role of emotion in moral deliberation. Decision-making is thus grounded in the core values of humankind's capacity to extend care to people who are vulnerable or in need.

Setting the context: society, beliefs and values

The delivery of mental health services occurs within the context of societies, their values and imperatives. As Layard (2005) points out, during the 20th century there has been a decline of religious belief in the Western world (see also Davie, 2002), a decline of confidence in secular systems such as socialism, and an increased suspicion of science. Paradoxically, there has been an increase in aspects and intuitions of spirituality (Hay, 2006). We are now in an era of what some call late modernity, others post-modernity, and what Zygmunt Bauman calls, in a luminous phrase, 'liquid modernity' (Bauman, 2000).

If individual consumerism and rampant individualism are the twin pillars of the dominant world ethos, then those who consume less – the poor and dispossessed, people with severe and enduring mental health problems, those with intellectual disabilities and older people with dementia, among others – have less value as citizens (Layard, 2005). There is also an impression of the loss of soul or spirit (Gilbert, in Coyte *et al*, 2007), which seems to be afflicting human beings struggling with a sense of disconnection from familiar landmarks. One aspect of all of this is a lessening of the sense of community. Chief Rabbi Jonathan Sacks sums up what community, including faith communities, may mean:

> A community is where they know your name and where they miss you when you are not there. Community is society with a human face [Sacks, 2005: p. 54].

191

The 20th-century spiritual care in mental health hospital services was modelled on a community model that itself was a copy of the parish system of the Church of England (Folland, 2006). The hospital chaplain would be ordained in the Church of England and was vicar to his parish that was the hospital. That his parishioners belonged to many faiths and none was not an unusual situation for a clerk in holy orders in the established church. Provision for Roman Catholics usually meant that a priest would visit to conduct weekly mass. Non-conformism, nominalism and mild antipathy to religion were, and still are, common fare to the English parson. Psychiatric hospitals were often villages in themselves, and religious life was self-contained. Staff would generally prefer their children to be baptised in the hospital chapel as it represented their community of belonging, and they were often resident in the vicinity.

As asylums closed, this model of spiritual care faltered. In Somerset, for example, no provision was made for chaplaincy with the redesign of services that accompanied the closure of the two large rural sites. The Somerset Spirituality Project (Mental Health Foundation, 2002) was a direct result of Church of England-led pressure to enquire of the new mental health trust what it intended to do with regard to its responsibilities in meeting the spiritual needs of patients and carers.

From the 1960s onwards, publications began appearing in North American and Australasian circles by professionals who found their education and training did not fit them to engage with service users and carers in this vital area that exercised them. The issue became prevalent much later in Britain and began to be taken forward by psychiatrists and nurses as a response not only to expressed user needs but also because the professionals themselves were increasingly multicultural and multi-faith. Ironically, social work, with its roots in religious philanthropy, remained more distant from this issue until recently (Moss, 2005), perhaps as a 1970s reaction against the institutional nature of the Church.

Drivers towards spiritual care

There are a number of policies, initiatives and influences that are driving the current agenda towards embedding a strong ethos of spiritual care in today's health and social care services.

Service users' and carers' views

The first of these is a desire by service users and carers, in the words of the Somerset Spirituality Project, 'to be taken seriously' (Mental Health Foundation, 2002). This is linked to three factors: the recovery movement, a dissatisfaction with a consumerist society and a greater complexity of belief systems in this country. Those who use services are making it clear they wish to be responded to as people. All the surveys of users/patients by the Commission for Health Inspection, the Commission for Social Care

Inspection and other bodies indicate that people desire something deeper than mere technical competence from staff.

Unfortunately, many users have strong reservations about revealing to professionals their spiritual and/or religious beliefs as they feel this may prejudice the professionals' perspective on them and lead to an increase in medication and confinement. A poet and service user, Sue Holt, writes:

> I have to behave myself today,
> No talking of God,
> And of his plans for me,
> [Holt, 2003: p. 93]

When Nigel Copsey, spiritual care coordinator for East London and the City Mental Health NHS Trust undertook his study for the Sainsbury Centre for Mental Health in 1997, he related the following:

> Many people to whom I spoke, drawn from all religions, said they dreaded going into a hospital or day centre, because there was nothing in those buildings which enabled them to express their faith. When I asked what they wanted, many said they wanted a place for prayer, contact with their religious community, and staff who wanted to talk to them about their faith. One person told me that, having been to a day centre once, she refused to return, as she felt so cut off from the things that mattered most to her [Copsey, 1997: p. 14].

Legislation and policies

The need to ensure that the faith and spiritual needs of all people – staff and service users alike – are addressed and that people are not discriminated against because of their religion or belief is enshrined in law. In 2000 Article 9 was introduced to the Human Rights Act 1998. It is concerned with 'freedom of thought, conscience or religion' and defines the right of the individual to religious observance. The matter of faith is also an important feature of the Equality Act 2006. One of the Act's main provisions makes it unlawful to discriminate 'on the grounds of religion or belief in the provision of goods, facilities and services'. Although this is written primarily to ensure that services are provided equally without faith or religion-related discrimination, faith needs for many service users are an intrinsic feature of their lives. Therefore those users who have declared a particular faith or spiritual belief should not be denied the right to equality as part of their treatment and care provision. As regards staff and employment, the Employment Equality (Religion and Belief) Regulations (UK Parliament, 2003) make discrimination, victimisation or harassment on grounds of religion or belief illegal. National policy, both generally and within the specific remit of mental health, brings spirituality, in its widest sense, centre stage. The *National Service Framework for Mental Health* (Department of Health, 1999), for example, sets two service standards. Standard one is promoting mental health for all, working with individuals and communities and combating discrimination against individuals and groups with mental health problems and promoting their social inclusion. Standard two takes into account the patients' individual requirements, their physical, cultural, spiritual and psychological needs and preferences.

In a more general sense, the White Paper on health and social care, *Our Health, Our Care, Our Say: A New Direction for Community Services* (Department of Health, 2006a), the 2007 *Commissioning Framework for Health and Well-Being* (Department of Health, 2007) and the Commission on Integration and Cohesion's Report *Our Shared Future* (2007) all point in the direction of increased choice and control for people who use services within a socially cohesive society. Additionally, the National Institute for Health and Clinical Excellence (NICE) guidelines in palliative care (2004) state that it is essential that health and social care staff have the necessary skills, knowledge and support to deliver sensitive spiritual care. They also highlight the spiritual and religious care competences for specialist palliative care developed by Marie Curie Cancer Care (2003). These could be adapted and provide a framework for mental health practice. NICE guidance (2005) on the short-term management of disturbed/violent behaviour in psychiatric in-patient settings and emergency departments has drawn attention to the recommendation of appropriate quiet space in in-patient settings for people who wish to pray or to reflect quietly.

Caring for the Spirit by the South Yorkshire Workforce Development Confederation (2003) is the key document to understanding how the Department of Health and faith communities have collaborated to form a strategic process to promote chaplaincy services. It sets out a framework for an understanding between trusts and religious bodies as to how religious, pastoral and spiritual care services should be delivered. There are five main sections: modernisation, quality and evidence, career development for chaplains, education and training programmes, and a plan for implementation.

A companion document for healthcare managers *NHS Chaplaincy: Meeting the Religious and Spiritual Needs of Patients and Staff* (Department of Health, 2003a) addresses the risk and cost issues involved in providing chaplaincy services and gives advice on staffing levels, making appointments, confidentiality, working with volunteers, providing worship space, training and development, bereavement services and major incident planning. The most recent update is the *Guide for Commissioners* (NHS Yorkshire and the Humber, 2007). The Scottish Executive produced its guidance on spiritual care in 2002 (NHS National Services Scotland, 2002), which has since been reviewed (NHS National Services Scotland, 2006; NHS Education for Scotland, 2007; NHS National Services Scotland & The Scottish Interfaith Council, 2007; The Scottish Government, 2009). Presently, the Scottish Partnership of Health and Faith Communities has the better reputation for cooperative working.

Audit evidence with spiritual assessment as a key performance indicator is also encouraged. The Healthcare Commission's acute in-patient mental health service review (Healthcare Commission, 2007) notably looked at this dimension for the first time in 2007. The second of its four criteria, 'the care and support provided appropriate to individual needs' involves staff receiving diversity training in religious awareness and service users assessment of, and access to, staff support for cultural and spiritual needs. The third criterion, 'service users and carers involved in how the ward is run' incorporates a welcome pack or information guide that is regularly reviewed and includes information about spiritual and cultural services, choices and support available on the ward. The fourth criterion, 'Is there a positive therapeutic environment that promotes safety and recovery?' includes the presence of a quiet room, and providing faith and spiritual activities, plus relaxation and meditation. In future, the 'annual health check' will also include the developmental standard that patients receive effective treatment and care that takes into account their individual requirements and meets their physical, cultural, spiritual and psychological needs and preferences.

Identity and diversity of ethnicity and belief systems

As human beings we have a number of spheres of identity, the more obvious being our ethnicity, belief systems, immediate and extended family, communities of meaning (Coyte et al, 2007, chapter 10) and profession and employment and friendship networks. These usually enhance, rather than undermine civil society. But the basis of one's identity can be complex with the history of immigration to the UK. Recent work carried out by the Mercia Group of researchers, based at the University of Warwick (Beckford et al, 2006: p.11) found that over the past fifty years, the discourse in Britain about 'racialised minorities' has mutated from colour, through race and ethnicity, to religion at the present time. This focus on religion has been driven by several phenomena. Major international events have highlighted the political demands associated with religious movements, and academics, policy makers and service providers have increasingly recognised the importance of religion in defining identity, particularly among Black and minority ethnic communities.

Interestingly, the national census of in-patients in mental health hospitals carried out by the Commission for Health Inspection, National Institute of Mental Health England (NIMHE) and the Mental Health Act Commission (Commission for Audit and Inspection, 2005) found a surprisingly high percentage of religious affiliation, even if this does not equate with religious belief. The chair of the Mental Health Act Commission, in launching the results of the survey, stated:

> If you don't know who I am, how are you going to provide a package of care for me, to deliver something? When you do not know how important my religion is to me, what language I speak, where I am coming from, how are you going to help me cope with my mental illness? And that is what I am trying to get over to people; the first step is about identity. It is absolutely fundamental to the package of care we offer an individual [Mulholland, 2005: p. 5].

195

Change in professional approaches and understanding

Many practitioners are working towards allowing users as much choice and control of their lives as possible, thus putting people at the centre of services (Department of Health, 2007: p. 18). This is all the more commendable when set against the background of a pendulum swing in mental health, where public safety appears to be a major preoccupation in some sectors of government and media circles. The recent position paper on the recovery approach in mental health (Care Services Improvement Partnership *et al*, 2007: p. vi) stresses as a core belief 'that adopting recovery as a guiding purpose for mental health services favours hope and creativity over disillusionment and defeat.'

From Values to Action (Department of Health, 2006*b*), the guidance by the Chief Nursing Officer on mental health nursing, recognises the relevance of spirituality and/or religion in mental healthcare and looks to nurses to recognise and respond to the spiritual and religious needs of service users. It also recommends that service providers ensure all mental health nurses have accessible sources of information/advice regarding religious/spiritual issues, including information directories and access to experts and/or faith community representatives. *Essence of Care* (Department of Health, 2003*b*) indicates that religious needs of patients are to be assessed and recorded, that there is coordination with chaplaincy for patient visiting and recommends that information about spiritual care be made available to service users and staff.

Mental Health Foundation

Following on from the Mental Health Foundation's report, *The Impact of Spirituality on Mental Health* (Cornah, 2006), a further report, *Keeping the Faith* (Lindridge, 2007) and its companion synopsis *Making Space for Spirituality* (Mental Health Foundation, 2007) aim to identify and understand positive practice in mental health from a spiritual perspective. Several mediating factors in the relationship between spirituality and mental health were discussed, including coping and attributional styles, locus of control, social support, physiological impact, culture and ethnicity. Eleven mental health initiatives that demonstrated positive practice were investigated and revealed specific themes pertinent to service users. It is interesting to note that all of these initiatives are run by agencies outside of the NHS. Definitions of spiritual practice from the Spirituality and Psychiatry Special Interest Group of the Royal College of Psychiatrists (2006) were used to map each initiative. This included a wide range of activities from religious to secular, such as belonging to a faith tradition, pilgrimage, music, acts of compassion, yoga, tai chi, contemplative reading, enjoying nature, and engaging in creative activities. The report also makes key recommendations for commissioners, service managers, clinicians and religious and spiritual leaders.

Engaging the spirit: the NIMHE spirituality and mental health project

In 2001, NIMHE established a national initiative to promote the integration of religious and spiritual considerations into the provision of mental health treatment and care. In 2003, this was made into a Partnership Project with the Mental Health Foundation. The project has four key aims set out in the joint publication *Inspiring Hope: Recognising the Importance of Spirituality in a Whole Person Approach to Mental Health* (Gilbert & Nicholls, 2003):

1   To collate current thinking on the importance of spirituality in mental health for individuals, groups and communities.
2   To evaluate the role of faith communities in the field of mental health.
3   To develop and promote good practice in whole-persons' approaches.
4   To liaise with external organisations and research communities.

Improving relations with faith communities can bring greater social cohesion and faith communities can play a positive role in family and community life (Cox *et al*, 2007; Gilbert & Kalaga, 2007). However, many people will not be signed up to a specific belief system, despite having faith in the divine; others move in and out of belief and different communities. One of the products of a multicultural society is that people will shift from one faith or denomination to another, or from faith to no faith and back again – especially at times of crisis. Some of the most desolate stories are from those who say that they have lost their faith and desperately want to believe, but feel they can no longer do so (Coyte *et al*, 2007).

One of the main lessons from the project's pilot sites is that work is best promoted when there are a number of interlinked factors: support from the board (with a board-level champion); a committed and imaginative head of spiritual and pastoral care working closely with the board champion and a senior operational manager; users, carers and front-line staff prepared to become engaged; and positive connections with community and voluntary sector partners. Unless this golden thread runs through the partnership, it is very difficult for isolated elements to keep the whole process moving.

Practising psychiatrists who wish to see the development of a 'bio-psychosocio-spiritual model of healthcare' (Powell, 2007) can find support from the Spirituality and Psychiatry Special Interest Group of the Royal College of Psychiatrists, partnership with chaplaincies, the regional support groups now being set up (2007) – in line with the NIMHE framework for the development of spiritual care in trusts (Aris & Gilbert, 2007) – and increasing support at a national policy level.

Putting spiritual care into practice

One of the authors (SE) set up a working group within her NHS mental health trust to oversee the provision of spiritual care. The trust has over

70 sites with only formal, part-time chaplaincy sessions remaining in two. The project was situated within the equalities and diversity group and attempted to have representatives from each in-patient site, users and a range of professions and faiths. A document was produced for the trust board (Central and North West London NHS Foundation Trust, 2007), outlining the importance of spirituality to service users and mapping current faith provision within the trust. The main emphasis was on one specific area of spiritual practice – faith and religion. To embed spirituality more strongly within services, minimum levels of provision had to be established and consistent partnerships with local chaplaincy services were needed to provide multi-faith support. The current provision varied greatly and often relied on an individual or small group with a particular interest to drive the agenda forward. Consequently, actions were recommended that may serve as a template for setting out minimum standards:

1   Statement of intent on faith and spirituality to be adopted by the trust.
2   Faith, belief and spiritual assessment form/process to be established and faith/religious information to be captured routinely and recorded on the assessment of all service users. Internal annual report on religious affiliations to be produced.
3   Multi-faith chaplaincy provision to be calculated by each directorate for its services, the cost to be included within budget-setting processes and negotiations with commissioners.
4   Faith visiting – the trust working towards developing and establishing local systems for the formal provision of faith visiting, with clear links to faith community and chaplaincy structures in line with the NHS chaplaincy guidelines.
5   Faith rooms to be established at all in-patient facilities that can be used by all faiths and to be available for use within in-patient facilities throughout the day and night.
6   Training of staff in appropriate faith and religious awareness and under-standing to be established within the equalities and diversity training, taking into account particular faith needs and local demographics.
7   Observance and involvement – guidance on religious festivals that may be celebrated within in-patient facilities, and a list of faith/religious books and other materials required. Staff to be aware of religious festivals and their significance, and service users to be involved in planning meetings with regard to the organising of faith observance.
8   Community links – all sites/services to have an available and regularly updated list of faith community contacts for service users who wish to attend external services or make their own informal contacts for support. Faith leaders to be involved in the process of faith awareness training at the local level.
9   Faith and spirituality groups – where practical and locally agreed, faith and spirituality groups to be established within service areas to take forward local initiatives. These would form part of local equality and diversity systems and processes.

10   Faith and spirituality policy and strategy to be developed by the trust and coordinator to be identified in order to implement it.

Implementing these recommendations has many ramifications and forms the basis of an action plan that requires involvement of all staff, from trust board members to estates departments. Although they are only initial steps for a trust that currently has very little faith and spirituality provision, other trusts are further developed, with spiritual care policies already written. Several trusts in England, such as Sussex (Sussex Partnership NHS Trust, 2006), Birmingham and Solihull, Bradford, Kent and others, have produced spiritual care strategies, and these all stress the importance of an overall approach rooted in governance arrangements that connect policy drivers with the reality of practice. Slay (2007), in describing the key to success for the Sussex trust strategy, says that it need not matter that there is often plenty of enthusiasm and usually little money; the imperative is for staff to see progress. To this end they have focused on a number of strategic objectives, including provision of sacred space, reviewing and revising service level agreements, a spirituality webpage on the trust site and training and mobile phones for spiritual care staff.

Whose responsibility?

The issue of establishing a trust-wide assessment process raises the question of whose responsibility is it to ensure it happens? McSherry (Orchard, 2001) argues that nurses could be regarded as the rightful custodians of all matters spiritual, by virtue of their continual presence. He also acknowledges, however, that there is a risk of the blurring of boundaries between all professional groups involved in the provision of spiritual care. This may result in fragmented or hindered spiritual care, lost in dispute over issues of role and responsibility. A more spiritually-orientated approach within supervision may be suggested by the role of reflective practice within the nursing profession. Wright (1998) maintains that a reflective journey may stimulate a spiritual journey, where the nurse not only undergoes a transformation of practice but also self-transformation.

Multidisciplinary team processes such as care programme approach documentation, including the health and social care assessment form, also can support spiritual care. A set of useful simple prompts in this area might include some or all of the following questions:

- What is important to you in your life?
- What helps and sustains you?
- Does faith or spirituality play a part in this, and how?
- Do you need support in relation to this, for example access to faith visitor, chaplaincy service, place of worship, or other form of spiritual support?

Another valuable supportive framework is the *Wellness and Recovery Action Plan – WRAP* (Copeland, 1997). It approaches spirituality as a dimension for empowerment and growth. It incorporates concepts such as meaning and purpose as goals for well-being and embraces the work of faith communities.

Clinical psychology services, too, have been developing models and interventions that include a spiritually oriented approach. Dialectic behaviour therapy (Linehan *et al*, 2007) has incorporated 'mindfulness' within a therapeutic approach that was originally developed for people with borderline personality disorders. This approach has been extended to other conditions (Hayes *et al*, 2004) and mindfulness therapy is now available in a number of centres. Based on Jon Kabat-Zinn's stress reduction programme at the University of Massachusetts Medical Center (Kabat-Zinn, 1990) and combined with techniques from cognitive therapy, mindfulness-based cognitive therapy has been used to help people stay well after recovery from depression (Teasdale *et al*, 2000). The Centre for Mindfulness Research and Practice at the University of Wales, and the Oxford Mindfulness Centre, University of Oxford Department of Psychiatry, are two of several places developing this approach in the UK. Isabel Clarke (2001) has been using a spiritually-based approach for people experiencing psychosis and transpersonal psychologist Elizabeth Wilde McCormick (2004, 2008) has described a mindfulness approach to cognitive analytic therapy. Secular approaches to psychotherapy may provide an alien values framework and a significant number of people would prefer an orientation more sensitive to a spiritual perspective (Bergin & Jensen, 1990).

Occupational therapists and activities coordinators are also in a unique position to contribute to the spiritual well-being of their patients (Johnston & Mayers, 2005). There are examples of occupational therapists successfully running patient spirituality groups in collaboration with chaplains and other members of the team (Phillips *et al*, 2002; Louis *et al*, 2007). Candlelight groups (weekly prayer groups) in old age services are also a way of bringing spirituality into the hospital setting (Higgins *et al*, 2004). Art, drama and music therapists all have a role in allowing people to express and explore their spirituality through creative means.

Spiritual care is, however, as much about an approach as it is about implementing policies. Psychiatrists can assist this process simply by enquiring into this area of their patients' lives (see chapter 2) and encouraging curiosity about spirituality among junior staff and team members. Our work is often 'soul' work, allowing love and kindness to flow back into people's lives. The very presence of a compassionate listener is, in essence, spiritual care. Being a role model in terms of delivering this kind of holistic care is one of the most powerful ways of humanising medicine.

Training of staff is crucial, but as yet there are only a few examples of this happening. It begins with undergraduate training, with about a third of UK medical schools reporting that teaching on spirituality is included in their curriculum (whether as an optional or compulsory element). Nevertheless, there is significant room for improvement (Neeley & Minford, 2008). The UK lags behind the USA, where over three-quarters of medical schools provide teaching on spirituality in medicine and this has risen from 13% in just over 10 years (Puchalski, 1998; 2006a).

Exploring people's spiritual needs has up until recently been overlooked, perhaps because the confidence and skills to do so within the workforce are lacking. Millison (1988) states that many professionals have, in the past, avoided spiritual aspects of mental healthcare 'for fear that they are unqualified, ill-equipped, or because they simply feel it is not a part of their job description' (p. 38). There have been attempts to redress this. In the USA, Puchalski (2006b: p. 230) has considerable experience of training doctors and other healthcare professionals at all levels on how to integrate spirituality (both their patients' and their own) into their professional practice and personal lives. Her curriculum includes the basis of compassionate care, the role of spirituality in health and illness, how to do spiritual assessments, how to collaborate effectively with spiritual care professionals, how to incorporate a patient's spirituality into their care plan and how to reflect on their own spirituality as it relates to their professional calling as healers.

An innovative training programme, 'Values in Healthcare: a Spiritual Approach' (Janki Foundation, 2004), has been positively received in some NHS trusts (Bendomir & Morrison, 2005; Ragbir-Day, 2005). These are not didactic lectures but facilitated, sequential, experiential workshops. Groups can explore their values using a learning style that draws upon 'appreciative inquiry' (Cooperrider et al, 2000) and other 'spiritual' learning tools such as visualisation, meditation, reflection and creativity. This educational approach allows healthcare professionals to explore their own ideas about spirituality and develop some of the skills necessary to come alongside people in order to support the patient journey.

The role of the chaplain

Some 100 chaplains are employed by 40 of the 75 mental health trusts in England and Wales. Less than half will work whole time in mental health. Chaplaincy[1] offers a considerable breadth of practice opportunity, with varying levels of task complexity. Thorough induction and effective continuing professional development are offered by the organisations responsible for chaplaincy services. Their shared aim is a workforce of chaplains able to fulfil and sustain their role with professional capacity. Where chaplaincy is resilient and lively, it is likely to be so because of its broad connections, positive support, quality resources, and openness to evidence and creativity. Career chaplains may expect to build competences on the basic foundation they have in practical theology, pastoral care and spirituality. They may also bring further skills from inter-faith studies,

---

1   Although chaplaincy has historically been associated with Christianity in the UK, the term is used here to denote representation of all major faith traditions in an increasingly multicultural Britain.

psychological therapies, sociology, education and health promotion. There is presently no national register specifically for mental health chaplains. Being a minority group within healthcare chaplains (itself a small professional body), there are risks associated with identity, purpose, self-esteem, effectiveness and support. The Mental Health Resource Group of the College of Healthcare Chaplains is able to offer resources and some support through its newsletter, network and training programme (see their website, www.healthcarechaplains.org).

In a review of theoretical models, Mark Folland differentiates four characteristic approaches to the task of being a chaplain (Folland, 2006). The 'hospital as parish' has already been described (p. 192). The 'priest or minister in the hospital', its natural successor, is about pastoral presence and professional style, but keeps its emphasis on religious, particularly sacramental ministry. In contrast, 'person-centred' chaplains, characteristic of the Clinical Pastoral Education movement, have influenced many others who centre their professional development on 'conversation and reflection'. Fourth, there are a growing number of chaplaincies where prominence is given to 'spiritual assessment', with the promotion and the normalisation of spirituality as an everyday dimension of human life.

The current and curious range of chaplaincy job titles illustrates how what was once a thoroughly religious occupation has become very much part of the NHS culture. Most chaplains will to some extent mix and match the designations that follow.

1   The specialist mental health chaplain takes patient referrals, conducts spiritual care assessments, runs support groups and builds opportunities for pastoral care. He or she can advise to better understand the religious context of a particular patient. The role is clinical to an extent that would not often be the case for other chaplains. Recognised qualifications and supervision are required to practise. Principle partners are clinical team members and multidisciplinary working is the key to effective practice.

2   The lead chaplain has adapted a nursing approach, developing best practice, working for modernisation, and keeping a brief for quality, risk and value for money. He or she is up to date with health culture change, partnership working and services in transition, for the empowerment of patients, carers and staff. Staff and patients are to be encouraged to share responsibility for their own spiritual needs, using the resources that are available within the service and in the wider community. Ward managers, modern matrons and leads in allied services are particularly important partners. Volunteers work with the lead chaplain to enable their best participation. Part-time chaplains are trained, supported and encouraged to work as healthcare professionals.

3   The team leader chaplain (also called head, presiding, trust, manager or coordinator chaplain) assesses needs, manages the service, evaluates and prioritises resources. In addition, he or she provides resources for

ethical process, education, induction, training courses and research. He or she is part of the trust governance system. A team leader chaplain shares in the trust's responsibility for the religious and non-religious alike and for ensuring that pastoral, religious and spiritual care is multi-faith and respectful to all, including offering protection from unwanted religious interest. He or she will meet with faith leaders to advise, inform and maintain links between the trust and the community.

4   The community chaplain works for the spiritual care of patients and carers by fostering social support, mental health promotion and combating stigma in partnership with faith communities. The places of work may depend on how voluntary (third sector) support for service users and carers is organised locally. Community chaplains will be encouraged by some faith communities and utterly frustrated by others, discovering the truth that religion can be both friend and foe to better mental health. It is essential for the community chaplain to have trusted links with crisis home treatment teams, community mental health teams and step-down services including rehabilitation units.

5   The chaplain (just plain chaplain) may still be greeted with 'Hello, vicar!', but more usually will simply be referred to by name. Clerical collared or not, the chaplain needs a strong spiritual tradition and a secure personal identity. The role of these chaplains is indivisible from, and dependent on, the connection they have with their own community of faith. Being 'in community' and 'building community' are terms from the wisdom of monastic life that evolved in response to the risks of the religious vocation. Though few chaplains are monks or nuns, a common duty to maintain the 'belonging' aspect of their spiritual lives remains. The result is the sustained capacity to love and respect those with whom life and work is shared, and to cope with, and hope for, that which is beyond and 'other' to ourselves. Another person's experience of mental illness is a holy 'other' place where it is a privilege to be invited. To an extent, those 'other worlds' of medicine, nursing, social care, psychological services and management also evoke the need to pause and consider. Willingness to listen to and learn from atheism, agnosticism and secular humanism is essential in mental health settings. Finally, in terms of otherness, religious diversity is the greater field for the chaplain's professional and theological working. Without a properly formed inter-faith intellectual framework, he or she will struggle with the NHS culture.

Chaplains have the opportunity to engage in the space beyond words. They can learn and absorb skills from music therapy, arts in health, meditation, relaxation, even circle dancing. Caring for the spirit can include activities such as picnics and music festivals. Indeed, the role of the chaplain should include having fun. When he or she has that aspect covered, things are probably going quite well. However, it is quite possible for chaplains to become intellectually lost, professionally and socially isolated, and spiritually disconnected. Poor-quality practice inevitably follows, and sometimes leads to loss of spiritual care services. The spiritual life of the chaplain is embedded in the faith community they belong to, as well as grown in the solitude, silence and stillness of the soul. The professional life of the chaplain is embedded in health and social care as well as arising from their training and experience in their communities of faith.

Working with chaplains

Sutherland (2008), as one of the UK's most experienced mental health chaplains, writes for psychiatrists in training with respect to the relationship between chaplains and the profession. Do chaplains have a common and recognisable clinical identity for the purposes of multidisciplinary working? Lack of uniformity of practice models or levels of training can be a problem when working alongside other health professionals. Sutherland's model requires working with patients' metaphoric, hermeneutic and relational structures in order to empower their social, emotional and cognitive worlds. If that sort of activity is seen as clinical, then chaplains and psychiatrists whose interests range beyond biological theories of causation of illness can work fruitfully together in a dialogue of sharing of theory and practice.

Mental health chaplains should be able to offer:

- empathic listening for those who want to relate experience to faith
- a reference resource for culturally competent care
- a means of access to appropriate spiritual practices and resources
- care for people in loss and bereavement
- connections with faith communities
- advocacy for patient, carer, staff and the organisation
- knowledge of spirituality for coping, recovery and well-being
- a partnership for dialogue regarding religious and spiritual matters
- complementary hermeneutics for human purpose, values and identity
- bridge building between the epistemologies of science and religion.

Chaplaincy responds to an extraordinarily wide group of recipients (Cumming, 2007), offering service benefits for patients, carers and relatives, for staff, for the organisation and for the community. Within these domains arise expectations for pastoral and spiritual care, religious and sacramental ministry, bereavement and end-of-life care, education, training and health awareness, advocacy for a spiritually responsible trust culture, and the promotion of culturally competent care and person-centred values. Realistically, such claims and aims are partly in place and partly aspirational. Holding it all together may seem an impossible task but steps are presently being taken through shared endeavour with other disciplines. Achieving a range of goals when there is a team of chaplains and a culture of openness to spiritual care is hard enough. Increasingly, chaplaincy departments, especially where there is only one chaplain, rely on clear demarcation between what they are principally responsible for, what it is they share a care in, and what they join with others in promoting.

Accountability for chaplains

Two umbrella groups of organisations connect to the work of chaplains. Faith groups and religious organisations are represented to trusts and the Department of Health through the Multi-Faith Group for Healthcare Chaplaincy and the Hospitals Chaplaincy Council. Their dominant paradigm is that of belonging to a faith community. This paradigm has significant implications for patient expectations: what they consider chaplains should deliver and the lines of authority. Whose chaplain is it anyway? From the faith community perspective, chaplains are expected to see their healthcare work as an extension of their primary calling and belonging. This is certainly not a sectarian view, for the person who is of another faith, or none, is responded to out of the universal values arising from the particular faith.

The College of Healthcare Chaplains, the Scottish Association of Chaplains in Healthcare and the Association of Hospice and Palliative Care Chaplains are the three main professional bodies. The College, the largest of the three, has over a thousand members. Their primary duty is service delivery according to need. However, some trusts are appointing spiritual care service managers who have no religious role themselves. This move is controversial as it may undervalue the traditional chaplaincy pathways and be driven by cost concerns. Despite the difficulties and conflicts of interests, chaplains' professional organisations, faith community representative bodies and the healthcare establishment are the three principle stakeholders in meeting religious and spiritual needs. Tripartite working must continue.

There is a perceived risk among chaplains that if spirituality for health becomes any further removed from the religious framework, secular models may claim to be able to fulfil the therapeutic role traditionally met by chaplains. In an era of sharing skills, one new role for the professional healthcare chaplain is to lead in this creative transition process, which is part of the contemporary shift in understanding healthcare. However, some chaplains will feel called to retain their clearly focused vocation of bearing God into the place of suffering. They have an ancient and effective tradition that is well-evidenced, patient-focused and certainly offers value for money. Both practice models should be endorsed and supported.

Where are we going?

When writing on experiences in mental health services in-patient care, hospital chaplain Mike Pritchard (Hardcastle et al, 2007) argues for 'the raising of spiritual awareness' in terms of an approach to people and the person's inner self. Spiritual care, he argues, 'moves us away from a cure and control culture, to one which is genuinely concerned with restoring

205

wholeness and could lead to a re-lighting of the candle in our current in-patient units' (Hardcastle, 2007: pp. 189–191; see also Moss & Gilbert, 2007).

Spiritual care is the shared responsibility of all who work in the NHS. Staff accept a duty of care which is understood in terms of compassion, and therefore give spiritual care without actually naming it. Responding to need in a caring manner and attending to the quality of care and the diversity of its recipients is at the heart of the spiritual approach. If the essence of spirituality in a healthcare context is about connecting people with their community of belonging, their creativity, the enjoyment of creation, their inner confidence and being helped to commune with the 'otherness' of life, then anyone prepared to listen and ask the right questions can contribute to spiritual care.

Anthony Suchman (2006) compares the 'quest for control' with an alternative clinical approach known as relationship-centred care. This, he believes, is more conducive to creative collaboration, especially in the field of healthcare. As we shift from a paternalistic (control) style to one based more on partnership (relationship), our attitudes, values and beliefs determine our capacity to be partners in any endeavour. The paradigm of relationship values the state of connection and belonging. One is part of a larger whole – a team, a community. The best outcomes are realised by emphasising the quality of process – the ability to be genuinely present – and involve being attentive to both the inner and outer experience. The clinician's role is to 'be with' patients, respecting their position as principal makers of values, meanings and decisions in their own lives. This also mirrors some ideas of the 'post-psychiatry' movement (Bracken & Thomas, 2005). Such a model underpins the idea of a person-centred approach but requires inner work on the part of both the organisation and individual practitioners. This reflects some of Swinton's concerns that spiritual care is not seen simply as a set of competences or a 'bolt on', but rather as a way of 'being' for both practitioners and patients (Swinton, 2001).

Conclusion

With massive and perpetual organisational pressures on the NHS, the humane imperatives of spirituality can easily be forgotten. It is a tribute to the dedication and perceptiveness of so many people that the spiritual dimension is now firmly on the agenda. There exists such a great deal of legislation, policy and guidance that NHS trusts can no longer ignore this aspect of patient care. Spiritual care can be seen as a unifying and encouraging presence in the NHS, but only if the whole approach is anchored to a clear system of governance and a set of values that celebrate cultural diversity. An inclusive approach that recognises users' self-identity in terms of mind, body and spirit is needed. Partnerships with many other professions and organisations are hugely important, as is the awareness that all participants are responsible for this aspect of patient care. What must be guarded against is the danger of it becoming yet another formulaic tick-box exercise.

The key question for anyone – psychiatrist, nurse, service user or chaplain – is one of engagement. The essential aspect of spirituality that cannot be escaped is that it is about all of us. Relationships, environment, creativity, otherness are truly common ground. Individual practitioners, as well as the organisations they work for, must ultimately take their own spirituality seriously, if patients are to benefit through spiritual care in the NHS.

References

Aris, S. J. & Gilbert, P. (2007) Organisation health: engaging the heart of the organisation. In *Spirituality, Values and Mental Health: Jewels for the Journey* (eds M. E. Coyte, P. Gilbert & V. Nicholls). Jessica Kingsley.

Bauman, Z. (2000) *Liquid Modernity*. Polity Press.

Beckford, J., Gayle, R., Owen, D., *et al* (2006) *Review of the Evidence Base on Faith Communities*. University of Warwick/OPDM.

Bendomir, A. & Morrison, S. (2005) The Janki Foundation: a values approach to spirituality and health. *Scottish Journal of Healthcare Chaplaincy*, **8**, 29–34.

Bergin, A. E. & Jensen, J. P. (1990) Religiosity of psychotherapists: a national survey. *Psychotherapy*, **27**, 3–7.

Bloch, S. & Green, S. A. (2006) An ethical framework for psychiatry. *British Journal of Psychiatry*, **188**, 7–12.

Bracken, P. J. & Thomas, P. (2005) *Postpsychiatry: Mental Health in a Postmodern World*. Oxford University Press.

Care Services Improvement Partnership, Royal College of Psychiatrists & Social Care Institute for Excellence (2007) *A Common Purpose: Recovery in Future Mental Health Services*. SCIE.

Central and North West London NHS Foundation Trust (2007) *Faith and Spirituality Provision within Central and North West London Mental Health NHS Trust: Report by the Faith and Spirituality Implementation Group*. Central and North West London NHS Foundation Trust.

Clarke, I. (ed.) (2001) *Psychosis and Spirituality: Exploring the New Frontier*. Whurr.

Cobb, M. & Robshaw, V. (1998) *The Spiritual Challenge of Healthcare*. Churchill Livingstone.

Commission for Audit and Inspection (now the Commission for Health Inspection) (2005) *Count Me In: Results for National Consensus of In-Patients in Mental Health Hospitals and Facilities in England and Wales*. Commission for Audit and Inspection.

Commission on Integration and Cohesion (2007) *Our Shared Future*. Commission on Integration and Cohesion.

Cooperrider, D., Sorensen, J., Whitney, D., *et al* (2000) *Appreciative Inquiry: Rethinking Human Organisation toward a Positive Theory of Change*. Stipes Publishing.

Copeland, M. E. (1997) *Wellness Recovery Action Plan – WRAP*. Peach Press.

Copsey, N. (1997) *Keeping Faith: the Provision of Community Mental Health Services Within a Multi-Faith Context*. Sainsbury Centre for Mental Health.

Cornah, D. (2006) *The Impact of Spirituality on Mental Health: a Review of the Literature*. Mental Health Foundation.

Cox, J., Campbell, A. & Fulford, K. W. M. (2007) *Medicine of the Person: Faith, Science and Values in Health Care Provision*. Jessica Kingsley.

Coyte, M. E., Gilbert, P. & Nicholls, V. (2007) *Spirituality, Values and Mental Health: Jewels for the Journey*. Jessica Kingsley.

Cumming, S. (2007) *How Chaplaincy Connects with the Services the Trust Offers*. East Midlands Strategic Health Authority.

Davie, G. (2002) *Europe: the Exceptional Case, Parameters of Faith in the Modern Word*. Darton, Longman and Todd.

Department of Health (1991) *The Patient's Charter*. HMSO.

Department of Health (1992) *HSG: The Provision of Spiritual Care to Staff, Patients, and Relatives*. Department of Health.

Department of Health (1999) *National Service Framework for Mental Health: Modern Standards and Service Models*. Department of Health.

Department of Health (2003*a*) *NHS Chaplaincy: Meeting the Religious and Spiritual Needs of Patients and Staff*. Guidance for Managers and Those Involved in the Provision of Chaplaincy–Spiritual Care. Department of Health.

Department of Health (2003*b*) *Essence of Care: Patient-Focused Benchmarks for Clinical Governance*. NHS Modernisation Agency, Department of Health.

Department of Health (2006*a*) *Our Health, Our Care, Our Say: A New Direction for Community Services*. Department of Health.

Department of Health (2006*b*) *From Values to Action: The Chief Nursing Officer's Review of Mental Health Nursing*. Department of Health.

Department of Health (2007) *Commissioning Framework for Health and Well-Being*. Department of Health.

Folland, M. (2006) *A Review of Some Theoretical Models of Healthcare Chaplaincy Service and Practice*. South Yorkshire NHS Strategic Health Authority.

Gilbert, P. & Kalaga, H. (2007) *Nurturing Heart and Spirit: Papers from the Multi-Faith Symposium*. Staffordshire University & Care Services Improvement Partnership.

Gilbert, P. & Nicholls, V. (2003) *Inspiring Hope: Recognising the Importance of Spirituality in a Whole Person Approach to Mental Health*. NIMHE & Mental Health Foundation.

Hardcastle, M., Kennard, D., Grandison, S., *et al* (eds) (2007) *Experiences of Mental Health In-Patient Care: Narratives from Service Users, Carers and Professionals*. Routledge.

Hay, D. (2006) *Something There: the Biology of the Human Spirit*. Darton, Longman and Todd.

Hayes, S., Follette, V. & Linehan, M. (2004) *Mindfulness and Acceptance: Expanding the Cognitive–Behavioural Tradition*. Guilford Press.

Healthcare Commission (2007) *Acute In-Patient Mental Health Service Review: Final Assessment Framework*. Commission for Healthcare Audit and Inspection.

Higgins, P., Allen, R., Karamat, S., *et al* (2004) *Candlelight Group: A Pilot Project for People with Dementia*. Royal College of Psychiatrists (http://www.rcpsych.ac.uk/PDF/higgins_8_4_04.pdf).

Holt, S. (2003) *Poems of Survival*. Chipmunka Publishing.

Janki Foundation (2004) *Values in Healthcare: a Spiritual Approach: A Personal and Team Development Programme for Healthcare Practitioners*. Janki Foundation.

Johnston, D. & Mayers, C. (2005) Spirituality: a review of how occupational therapists acknowledge, assess and meet spiritual needs. *British Journal of Occupational Therapy*, **68**, 9.

Kabat-Zinn, J. (1990) *Full Catastrophe Living: How to Cope with Stress, Pain and Illness Using Mindfulness Meditation*. Delacorte.

Layard, R. (2005) *Happiness: Lessons from a New Science*. Allen Lane.

Lindridge, A. (2007) *Keeping the Faith: Spirituality and Recovery from Mental Health Problems*. Mental Health Foundation.

Linehan, M., Dimeff, L. & Koerner, K. (2007) *Dialectical Behaviour Therapy in Clinical Practice: Applications across Disorders and Settings*. Guilford.

Louis, E., Jones, N., Green, C., *et al* (2007) Exploring your spiritual side. In *Occupational Therapy News*, pp. 34–35. College of Occupational Therapists.

Marie Curie Cancer Care (2003) *Spiritual and Religious Care Competencies for Specialist Palliative Care*. Marie Curie Cancer Care.

Mental Health Foundation (2002) *Taken Seriously: Report of the Somerset Spirituality Project.* Mental Health Foundation.

Mental Health Foundation (2007) *Making Space for Spirituality: How to Support Service Users.* Mental Health Foundation.

Millison, M.B. (1988) Spirituality and the caregiver: developing an underutilized facet of care. *American Journal of Hospice Care,* **5**, 37–44.

Moss, B. (2005) *Religion and Spirituality.* Russell House Publishing.

Moss, B. & Gilbert, P. (2007) Flickering candles of hope: spirituality, mental health and the search for meaning. *Illness, Crisis and Loss,* **15**, 179–191.

Mulholland, H. (2005) Counting on change. *Society Guardian,* 7th December.

Murray, S., Kendall, M., Boyd, K., *et al* (2004) Exploring the spiritual needs of people dying of lung cancer or heart failure: a prospective qualitative interview study of patients and their carers. *Palliative Medicine,* **18**, 39–45.

National Institute for Health and Clinical Excellence (2004) *Improving Supportive and Palliative Care for Adults with Cancer: the Manual.* pp. 93–103. NICE.

National Institute for Health and Clinical Excellence (2005) *The Short-Term Management of Disturbed/Violent Behaviour in Psychiatric In-Patient Settings and Emergency Departments.* NICE.

Neely, D. & Minford, E. J. (2008) Current Status of Teaching on Spirituality in UK Medical Schools. *Medical Education,* **42**, 176–182.

NHS Education for Scotland (2007) *Standards for NHS Scotland Chaplaincy Services.* NHS Scotland.

NHS National Services Scotland (2002) *Spiritual Care in NHS National Services Scotland.* NHS Scotland.

NHS National Services Scotland (2006) *Spiritual Care in NHS National Services Scotland: Statement of Intent.* NHS Scotland.

NHS National Services Scotland & The Scottish Interfaith Council (2007) *Religion and Belief Matter: an Information Resource for Healthcare Staff.* NHS Scotland.

NHS Yorkshire and the Humber (2007) *Improving Healthcare Chaplaincy Services: a Guide for Commissioners.* NHS Yorkshire and the Humber.

Orchard, H. (2001) *Spirituality in Health Care Contexts.* Jessica Kingsley.

Phillips III, R. E., Larkin, R. & Pargament, K. (2002) Brief report: development and implementation of a spiritual issues psycho-educational group for those with serious mental illness. *Community Mental Health Journal,* **38**, 487–495.

Powell, A. (2007) Spirituality and psychiatry: crossing the divide. In *Spirituality, Values and Mental Health: Jewels for the Journey* (eds M. E. Coyte, P. Gilbert & V. Nicholls), pp. 161–171. Jessica Kingsley.

Pulchalski, C. M. (2006*a*) Spirituality and medicine: curricula in medical education. *Journal of Cancer Education,* **21**, 14–18.

Puchalski, C. M. (2006*b*) *A Time for Listening and Caring.* Oxford University Press.

Puchalski, C. M. & Larson, D. B. (1998) Developing curricula in spirituality and medicine. *Academic Medicine,* **73**, 970–974.

Ragbir-Day, N. (2005) Values in healthcare: is a values-based approach practical? In *The Economics of Health Reforms* (ed. J. N. Yfantopoulos). ATINER.

Sacks, J. (2005) *To Heal a Fractured World: The Ethics of Responsibility.* Continuum.

Slay, G. (2007) Let's get spiritual. *Mental Health Practice,* **11**, 26–28.

South Yorkshire Workforce Development Confederation (2003) *Caring for the Spirit: A Strategy for the Chaplaincy and Healthcare Workforce.* South Yorkshire Workforce Development Confederation.

Speck, P. (2005) The evidence base for spiritual care. *Nursing Management,* **12**, 28–31.

Spirituality and Psychiatry Special Interest Group (2006) *Spirituality and Mental Health* (*Help is at Hand* series). Royal College of Psychiatrists.

Suchman, A. (2006) Control and relation: two foundational values and their consequences. *Journal of Interprofessional Care,* **20**, 3–11.

Sussex Partnership NHS Trust (2006) *Spiritual and Religious Care Strategy*. Sussex Partnership NHS Trust.

Sutherland, M. (2008) The contribution of chaplains in the psychiatric setting. In *Handbook for Psychiatric Trainees* (ed. D. Bhugra & O. Howes). Royal College of Psychiatrists.

Swinton, J. (2001) *Spirituality and Mental Health Care: Rediscovering a 'Forgotten' Dimension*. Jessica Kingsley.

Teasdale, J. D., Segal, Z. V., Williams, J. M. G., *et al* (2000) Prevention of relapse/recurrence in major depression by mindfulness-based cognitive therapy. *Journal of Consulting and Clinical Psychology*, **68**, 615–623.

The Scottish Government (2009) *Spiritual Care and Chaplaincy*. The Scottish Government (http://www.scotland.gov.uk/Resource/Doc/259076/0076811.pdf).

UK Parliament (2003) *Employment Equality Regulations (Religion and Belief)*. TSO (The Stationery Office).

Wilde McCormick, E. (2004) Mindfulness and cognitive analytic therapy in reformulation. *Journal of the Association for Cognitive Analytic Therapy*, **23**, 5–10.

Wilde McCormick, E. (2008) *Change for the Better* (3rd edn). Sage Publications.

Wright, S. (1998) The reflective journey begins a spiritual journey. In *Transforming Nursing Through Reflective Practice* (ed. C. Johns & D. Freshwater). Blackwell.

Resources for spirituality in UK mental health services

Royal College of Psychiatrists

Spirituality and Mental Health (web leaflet), by Spirituality and Psychiatry Special Interest Group (2006) *Help is at Hand* series, Royal College of Psychiatrists (http://www.rcpsych.ac.uk/mentalhealthinformation/therapies/spiritualityandmentalhealth.aspx)

Mental Health Foundation

Mental Health Foundation: http://www.mentalhealth.org.uk/information/mental-health-a-z/spirituality/
Search for spirituality at: http://www.mentalhealth.org.uk/publications/

Taken Seriously, report (2002)
The Impact of Spirituality on Mental Health: A Review of the Literature, by D. Cornah (2006)
Keeping the Faith: Spirituality and Recovery from Mental Health Problems, by A. Lindridge (2007)
Making Space for Spirituality: How to Support Service Users, booklet (2007)

CSIP/NIMHE

Facilitating spirituality, resources: http://www.nimhe.csip.org.uk/our-work/spirituality-in-mental-health/spirituality-resources.html

Inspiring Hope: Recognising the Importance of Spirituality in a Whole Person Approach to Mental Health, by P. Gilbert & V. Nicholls (2003) (http://www.nimhe.csip.org.uk/our-work/spirituality-in-mental-health/spirituality-resources.html)
Promoting Mental Health: A Resource for Spiritual and Pastoral Care, published jointly (2004) by the Church of England, the National Institute of Mental Health in England, and Mentality (http://www.cofe.anglican.org/info/socialpublic/homeaffairs/mentalhealth/parishresource.pdf)
Guidelines on Spirituality for Staff in Acute Care Services, by P. Gilbert, R. Merchant and L. Hayes (2008), NIMHE Acute Care Programme/Staffordshire University; booklet, leaflet, poster and evidence resource (http://www.virtualward.org.uk/recovery/improving-recovery-.html)

Department of Health

NHS Chaplaincy (2003) (http://www.dh.gov.uk/en/Publicationsandstatistics/Publications/
PublicationsPolicyAndGuidance/DH_4062016)

NHS Chaplaincy Meeting the Religious and Spiritual Needs of Patients (2003) (http://www.
dh.gov.uk/en/Publicationsandstatistics/Publications/PublicationsPolicyAndGuidance/
DH_4073108)

Religion or Belief: A Practical Guide for the NHS, by the Department of Health Equalities and
Human Rights Group (2009) (http://www.dh.gov.uk/en/Publicationsandstatistics/
Publications/PublicationsPolicyAndGuidance/DH_093133)

National Health Services Scotland

Religion and Belief Matter: An Information Resource for Healthcare Staff, by NHS National
Services Scotland and The Scottish Interfaith Council (2007) (http://www.
scottishinterfaithcouncil.org/resources/Religion+and+Belief.pdf)

Spiritual Care Matters – An Introductory Resource for all NHS Scotland Staff, published by NHS
Education for Scotland (2009) (http://www.nes.scot.nhs.uk/documents/publications/
classa/030309SpiritualCareMatters.pdf)

Spiritual Care and Chaplaincy, by The Scottish Government (2009) (http://www.scotland.
gov.uk/Resource/Doc/259076/0076811.pdf)

Chaplaincy

Multi-Faith Group for Healthcare Chaplaincy, resources: http://www.mfghc.com/
resources/resources_docindex.htm

The College of Healthcare Chaplains CHCC, Mental health resource group: http://www.
healthcarechaplains.org/

The UK Board of Healthcare Chaplaincy (UK BHC): http://www.ukbhc.org.uk/

The Scottish Association of Chaplains in Healthcare (SACH): http://www.sach.org.uk/
index.htm

NHS Chaplaincy Collaboratives: http://www.nhs-chaplaincy-collaboratives.com/index.
htm

*The Potential for Efficacy of Healthcare Chaplaincy and Spiritual Care Provision in the NHS (UK).
A Scoping Review of Recent Research*, by H. Mowat (2008). Mowat Research (http://www.
mfghc.com/cfts/efficacy_0801.pdf)

Mindfulness

The Centre for Mindfulness Research and Practice at the University of Wales, Bangor:
http://www.bangor.ac.uk/mindfulness

Mindfulness Based Cognitive Therapy, University of Oxford, Department of Psychiatry,
Warneford Hospital, Oxford: http://www.mbct.co.uk

University of Oxford Centre for Suicide Research: http://cebmh.warne.ox.ac.uk/csr/
mbct.html

Oxford Mindfulness: http://www.oxmindfulness.org/home/

CHAPTER 11

The transpersonal perspective

Tim Read and Nicki Crowley

The transpersonal concept of consciousness may be unfamiliar to many psychiatrists and some of its tenets may not receive widespread acceptance, yet it could potentially be applied to psychiatric treatment. William James first coined the term 'transpersonal' over one hundred years ago. Meaning 'beyond the personal', the transpersonal perspective adds a deeper layer of appreciation to the individual and collective psyche. The term was reintroduced in the 1960s by Abraham Maslow and Stanislav Grof to describe an emerging model of mind that attempts to integrate science with the world's wisdom and spiritual traditions, as well as introducing a more complete model of consciousness than the one derived from traditional science, psychology and psychiatry (Vich, 1988).

Transpersonal experience is all human experience beyond the ego (Scotton, 1996a). If it occurs in a religious context, it will indeed be felt to be a religious epiphany. However, many spiritual and transpersonal experiences occur outside of religion and seem to represent a universal aspect of human consciousness.

The transpersonal field is multidisciplinary, incorporating insights from anthropology, theology, mythology, thanatology and parapsychology. It includes the empirical study of unusual mental states and psychological experiences which do not easily fit traditional psychiatric diagnostic categories.

Of the psychiatrists who have led the transpersonal field over the past hundred years, Carl Jung and Stanislav Grof have made especially important contributions. Both men drew deeply on their personal experience of non-ordinary states of consciousness (NOSC), which informed and drove their clinical and theoretical work. Jung's transpersonal perspective and insistence on the importance of spirit was a major factor in his split with Sigmund Freud. Where Freud focused his attention on the personal unconscious and the ego, Jung emphasised the importance of the collective unconscious[1] and

---

1   Jung, like Freud, used the term 'unconscious' to describe mental contents that are inaccessible to the ego and to delineate a psychic space with its own character, laws and functions. He considered the personal unconscious to include repressed, infantile and personal experience, but extended this concept to define a collective

the self.[2] The tensions between these two schools of thought continue to this day.

The work of Carl Jung

The Swiss psychiatrist Carl Jung had a crisis in mid-life, with many unusual experiences that could be considered psychotic. This 'creative illness' lasted from 1912 to 1917, during which time he allowed himself to open to the contents of his deep psyche, becoming almost overwhelmed by the visions, dreams and intensity of feeling that followed. Jung felt his consciousness was flooded by forces which he called archetypal[2] but which in previous ages may have been regarded as divine or demonic. The key features of his illness were (Jung, 1961):

- surrendering to the emergence of material from the unconscious
- willingness to explore the symbolic meaning of his experiences as part of a journey towards growth
- reports of journeying to non-physical domains
- communication with 'non-physical beings', named Basilides and Philemon
- partial withdrawal from the demands of everyday life to provide a suitable and supportive environment where he could try to integrate his experiences by various artistic and expressive pursuits such as carving, painting mandalas, writing poetry, building and sand play.

It is difficult to apply a DSM–IV or ICD–10 diagnostic category to Jung's condition, which showed many of the classical features of 'spiritual emergency' (see pp. 227–230) and had a positive rather than a negative outcome (cf. the quote on p. 221). Most commentators agree that Jung did not have psychosis in the accepted sense, but this was a 'near miss' and he could well have developed a chronic disabling psychiatric disorder, if it were not for his ability to work deeply on his internal processes and the degree of support he had from his circle of intimates (McLynn, 1996). Jung's 'illness' did not recur and he regarded it as a crucial part of his individuation.[3] He later said about his crisis:

> I loved it and hated it but it was my greatest wealth ... I have never lost touch with those initial experiences ... All my works, all my creative activity came from those initial fantasies and dreams beginning in 1912 [Jung, 1961: pp. 194–225].

---

unconscious that differed from it and was related directly to the phylogenetic and instinctual basis of the human race (see Samuels *et al*, 1986).

2   Jung considered archetypes to be pre-existent, primordial images or universal symbols based in the unconscious and influencing a person's functioning (Jung, 1981).

3   Individuation is a Jungian concept, being the maturational task of the second half of life. The pursuits of the ego give way to the goal of self-realisation, in which a person becomes fully conscious of what it means to be a unique human being and yet, at the same time, remaining a common man or woman (see Samuels *et al*, 1986).

Jung could not explain his experiences using the model of the mind provided by Western science. He studied mythical and mystical traditions from Africa, Asia and America and wrote about the psychological significance of the history of Western alchemy, the I Ching, the *Tibetan Book of the Dead* and the *Great Liberation* as well as zen Buddhism (Jung, 1958). He proposed that these works gave important information about the structure of the mind and the nature of consciousness, which included a collective unconscious containing archetypes as universal forms of meaning. Jung developed the idea of the self as driving the process of individuation and as representing a more complete version of the psyche than the ego.

Jung also developed the concept of synchronicity (Jung, 1972). By this, he refers to an 'acausal' connecting principle, revealing 'meaningful coincidence' between the inner world and external reality (i.e. the occurrence of two significant but seemingly unconnected events which are yet connected by a sense of meaning for the individual experiencing them). Such dramatic coincidences often seem to occur in periods of crisis or spiritual growth and Jung felt that they provided, like dreams, an impetus towards greater wholeness of the personality (or individuation).

It is crucial that psychiatrists should be able to distinguish between synchronicities and psychosis, so as to avoid treating all unusual mental phenomena as mental illness (case study 11.1, p. 215).

Pioneers of transpersonal psychology

In the work of Ken Wilber, Abraham Maslow, Roberto Assagioli and others, transpersonal development is part of a continuum of consciousness, ranging from pre-personal (before the growth of the ego) to the personal (having a functioning ego) and beyond to the transpersonal. This schema of development involves first differentiating an independent functional ego and then transcending attachment to the ego (Scotton, 1996a).

Maslow (1964) studied self-actualised individuals who had mystical or 'peak' experiences. He demonstrated that these were frequently beneficial and should not necessarily be understood as representing psychopathology. These experiences put individuals in touch with 'the sacred', often when emerging from previously difficult and painful self-confrontations. This contrasts with the New Age trap of narcissistic self-absorption, where spiritual practice can potentially be used as an escape from everyday life and subsequently, owing to lack of healthy ego development, reveal an intolerance of conflict.

Assagioli (1975) developed psychosynthesis as a treatment that would address both personal and transpersonal issues. He recognised that a psychological crisis could be the natural and potentially healthy accompaniment to spiritual development. His approach was to first address problematic personal issues and then to explore the transpersonal dimension.

The third pioneer of transpersonal psychology, Ken Wilber (1977), considers consciousness as a spectrum. He describes how various schools

Case study 11.1

In AD 386, at a time of spiritual crisis, St Augustine heard a child's voice saying 'pick up and read'. He opened at random St Paul's epistles and there read words that spoke with uncanny precision to the nature of his lifelong conflict so that 'the light of certainty flooded my heart and all dark shadows fled away' (Tarnas, 2006).

Jumila, a 35-year-old legal executive, told her psychiatrist that she was experiencing synchronicities. She described advertisement hoardings lighting up when she passed them and that streets signs were featuring the initials of her name. She believed this indicated her mission to educate the world about global warming. She was treated for a relapse of bipolar disorder.

of psychology address different portions of this spectrum and that each part, whether pre-personal, personal or transpersonal, can have its own pathology, and may require different treatments. He recommends pharmacological treatments for psychosis related to early developmental failures and traditional cognitive or explorative psychotherapies for personality and neurotic disorders; for transpersonal disorders he recommends a combined treatment based on spiritual and psychotherapeutic traditions (Wilber et al, 1986). The underlying rationale for Wilber's different therapeutic recommendations is based on the concept of the pre/trans fallacy (Wilber, 1980). 'Pre' stands for pre-rational and 'trans' stands for transpersonal, the fallacy being a failure to distinguish between integrated and non-integrated states of mind. For example, it is important to differentiate between psychotic and mystical experiences, though they may at times be similar. Healthy transpersonal phenomena rest on a secure psychological foundation, whereas psychotic phenomena, being 'pre-rational', are an expression of a poorly integrated or underdeveloped psychological self.

The work of R. D. Laing and David Lukoff

Epiphany experiences (case study 11.2) have been well described by the British psychiatrist R. D. Laing (1965a), who noted that they seemed to be the original fount of all religion and that they occur in psychotic states as well as in 'the sane experience'. Subsequent authors (Goodwin & Jamison, 1990; Clarke, 2001) suggest that psychotic disorders frequently contain a religious or spiritual component. The psychologist David Lukoff (1996b) proposes a separate diagnostic category of psychotic episode with mystical features.

Laing proposed that some forms of psychosis could lead to breakthrough rather than breakdown, but that exploring the inner world without guidance could lead to confusion between inner and outer reality (Laing, 1965b). His psychological approach to psychosis was controversial and never gained credibility within the profession as a whole. However, his work invited a fresh way to view psychosis as holding significance and meaning.

> Case study 11.2
>
> A liaison psychiatrist assessed Margaret, a 42-year-old housewife and mother who had jumped in front of a train, sustaining multiple fractures. She described an experience 2 years previously, while on holiday in a place of outstanding natural beauty, of a sudden epiphany, an experience of clarity, universal love and bright light. She had continued her working life without any evidence of psychiatric disorder until the suicide attempt. She said she had wanted to dispense with her physical body to become one with the Divine. Owing to some elation of mood and reduced need for sleep, a tentative diagnosis of hypomania was made. The relationship between the epiphany experience and her mental illness was unclear.

Thirty years after Laing's work was first published, Lukoff succeeded in getting 'religious or spiritual problem' entered as a new diagnostic category (V62.89) in the DSM–IV (American Psychiatric Association, 1994), the V Code denoting a state as the focus of clinical attention but not considered a disorder. He describes how his first-hand knowledge of hallucinogen-induced psychosis contributed greatly to his ability to work with patients experiencing psychotic episodes in clinical practice, and makes the important point (Lukoff, 1996a) that the post-psychotic integration phase lasts much longer than the psychotic phase. He also argues that milder forms of spiritual disturbance should not be diagnosed or treated as mental disorders but rather as spiritual or religious problems (Lukoff, 1996b).

Stanislav Grof: holotropic breathwork and the perinatal domain

The Czech psychiatrist Stanislav Grof has extended Jung's work with 'active imagination'[4], making two important contributions to the transpersonal field: the development of holotropic breathwork and the understanding of the perinatal and birth experience as being relevant to the development of the individual, as well as a portal to the transpersonal dimension.

Holotropic breathwork

Grof (1975, 1985) claims to have discovered reliable and safe methods for the induction, amplification and integration of therapeutic non-

---

4   Jung used this term in 1935 to describe a process of dreaming with open eyes. In doing so, a new situation is created in which unconscious contents are exposed in the waking state. Awareness is heightened and following integration, maturation is quickened. Active imagination differs from day dreaming, which is more or less of one's own invention, and remains on the surface of personal and daily experience. It is the opposite of conscious invention, but does require the active and creative participation of the ego, as opposed to dreams, which are experienced passively.

ordinary states of consciousness (NOSC). Grof first used lysergic acid diethylamide (LSD) to study NOSC during the 1960s era of research into psychedelic drugs (entheogens[5]), before developing the technique of holotropic breathwork, which he believes allows to access the same part of the psyche as LSD.

The term 'holotropic' derives from the Greek and means 'moving towards wholeness'. Key components of holotropic breathwork are:

- accelerated breathing to initiate the NOSC
- powerful, evocative music
- focused bodywork[6] where appropriate, to work through unresolved process
- a highly supportive and integrative setting
- an international training organisation.

Grof considers that without the use of these techniques, a deep area of the psyche would remain relatively inaccessible. Individuals who have experienced these unusual states of consciousness frequently report that they have entered new, authentic domains of reality that seem to be supraordinate to everyday consciousness.

The holotropic breathwork technique has important differences to a drug-enabled NOSC, in that the depth of the experience is largely under conscious control and can be lightened or terminated at any time. A key feature of the experience is the intensity of the emotional experience. Participants are encouraged to maintain the intensity, bringing it completely into awareness until it reaches a critical threshold and then dissolves, allowing some resolution (Grof, 1988). The setting, with help from trained facilitators, is a crucial determinant of outcome.

For many people, holotropic breathwork has been a profoundly healing and transformative experience (Grof, 1985). However, the method has been described here to illustrate how consciousness may be beneficially expanded without the use of mind-altering substances, particularly relevant in today's drug-abusing culture.

Perinatal domain and perinatal matrices

Grof reports that in a non-ordinary state of consciousness, people often experience moving beyond the level of memories from childhood and infancy to encountering emotions and physical sensations of extreme intensity which hold a strange mixture of themes of birth and death. These include images, emotions and physical experiences that seem

---

5   The word 'entheogen' drives from the Greek 'theo' meaning God or spirit and 'gen' meaning creation and can be applied to a psychoactive sacrament – a plant or chemical substance taken to occasion a spiritual or mystical experience.

6   'Bodywork' describes a range of body-based approaches emphasising manipulation and realignment of the body's structure. 'Focused bodywork' refers to working with a specific part of the body causing pain or tension, with the aim of processing associated psychological issues (Grof, 1985).

related to the birth process itself and which have been in some instances veridically confirmed. Grof named this the perinatal domain (1975) and described four basic perinatal matrices (Fig. 11.1), each having a physical and a transpersonal component. Grof (1975, 1985) suggests that some psychopathology in adult life may be related to unresolved perinatal trauma, possibly in resonance with traumas or challenges arising at other stages of psychological development.

1   The first basic perinatal matrix[7] (BPM I)
     This represents the gestational period until the onset of labour. In a corresponding NOSC, the perception of oceanic feelings of ecstasy and cosmic unity are thought to correspond to a 'good womb' experience. Similarly, toxic feelings and paranoia equate with a 'bad womb' experience.

2   The second matrix (BPM II)
     This represents the physical onset of labour, where the uterus contracts against a closed cervix. During the NOSC this can be a challenging process, with personal and archetypal feelings of stasis and despair. Grof believes that a successful working through of this phase is fundamental to recovery from some neurotic disorders (Grof, 1975).

3   The third matrix (BPM III)
     This represents the physical process of movement out of the 'stuckness' of a constricted womb and the start of the journey towards birth. The theme is of tumultuous forces and a perilous journey towards the outside world. In a corresponding NOSC there may be an archetypal encounter with death, corresponding with this actual physical struggle to be born.

4   The fourth matrix (BPM IV)
     This represents the completion of birth, the emergence into a new world and the recovery phase for mother and baby. The themes of this phase are triumph, fortuitous escape from danger, revolution, decompression and expansion of space, radiant light and colour; unitive experiences may occur.

Wilber and Grof disagree about the significance of the perinatal experience. Wilber (1995) views the perinatal layer as a pre-personal state, without true transpersonal quality, and as such having little impact on human development. Grof (1975) views the perinatal layer as a portal to transpersonal experience and holds that consciously accessing previously unconscious, traumatic material related to birth (and subsequent life traumas) is integral to resolving psychopathology and promoting personal growth.

---

7   The word 'matrix' is defined in the *Oxford English Dictionary* as a 'place in which a thing is developed', and in this context denotes a typical pattern or dynamic constellation of experience.

Fig. 11.1   Four basic perinatal matrices (Grof, 1975)

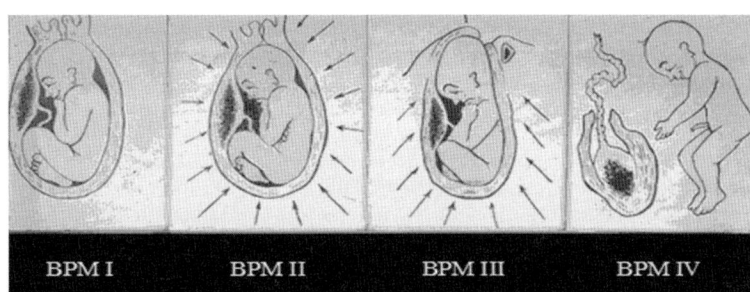

This illustration is reproduced with kind permission of Stanislav Grof.

The therapeutic uses of NOSC

Grof (1985) claims that people with various psychiatric disorders (particularly post-traumatic states, depression, anxiety, phobic states and some psychosexual and psychosomatic conditions) have improved as a result of practising holotropic breathwork. He reports that mood disorders have a specific connection to unresolved perinatal, emotional trauma and suggests that inhibited depression is related to BPM II, agitated depression to BPM III and manic episodes to an incomplete transition between BPM III and BPM IV.

The following case vignette (case study 11.3, p. 220) illustrates the complex relationship between past trauma and current mental state, and how skilful work with NOSC can be a helpful step towards a person's recovery.

Transpersonal experience in holotropic breathwork

The experiences triggered by holotropic breathwork are of interest to the psychiatrist because many of those phenomena resemble those described by patients with psychosis. The clinician with an interest in the transpersonal dimension will be concerned with helping the patient find meaning in their experience of illness, just as the person exploring holotropic breathwork seeks to do. The crucial difference between a therapeutic NOSC and a spontaneous psychotic disorder or spiritual emergency (pp. 227–230) is the ability to utilise and integrate the emerging unconscious material into everyday consciousness.

The phenomena that can be experienced in a NOSC include:

- experiences beyond spatial boundaries, including the powerful sense of being other than oneself
- experiences of a 'micro world', such as an experience of cellular consciousness, DNA or subatomic particles
- a transcendence of temporal boundaries including foetal, ancestral or experiences of life in a different historical period

219

> ### Case study 11.3
>
> Jennifer is a psychotherapist in her fifties who sought holotropic breathwork due to chronic low mood that had not responded to psychoanalytic psychotherapy or antidepressant medication. She had a history of childhood emotional and physical abuse. Her breathwork sessions often involved a painful revisiting of her childhood traumas followed by an apparent perinatal memory of being stuck in the birth canal feeling terrified and helpless. On several occasions she reported a profound spiritual experience after the perinatal experience. The facilitators encouraged her to intensify these feelings and after a number of sessions, with the aid of some focused bodywork, she felt symptomatically and functionally improved.

- visions of archetypal beings, communication with spirits or extra-terrestrial beings (Grof, 2000).

Because of the fragmented nature of the psyche in someone who has a psychosis, the task of subsequently making sense of the psychotic episode may take lengthy and systematic psychotherapeutic work, in those patients for whom it is advisable. A doctor's account of a holotropic breathwork session follows (case study 11.4).

A theoretical contribution to the understanding of psychosis

Grof's work also contributes to a broader understanding of psychosis, not just as a neurobiological malfunction leading to illness, but as an expression of an altered state of consciousness. Nelson has defined psychosis as 'any one of several altered states of consciousness, transient or persistent, that prevent integration of sensory or extrasensory information into reality models accepted by the broad consensus of society, and that lead to maladaptive behaviour and social sanctions' (Nelson, 1994: p. 3).

> ### Case study 11.4
>
> The initial impression was that nothing much was happening, but I enjoyed the music and continued to breathe. Then I started to feel intense fear and needed to struggle. I felt I was being choked and my head felt crushed. Part of me wondered whether this was a re-enactment of the birth process, but my thinking was not as strong as the sensations I was experiencing. I knew that there was help nearby from the facilitators if I needed it and I was able to stay with the sensations. Then, to my surprise, this was followed by an intense spiritual experience where I found myself in 'another place', permeated by love and peace. I felt deeply at one with myself and all things. I do still wonder if the perinatal experience may have been triggered by a lecture on the subject earlier that day. But the mystical experience felt so strong and authentic to me. It has led to a subtle reorganisation of my life-style, which now includes regular spiritual practice.

Transpersonal concepts

Key transpersonal concepts:
1   Consciousness as primary, not confined to neural process and existing independently of the brain.
2   There exist deeper layers of personal and collective consciousness imbued with spiritual meaning.
3   Psychological development continues throughout life, with the potential to open to higher levels of consciousness.
4   Each person has, under the right conditions, access to a 'higher' or 'transcendent' self.
5   Non-ordinary states of consciousness are not to be assumed to be merely pathological; they may hold profound therapeutic possibilities.

Levels of consciousness

The transpersonal perspective is uniquely placed to bring together the Eastern and Western concepts of mind. In the West, depth psychologies have provided a schema for healthy maturational development and its psychopathology. Eastern metaphysics offers its own developmental schema for levels of consciousness, which includes the concept of the chakras. This concept is pivotal both to the ancient Ayurvedic healing tradition and to Oriental medicine, where chakras are considered to be vortices of subtle energy, depicted as lotus-like 'wheels', each with a specific mid-line location in the body. They are held to be conduits for drawing vital life force inward from a universal ambient field by interfacing between the physical and subtle energy realms. It is postulated that they also represent psychological archetypes (Nelson, 1994).

In considering psychosis to be a non-ordinary or altered state of consciousness, this expansive model of the psyche enables us to contrast the level of consciousness in a malignant psychotic regression with that of an adaptive 'psychotic' regression that may precede spiritual growth and/or the healthy capacity to enter into a transcendent or higher state of consciousness. To this end, Nelson (1994) has put forward four essential questions aimed at refining the psychiatrist's ability to categorise 'psychotic' altered states of consciousness in ways that helpfully complement those currently employed in the West:
1   At what level of consciousness did psychotic regression begin?
2   At what level did it end?
3   What is the highest level of consciousness ever attained by the person?
4   Do the symptoms resemble those of an emerging spiritual realisation?
The following schema presents a model of consciousness with different octaves of meaning and significance, from the mundane to the numinous (Powell, 2003). There are held to be seven levels, each with its own chakra:

1 The first (or root) chakra represents the basic, instinctive drive to survive, connect and thrive. It concerns response to danger and binds consciousness into the demands of everyday reality. The counter-current is the innate drive to dissolve, disconnect and to 'not-be'. For people predominantly centred at this chakra, relationships with others are dependant and based on need.

2 The second chakra represents sexual energy, appetite, generativity and the pleasure principle. The expression of this energy will vary according to time of life and the modifying effect of other physical and psychological factors. Freud's early work on the sexual aetiology of neurosis approached the world through the lens of this level. Relationships borne out of this level of consciousness tend to be idealised and tinged with fantasy.

3 The third chakra represents action in worldly life, in which the ego is most highly developed. It involves power, will, hierarchy and issues of social organisation of individuals and groups. Issues arising from this level of consciousness concern role, status and station in life. A person focused solely at this level of consciousness will be involved in competitive and manipulative relationships.

4 The fourth or heart chakra represents the crucial transitional point between the personal and transpersonal, where further development depends less on intellect and more on 'gnosis kardias', the knowledge of the heart (Hoeller, 1982.) It is the level represented by the Christ archetype of compassion, suffering and altruistic love. There is often a crisis and a personal paradigm shift when this is manifested in a person's life. As survival, procreation and status no longer dominate the agenda, different values are sought and the demands of the ego begin to recede. Consciousness increasingly takes up the position of an observer and witness of the mind, and becomes less identified with it. Relationships borne out of this level of consciousness are selfless and magnanimous.

5 The fifth chakra level represents a quickening towards the energy of the collective unconscious. With dis-identification of the ego comes an influx of higher consciousness that seeks creative expression. Huxley (1961) describes an experience of these higher levels of consciousness as a positive transfiguration of the external world, so that it seems over-whelmingly beautiful, alive and shining. Creative genius may flow from access to this level, and relationships formed at this level are characterised by a shared commitment to higher goals. Western psychology has generally assumed that this is the highest stage a person can reach in life, and pathologises the next two stages, which are recognised and valued only in the Eastern way of thinking (Nelson, 1994).

6 The sixth chakra, also known as the 'third eye', represents a more complete opening to the transpersonal. It is the vehicle of extra-sensory perceptions and accesses the highest spiritual realm of the phenomenal world.

7   The seventh (or crown) chakra represents the numinal world of non-duality and marks a return of self to Source. There is no observer and no observed; there are no boundaries, no thoughts and no words; the experience is beyond time and space. This is Samadhi as described by mystics and contemplatives, who have attained a numinous, ineffable state, where the significance of all things is experienced at its most meaningful and subtle.

Experiences of the higher three levels (5, 6 & 7) may be so different to our Western consensual reality that the distinction from psychosis can be problematic (Scotton, 1996b). Such unitive mystical states may be confused with psychotic regression. Indeed, appreciating the difference between the ego's need to attach to a secure parental figure and the possibility of a transcendent aspect of oneself joining in oneness with God is a continuing point of disagreement between traditional and transpersonal schools of psychology. Psychoanalysis has traditionally seen meditation as a search for the gratification of primary narcissism, although more recently there has been a shift towards recognition that there are different types of 'oneness experience', some of which can be healthy and can lead to a shift in the internal organisation of the psyche (Falkenstrom, 2003).

Philosophy, physics and parapsychology

> The universe is more like a great thought than a great machine.
>
> Sir James Jeans (1931)

The nature of reality and how it is experienced by our conscious mind has been one of the crucial questions pondered by philosophers. Plato suggested in *The Republic* that our interpretation of reality is but a pale shadow of the underlying reality. Kant's central thesis was that the mind imposed its own cognitive structure on the world it experienced; thus humankind's knowledge of the world through scientific observation is never a description of external reality as such, but always the product of man's cognitive apparatus (Tarnas, 1991). The physicist and Nobel Prize winner David Bohm (1980) hypothesised that there exists an underlying reality, the 'implicate order'. He believed that it had holographic properties, so that accessing a part of it allows access to the whole. The implicate order unfolds into the 'explicate order', which is our world of perceived reality. Further, the implicate order is a unity and is not understandable according to the rules of space–time. The primary organising structure of the implicate order is meaning, thus matter and meaning are inseparable. Bohm used the term 'soma significance' to emphasise this unity between consciousness and matter.

According to Bohm, it is possible that meaning and significance can be infinitely extended to ever greater levels of subtlety and complexity that go far beyond the capacity of the brain as a finite structure. In the same way that there are light frequencies that the eye cannot see and sound frequencies that we cannot hear, there may be meanings and ranges of meaning that the psyche, as a sense organ, cannot usually gather. One way of understanding a NOSC is that this subtle informational field becomes more accessible. In this way transpersonal experience may be related more to the implicate order than to our ordinary waking reality.

Fritz Capra (1976) and Gary Zukav (1979) were the first to popularise the similarities between quantum physics and the emerging mystical and transpersonal synthesis of the 1960s. The 'new physics' challenged the certainties of the Newtonian era. For example, the notion of a fixed objective reality had been overturned, since quantum physics had shown that what we take to be 'reality' is the product of consciousness. Experiments with photons showed that once entangled, they remain connected even when widely separated in space, providing evidence for the interconnected nature of the universe. The strangeness of the new physics seemed in tune with the transpersonal paradigm, fostered a flowering of conceptual thinking and renewing a sense of the unknowable. In this vein, Lynne McTaggart (2001) and Ervin Laszlo (2004) have argued the case for the zero point field as the substrate for consciousness, the explanation for psychic phenomena (psi) and the location of the collective unconscious.

At the same time, there has been criticism of the inappropriate adoption of physics to suit favoured concepts. Wilber (1984) studied the writings of the world's great physicists to find that they considered physics and mysticism as essentially addressing different domains despite there being significant parallels, and that quantum physics does not definitely confirm mystical insights. Chris Clarke and Michael King (2006) also disagree with Laszlo and McTaggart's interpretation of the zero point field, noting that these claims do not seem to be supported by hard science and that such approaches actually close down the essentially paradoxical nature of the new physics.

Such a clash of viewpoints is hardly surprising, given the enormous significance of whether consciousness is produced by the brain or exists independently of the brain. This is why parapsychological research is so hotly debated. Among many varieties of psi, the strongest scientific evidence has been presented for psychokinesis and telepathy. Psychokinesis involves the ability of mind to influence matter. Robert Jahn and colleagues (1997) have accumulated a robust database showing small but measurable results in favour of psychokinesis using random number generators. Ganzfeld studies measure how people under mild sensory deprivation can accurately visualise unseen objects at a distance (remote viewing or clairvoyance) and meta-analysis again shows positive results, especially with visual targets (Radin, 2006). The conclusion is that psi must be a plausible theory.

Shamanism and shamanic states of consciousness

Non-ordinary states of consciousness have played an important role in shaping the cultural and spiritual life of our species, with shamanism, meditation and the use of entheogens or sacred medicine having been part of human society for thousands of years.

'Shaman' is a term used by anthropologists for a special kind of medicine man or woman who deliberately enters non-ordinary states of consciousness in order to journey to 'other realities' and encounter 'other entities', both human and animal, to bring about the required healing for an individual or community. Shamans consider the content and nature of these experiences to be an authentic expression of the psyche in direct connection with the cosmos. Even in shamanic cultures, becoming a shaman is a hazardous calling, involving a rite of passage often initiated by a serious physical illness or difficult and unusual transpersonal experiences. These cultures make a clear distinction between people who are shamans and those who are mentally ill (Kalweit, 1989).

Harner (1980) has identified certain core features of shamanism that are similar the world over, even when the cultures are very different in other respects. He reports that the shamanic states of consiousness can be readily accessed by listening to a drum beat of 200 to 220 beats per minute; in the West this technique is increasingly being used as a method of personal growth and exploration.

Shamanic rituals have been largely dismissed as primitive by Western medicine, but indigenous practice continues in many parts of the world and psychiatrists need to find ways of working with these belief systems, if they want to be able to work in a transcultural context.

Within indigenous cultures, the sacred practice of expansion of consciousness would be undertaken as part of a ritual imbued with meaning and within the context of a stable cultural tradition. In today's Western culture, the chaotic and irreverent use of illicit drugs has replaced this. However, far from bringing about integration of aspects of the psyche, it produces fragmentation, both within the individual and within the global community.

In recent years, further non-drug methods have been developed which can readily induce non-ordinary states with the use of audio sound patterns. Robert Munroe sums up a vast body of research on 'out-of-body experiences' in his three books (Munroe, 1971, 1985, 1994) that essentially describe the uncovering of an aspect of a transcendental or higher self, aided by listening to specific sound frequencies. However, application of these techniques does not confer instant enlightenment. Bache (2003) suggests, rather, that permanent change becomes ingrained through the repeated immersion in higher levels of consciousness and by integrating the experience through regular spiritual practice.

There is a natural propensity for human beings to seek spiritual experience. Psychiatrists are all too aware of the devastating consequences of psychotic breakdown when people seek escapism into NOSC outside of a safe setting, yet they also need to be informed about research that highlights the positive transformational potential of mystical experiences.

Researching the transpersonal field

There have been many anecdotal reports describing the transformative potential of mystical experience (case study 11.5), but such spontaneous events are notoriously difficult to research. Mystical experiences are common, reported overall by about a third of the population in the UK and the USA (McCready & Greeley, 1976; Hay, 1987) and although these experiences are transient, they may have lasting effects.

In the 1960s, research focused on inducing mystical states of mind through the use of entheogens to see whether this could provide a more informative evidence base. Many pioneers devoted their careers to this field, hoping that entheogenic drugs could become to psychiatry what the microscope is to biology or the telescope to astronomy – an essential tool to explore the parts of the internal world that are usually inaccessible (Sessa, 2005). Despite the volume of publications from this period, most of the published material refers to anecdotal case reports that are of limited value by contemporary research standards because they lack sufficient follow-up and controls (Grob, 1994). Nevertheless, one of the main lessons from research into individual case studies has been the importance of 'set' and 'setting', the set being the mental and developmental state of the participant and the setting being the nature of the environment. A gentle, contemplative, spiritually-orientated setting with the intention of opening to higher levels of consciousness predisposes to a beneficial spiritual experience.

Entheogens may be particularly useful for those facing death. A study of LSD usage in people who were terminally ill found a reduced need for analgesics, with improved mood and reduced fear of death in 60–70% of participants. The treatment response seemed to be correlated with the extent to which the participants experienced a mystical or transcendent state (Kast, 1966; Pahnke *et al*, 1969; Grof *et al*, 1973). In another study. S. W. Holmes *et al* (1996) concluded that holotropic breathwork led to significant reductions in death anxiety and increases in self-esteem relative to traditional, verbally oriented psychotherapy.

Case study 11.5

Robert, a 35-year-old fireman, had a 5-year history of severe post-traumatic stress disorder causing severe occupational and social disability. He swam out to sea as a suicide attempt and was on the point of drowning when he experienced an overwhelming experience of joy, peace and unity accompanied by a bright light. He was rescued and reported that the symptoms of his post-traumatic stress disorder went into remission. He was able gradually to discontinue psychotropic medication. He told his psychiatrist that the spiritual experience had given him a new perspective and transformed his life.

More recently, R. R. Griffiths *et al* (2006) performed a double-blind study administering either psilocybin or methylphenidate in a non-clinical and supportive setting to volunteers who had not previously taken mind-altering substances and who had a regular spiritual or religious activity. Of the 36 participants, 22 described a mystical experience following the use of psilocybin, compared with 4 after methylphenidate; 8 felt significant anxiety or dysphoria during the session, which did not, however, persist and was felt to be of no lasting importance. At the 2-month follow-up, 67% rated the psilocybin experience as either the single most meaningful or in the top five meaningful experiences of their lives, compared with only 8% with methylphenidate. These participants reported that psilocybin enhanced their attitudes about life in general, their mood and their relationships with others and this was confirmed by independent ratings from family and friends. This well-designed study shows the potential of a pharmacologically induced NOSC, in sharp contrast to the cultural abuse of such drugs.

Spiritual emergency

Spiritual emergency is a term first coined by Stanislav and Christina Grof (1989) to describe a range of dramatic experiences and unusual states of mind that suggest both a crisis and an opportunity of rising to a new level of awareness or 'spiritual emergence'.

Symptoms of a spiritual emergency often involve an intensification of feeling, visions and perceptual changes, unusual thought processes and a variety of physical sensations often in combination with spiritual themes. The presentation of spiritual emergencies ranges from a simple yet profound experience of psychological renewal and individuation, through to 'peak experiences' (episodes of unitive consciousness), 'the shamanic crisis', 'past life experiences', 'near death experiences', 'possession states' and the awakening of 'kundalini' (see pp. 228–229) (Grof & Grof, 1989).

Among the causes of the spiritual emergency are physical factors such as accidents, operations, extreme physical exertion, fasting, sleep deprivation, childbirth, miscarriage, abortion or powerful sexual experience; psychological factors such as traumatic emotional experiences involving devastating loss or failure; and spiritual factors such as partaking in shamanic ritual, the practice of yoga (kundalini, tantra, hatha, raja), Sufi Zikr, Kabbalistic practice, Christian prayer (monastic contemplation and Hesychasm in the Orthodox church), Buddhist meditation (zen, vipassana, vajrayana) and Taoist meditation (Grof & Grof, 1989). In fact, meditation can cause a variety of symptoms as side-effects, including agitation, depression and euphoria, as well as psychotic symptoms (Epstein & Lieff, 1981).

Case study 11.6 describes a brief, transient psychotic episode, which also fits the description of a classical kundalini experience and usefully illustrates Assagioli's four stages of spiritual transformation (Assagioli, 1989):

1   Crisis preceding the spiritual awakening – existential conflict.
2   Crisis of spiritual awakening – inrush of energy, ego inflation, 'psychotic' symptoms.
3   Reactions following spiritual awakening – the 'dark night of the soul'.
4   The processes of transmutation, integration and assimilation.

Assagioli notes that spiritual awakenings are usually associated with psychological disturbance and that pre-existing problems in personality development and emotional conflicts tend to be brought to the surface (Assagioli, 1989). The crucial point here is that spiritual development alone, without due attention being paid to intra-psychic and interpersonal issues, can lead to psychological imbalance. The initial inflow of spiritual energy experienced in a spiritual emergency may cover the sharp edges of personality with a veneer of peace and love; but as the spiritual energy ebbs, the personality reverts to the previous state. What remains is a memory of the 'spiritual awakening' and, ideally, a model to help articulate what has happened for the person and a signpost for subsequent spiritual growth, grounded within a balanced, maturing personality.

The term 'dark night of the soul' is taken from the writings of the Spanish poet and Roman Catholic mystic Saint John of the Cross, a Carmelite priest living in the 16th century, who experienced profound loneliness and desolation while in prison. He wrote *The Dark Night of the Soul* on a scroll smuggled to him by one of his guards and it has come to stand for the ultimate expression of the journey from estranged despair towards blissful union with the Divine (Starr, 2002).

Assagioli writes about the dark night of the soul as a crucial stage in the crisis of spiritual development. He asserts that 'the therapist can give much

---

Case study 11.6

Rebecca became profoundly unhappy in mid-life, with an acute and painful tension between her outwardly successful life and a sense of not living the life that was right for her. She disengaged from her job and marriage to 'make space'. A crisis developed over a 2-week period with a massive energy snaking around her body, the sensation of heat coming out of her feet and extraordinary spontaneous orgasms. She thought she was dying. She started to see colours and miniature angels. She then had an experience of feeling cosmic unity and seeing white light and experienced an archangel telling her she was to give birth to Christ.

For 5 days Rebecca was convinced she was the Virgin Mary, after which her awareness shifted back into ordinary day-to-day reality. Following this experience, she underwent prolonged transpersonal psychotherapy (psychosynthesis) to integrate and understand her experiences. She had a subsequent experience of a similar energy which was not overwhelming. She came to see her experience of carrying Christ as a symbolic opening of the heart chakra and now believes that she lives her life transformed by an experience of universal love.

help by assuring him [the patient] that his present condition is temporary and not in any sense permanent or hopeless as he seems compelled to believe' (Assagioli, 1965: p. 56).

The word *kundalini* derives from the yoga tradition and is described as an energy that can be awakened either spontaneously or intentionally as part of a spiritual practice. Kundalini has long been recognised in India. In the West it is now being seen increasingly by clinicians and is associated with both positive and negative outcomes (Scotton, 1996b; Galbraith, 1999; Thomas, 2000; Lane 2003). A classic kundalini experience (Sanella, 1978) begins with the energy (*prana*) arising 'like a coiled serpent' from the base of the spine (root chakra) and ascending through each chakra in turn, overcoming 'impurities' as part of a process of spiritual purification. The rising energy can be experienced as powerful and terrifying, or ecstatic. Uncontrolled kundalini can cause an excited, quasi-psychotic state that needs careful differentiation from a functional psychosis.

Scotton (1996b) and House (2001) suggest that interventions designed to treat kundalini without suppressing symptoms with conventional psychiatric treatment produce better outcomes. Sanella (1978) suggests that kundalini is a psycho-spiritual state unfolding with the following characteristics:

- motor phenomena including automatic body movements and postures, unusual breathing patterns and occasionally paralysis
- sensory phenomena including tickling, heat and cold sensations, inner lights and visions, inner sounds
- interpretive phenomena such as unusual or extreme emotion, distortions of thought processes, detachment, dissociation
- neurophysiological phenomena such as out-of-body experiences and paranormal experiences.

Strategies for treating spiritual emergency

Therapeutic interventions for a person experiencing an adaptive altered state of consciousness can include (from Lukoff, 1996b):

- normalisation (a framework of understanding)
- 'grounding' (includes exercise, whole-food diet)
- reduction of environmental and interpersonal stimulation
- temporary discontinuation of spiritual practices
- encouragement of creative therapies (art, music, writing, poetry, dance)
- creation of a therapeutic encounter/transpersonal psychotherapy
- consideration for specific bodywork (e.g. biodynamic massage)
- evaluating for medication (a necessary clinical decision may need to be made between allowing the 'psychotic' experience full expression with natural resolution or using medication to suppress symptoms in order to alleviate damaging psychological distress).

Conclusion

The aim of this chapter has been to introduce the transpersonal perspective: its short history; its expansion of our understanding of the human psyche to include the transpersonal and perinatal domains; the therapeutic value of mystical experiences; and how adaptive psychotic symptoms such as those experienced in a spiritual emergence or emergency can be recognised as such, and if properly facilitated, enable personal growth and maturation.

At the root of the transpersonal perspective is the idea that there is a deep level of subjectivity, consciousness or pure spirit that infuses matter and every event. It is necessary for all sentient life, experience and awareness only being possible through activating the life force that flows from this Source (Nelson, 1994).

Pioneering work into the nature of consciousness has been controversial. However, its findings are relevant to a psychiatry that extends itself beyond the bio-mechanical model and includes the concept of consciousness in its understanding of the mind–brain–body continuum.

If consciousness is recognised to be more than just secondary to brain function and the concept of levels of consciousness is acknowledged as relevant to understanding unusual mental states, then the transpersonal perspective affords us an opportunity to build a modern scientific theory of mental illness around a radically expanded view of consciousness. The case for a deeper understanding of non-ordinary, or altered, therapeutic states of consciousness becomes, once again, relevant for psychiatry.

References

American Psychiatric Association (1994) *Diagnostic and Statistical Manual of Mental Disorders* (4th edn) (DSM–IV). APA.

Assagioli, R. (1965) *Psychosynthesis*. Hobbs Dorman.

Assagioli, R. (1975) *Psychosynthesis: A Collection of Basic Writings*. Turnstone Press.

Assagioli, R. (1989) Self-realization and psychological disturbances. In *Spiritual Emergency – When Personal Transformation Becomes a Crisis* (eds S. Grof & C. Grof), pp. 27–48. Penguin Putnam.

Bache, C. M. (2003) Is the sacred medicine path a legitimate spiritual path? *Scientific and Medical Network Review*, **81**, 19–22.

Bohm, D. (1980) *Wholeness and the Implicate Order*. Routledge.

Capra, F. (1976) *Tao of Physics*. Fontana.

Clarke, C. & King, M. (2006) Laszlo and McTaggart – in the light of this thing called physics. *Scientific and Medical Network Review*, **92**, 6–11.

Clarke, I. (2001) *Psychosis and Spirituality*. Whurr.

Epstein, M. & Lieff, J. (1981) Psychiatric complications of meditation practice. *Journal of Transpersonal Psychology*, **13**, 57.

Falkenstrom, F. (2003) A Buddhist contribution to the psychoanalytic psychology of self. *International Journal of Psychoanalysis*, **84**, 1551–1568.

Galbraith, J. (1999) Is spiritual emergence up the spine always a benign process? *Scientific and Medical Network Review*, **71**, 11–14.

Goodwin, F. & Jamison, K., (1990) *Manic Depressive Illness*. Oxford University Press.

Griffiths, R. R., Richards, W. A., McCann, U., *et al* (2006) Psilocybin can occasion mystical-type experiences having substantial and sustained personal meaning and spiritual significance. *Psychopharmacology*, **11 July**, 41–50.

Grob, C. (1994) Psychiatric research with hallucinogens: what have we learned? In *Yearbook for Ethnomedicine* (eds C. Ratsch & J. Baker). Verlag für Wissenschaft und Bildung.

Grof, S., (1975) *Realms of the Human Unconscious: Observations from LSD Research*. Viking Press.

Grof, S. (1985) *Beyond the Brain*. State University of New York Press.

Grof, S. (1988) *The Adventure of Self Discovery*. State University of New York Press.

Grof, S. (2000) *Psychology of the Future*. State University of New York Press.

Grof, S. & Grof, C. (1989) *Spiritual Emergency: When Personal Transformation Becomes a Crisis*. Penguin Putnam.

Grof, S., Goodman, L. E., Richards, W. A., *et al* (1973) LSD-assisted psychotherapy in patients with terminal cancer. *International Pharmacopsychiatry*, **8**, 129–144.

Harner, M. (1980) *The Way of the Shaman*. Harper & Row.

Hay, D. (1987) *Exploring Inner Space* (2nd edn). Penguin.

Hoeller, S. A. (1982) *The Gnostic Jung*. Quest.

Holmes, S. W., Morris, R., Clance, P. R., *et al* (1996) Holotropic breathwork: an experiential approach to psychotherapy. *Psychotherapy: Theory, Research, Practice, Training*, **33**, 114–120.

House, R. (2001) Psychopathology, psychosis and kundalini. In *Psychosis and Spirituality* (ed. C. Clarke). Whurr.

Huxley, A. (1961) Visionary experience. In *Moksha*. pp. 190–209. Park Street Press.

Jahn, R. G., Dunne, B., Nelson, R. D. *et al* (1997) Correlations of random primary binary sequences with pre-stated operator intention: a review of the 12-year programme. *Journal of Scientific Exploration*, **11**, 345–367.

James, W. (1902) *The Varieties of Religious Experience: A Study in Human Nature*. Collins Fontana Library.

Jeans, J. (1931) *The Mysterious Universe*. Cambridge University Press.

Jung, C. (1935) *Analytical Psychology in Theory and Practice – The Tavistock Lectures*. Routledge Kegan Paul.

Jung, C. (1958) *Foreword to the I Ching, Commentary on The Tibetan Book of the Great Liberation, Commentary on the Tibetan book of the Dead and Forward to Introduction to Zen Buddhism*. Collected works. Princeton University Press.

Jung, C. (1961) *Memories, Dreams, Reflections*. Random House.

Jung, C. (1972) *Synchronicity: An Acausal Connecting Principle*. Routledge & Kegan Paul.

Jung, C. (1981) *The Archetypes and The Collective Unconscious (Collected Works of C. G. Jung*, Vol. 9) (2nd end) (transl. G. Adler & R. F. C. Hull). Princeton University Press, Bollingen series.

Kalweit, H. (1989) When insanity is a blessing: the message of shamanism. In *Spiritual Emergency: When Personal Transformation Becomes a Crisis* (eds S. Grof & C. Grof). Tarcher Putnam.

Kast, E. (1966) LSD and the dying patient. *Chicago Medical School Quarterly*, **26**, 80–87.

Laing, R. D. (1965a) *The Divided Self: An Existential Study in Sanity and Madness*. Penguin.

Laing, R. D. (1965b) Transcendental experience in relation to religion and psychosis. *Psychedelic Review*, **6**, 7–15.

Lane, S. (2003) Kundalini – experiential and theoretical aspects. *Scientific and Medical Network Review*, **81**, 26.

Laszlo, E. (2004) *Science and the Akashic Field*. Rochester.

Lukoff, D. (1996a) Transpersonal psychotherapy with psychotic disorders and spiritual emergencies with psychotic features. In *Textbook of Transpersonal Psychiatry and Psychology* (eds B. Scotton, A. Chinon & J. Battista). Basic Books.

Lukoff, D. (1996*b*) Diagnosis: a transpersonal clinical approach to religious and spiritual problems. In *Textbook of Transpersonal Psychiatry and Psychology* (eds B. Scotton, A. Chinon & J. Battista). Basic Books.

Maslow, A. (1964) *Religions, Values and Peak Experiences*. Ohio State University Press.

McCready, W. C. & Greeley, A. M. (1976) *The Ultimate Values of the American Population*. Sage.

McLynn, F. (1996) *Carl Gustav Jung*. pp. 233–252. St Martins Griffin.

McTaggart, L. (2001) *The Field*. HarperCollins.

Munroe, R. (1971) *Journeys Out of the Body*. Bantam Doubleday Dell.

Munroe, R. (1985) *Far Journeys*. Bantam Doubleday Dell.

Munroe, R. (1994) *The Ultimate Journey*. Bantam Doubleday Dell.

Nelson J. (1994) *Healing the Split*. State University of New York Press.

Pahnke, W. N., Kurland, A. A., Goodman, L. E., *et al* (1969) LSD-assisted psychotherapy with terminal cancer patients. *Current Psychiatric Therapies*, **9**, 144–152.

Powell, A. (2003) *Love and the Near Life Experience*. Royal College of Psychiatrists (http://www.rcpsych.ac.uk/pdf/Andrew%20Powell%20Love%20and%20the%20Near%20Life%20Experience.x.pdf).

Radin, D. (2006) *Entangled Minds*. Paraview.

Samuels, A., Shorter, B. & Plaut, F. (1986) *A Critical Dictionary of Jungian Analysis*. Routledge.

Sanella, L. (1978) *Kundalini: Transcendence or Psychosis?* Dakin.

Scotton, B. W. (1996*a*) Introduction and definition of transpersonal psychiatry. In *Textbook of Transpersonal Psychiatry and Psychology* (eds A. B. Chinen, J. R. Battista & B. W. Scotton). pp. 2–8. Basic Books.

Scotton, B. W. (1996*b*) The phenomenology and treatment of kundalini. In *Textbook of Transpersonal Psychiatry and Psychology* (eds A. B. Chinen, J. R. Battista & B. W. Scotton). pp. 261–270. Basic Books.

Sessa, B. (2005) Can psychedelics have a role in psychiatry once again? *British Journal of Psychiatry*, **186**, 457–458.

Starr, M. (2002) *Dark Night of the Soul*. Random House.

Tarnas, R. (1991) *The Passion of the Western Mind*. Crown.

Tarnas, R. (2006) *Cosmos and Psyche*. Penguin, p. 53.

Thomas, K. (2000) *The Kundalini Phenomena*. New Media Books.

Vich, M. A. (1988) Some historical sources for the term 'transpersonal'. *Journal of Transpersonal Psychology*, **20**, 107–110.

Wilber, K. (1977) *The Spectrum of Consciousness*. Quest.

Wilber, K. (1980) The pre-trans fallacy. *Revision*, **3**, 64.

Wilber, K. (ed.) (1984) *Quantum Questions: Mystical Writings of the World's Great Physicists*. Shambhala.

Wilber, K. (1995) *Sex, Ecology and Spirituality*, Vol. 1. Shambhala.

Wilber, K., Engler, J. & Brown, D. (eds) (1986) *Transformations of Consciousness*. Shambhala.

Zukav, G. (1979) *The Dancing Wu Li Masters*. William Morrow.

CHAPTER 12

Religion and religious experiences

Mohamed Omar Salem and John Foskett

In this chapter we aim to show how religious beliefs relate to the wider concept of spirituality and to the practice of psychiatry. We concur with the definition of spirituality given in chapter 1, where it was stated that for the purpose of this book 'it might be helpful to emphasise that religion is concerned with socially and traditionally shared beliefs and experience' (p. 4).

Spirituality comprises a major part of religious tradition and practice, along with doctrine, scripture, ritual and worship. Within the broad spiritual tradition of each religion, there is the personal and unique spirituality of each adherent. Yet there is also the possibility of someone being religious in name only, as when someone has been raised in a religious community, but rejects its spiritual component. We are distinguishing here between intrinsic religiosity, which implies taking the teachings of religion seriously, and extrinsic religiosity that involves a 'selfish and instrumental' use of religion (Hunt & King, 1972). Batson *et al* (1993) suggested a positive relationship between intrinsic religiosity and a number of measures of mental health, while extrinsic religiosity related to poor mental health.

We wish to see an open-mindedness in mental healthcare that enables the acquisition of a wider knowledge base through learning from the experiences brought by our patients – the best possible way to gain confidence and skills. We will identify the often under-used resources for this work within the health service in relation to multidisciplinary teams, provisions for chaplaincy and spiritual care departments, and with religious organisations in the community at large. We will look at how service outreach can be supported, using religious buildings as less stigmatising and more user-friendly places for care and treatment.

Psychiatrists should know about the world views held by their patients, as they affect decision-making in health and illness; religious concepts and experiences contribute importantly to such world views. For example, knowing the religious affiliation of a person with a suicidal intent, including his or her concept of the afterlife, can help the psychiatrist evaluate risk (Hassan, 1983; Mahy, 1993). However, mental health professionals have only limited time to engage with and understand the religious beliefs of their patients when faced with the increasingly complex ideas, practices and traditions of the many faiths in our growingly multicultural societies. The only way forward for the mental health specialist is not to assume an understanding of what a person's faith means to them, but rather to ask and learn from that individual.

From theory to practice

> The community nurse was terrific. Although he was not a Christian, he asked me very pertinent questions about how I reconciled my faith with what was happening to me and what God meant to me. He was very helpful and made me think a lot [Nicholls, 2002: p. 25].

How, what and why we believe is unique to each of us. Thus we would emphasise the central importance of the patient's experience.

> Ultimately, the lesson to be learnt from our patients is that each one of them – is a human being in his/her entire dignity – is the teacher at the point we meet him/her ... And the teacher is in pain. S/he will use his/her own language to express this pain, one that the professional can decode more effectively with a change of attitude, practice and wider knowledge base [Lawrence, 2003: p. 18].

For this reason, although it is important for psychiatrists to be informed about the major faith traditions, we advocate a broad-based generic approach to religion in clinical psychiatric practice. We believe such an approach is the most practical way to help busy professionals think about the religious beliefs of their patients and react creatively and therapeutically to them. This approach is concerned with all religions. Research in this field is still in its infancy (Cornah, 2006), but we shall explore the implications for mental healthcare in relation to its wider social aspects and in particular working with multi-faith communities.

We recognise the historical residue of suspicion between psychiatry and religion and its effect upon this area of work (Levin, 1994; Loewenthal, 1995). For many in the health service, religion remains psychiatry's last taboo and many religious believers still think most psychiatrists regard religion as being at best irrelevant to mental health, and at worst delusional and a symptom of mental illness. Both views have inclined professionals to keep their distance (Neeleman & King, 1993; Neeman & Persaud, 1994; Foskett et al, 2004) and for the most part it has been patients who have taken the lead in bringing about a change of attitude (Macmin & Foskett, 2004). We will be paying special attention to patients' experiences in this chapter and discuss at length the poems of Premila Trivedi, who has made a major contribution to the body of work of mental health services users and survivors. Two of her poems help to illustrate the place that religion played in her story and the stories of so many fellow patients.

In the following poem, Trivedi explores her complex relationship with her Hindu faith. In childhood, it overwhelmed her and she had to free herself from its demands:

> Growing up, I constantly saw it in front of me,
> My Hindu faith
> Holding us in, controlling us
> Dictating every aspect of our lives.

[Trivedi, 2007: p. 67]

Many patients have a similar experience of how their faith repressed and controlled them and how they had to free themselves in order to define their own spirituality, either separately or within the tradition in which they grew up. Mental health crises can be times of such freeing and rediscovering, if time, space and attention are given to this process. As Trivedi grew away from and 'bypassed' her faith she did not realise how 'embedded it remained in her soul'. Following a breakdown, she was hospitalised and had a different experience of oppression, which she illustrated in an untitled poem:

> Valium, psychiatrists, falling more into the abyss
> Of white man's medicine
> Hospital, enforced activity, constant cajoling
> To fit their characterisation of me,
> All the time denying me; my pain, my hurt, my confusion.

> And in the end I saw it their way, the guilt was mine.
> So I have the privilege of existing in their world –
> Of experiencing their values, their beliefs
> Their prejudice, their power.
> What does it matter that I died in the process.

[Trivedi, 1992: p. 82]

Returning to Trivedi's first poem, in the second part she speaks of her rediscovery of her Hindu faith and its place in a time of tragedy. When her sister died, the family found in their religious tradition a vehicle for mourning:

> And we came together in our grief
> To say prayers and sing bhajans,
> To help her on her journey into the next life
> And then, gathered together once more,
> Our hearts ached and our tears flowed freely
> As the pundit lit a holy fire to purify the air
> And said some final prayers
> Completing my sister's ceremony
> Enabling her to move on.

[Trivedi, 2007: p. 69]

For many patients, this story will resonate with their own experience of ambivalence about their faith tradition, and how the mental health services can compound their problems by ignoring or belittling its importance.

Trivedi found a companion in her search for meaning in an unlikely place – the chaplain helped her talk through her grief in his acknowledgement of her soul. The fact she was Hindu and he was Christian was irrelevant. How people are received by their religious and mental health professionals can make an enormous difference to the outcome of their crisis and their eventual well-being.

Religion and mental health

Religion plays a central role in the lives of people across the world. Patients seek healing not just for physical or emotional pain but also for a sense of wholeness and wellness. They turn to psychiatrists both for help with their conflicts and symptoms and to find meaning and purpose in their lives as they struggle with difficult situations. Such themes interleave with the patient's world view, including his or her religion. Psychiatrists and psychologists previously neglected this important area (Sims, 1994; Pargament, 1997), but in recent years there has been a growing number of published studies examining the relationship of religion to health in general and to mental health in particular (Salem, 2006).

Recent empirical research has shown convincingly that religious devoutness and commitment is usually positively associated with healthy physical, emotional and social functioning. It extends the individual's coping resources, offers hope and helps give meaning to suffering. Depression, alcohol misuse, drug misuse, anxiety disorders and suicide have been found at lower rates among persons who are more involved with religion (Khavari & Harmon, 1982; Koenig *et al*, 1992, 1993, 1994; Stack, 1983). Also, there are biological data suggesting that those who are active in religion may have a stronger immune system (Koenig, 1997). Religious conversion has been associated with major transformations in pathological social conduct, showing that religion can powerfully shape an individual's identity (Paloutzian *et al*, 1999).

The world's major faith traditions

The three major monotheistic faiths today are Judaism, Christianity and Islam. Together, they are also sometimes referred to as the 'Abrahamic' religions, reflecting their common tradition of Abraham as ancestor (taken literally in Judaism and Islam and as a 'father of the faithful' in Christianity). These three religions all originated in the Near and Middle East.

'Eastern' religions include Hinduism, Sikhism, Jainism, Buddhism, Shintoism and Taoism. Of these, Buddhism, Taoism and Shintoism do not hold to the concept of belief in a personal, eternal God. Shintoism (2.8 million believers)[1] is indigenous to Japan and entails a reverence for

---

1   The figures cited in this chapter are from the *World Christian Encyclopedia* (Barrett *et al*, 2001).

family traditions, cleanliness and nature, all of which is regarded as infused with sacred powers, spirits or divine beings known as *kami*. Taoism (2.7 million),[2] the main subset of Chinese traditional religion, has influenced various other religions, especially Buddhism. The *tao* (translated as 'path' or 'way') emphasises 'wu-wei' or 'effortless doing', through finding harmony with the natural balance of nature, with the 'three jewels' of compassion, moderation and humility, but the *tao* is also understood to be the source and ground of all things. The *Tao Te Ching*, probably written sometime between the 5th and 3rd centuries BCE by the Chinese sage Lao Tzu, is regarded as the foundation text.

The Abrahamic traditions

Judaism

Although a relatively small religion when considering the number of followers (14.4 million), Judaism is the historical foundation stone of the Abrahamic faiths. The Hebrew Scriptures, which form the *Old Testament* of the Christian *Bible*, describe the creation of the world by one God and give an account of the history of the Hebrew people as the offspring of the patriarchs: Abraham, Isaac and Jacob (later called Israel). To these people, as Jews, Christians and Muslims believe, God gave the 'Torah' or law. Today, a distinction is often made between cultural Judaism, which does not necessarily observe traditional religious beliefs, and religious Judaism, which accepts the teachings of the Torah. Jewish scriptures comprise the Torah, the Nevi'im (prophets) and the Kethuvim (writings). A defining event in the Hebrew Scriptures is that of the exodus of the Hebrew people under the leadership of Moses from slavery in Egypt to freedom in the 'promised' land of Canaan. This account attributes deliverance from slavery to the miraculous intervention of God, notably by parting of the waters of the sea that had prevented the escape of the Hebrews from Egypt. Hebrew scripture thus gives testimony to an ongoing relationship between God and human beings, and particularly to an ongoing relationship between God and the Jewish people. Contemporary Judaism is expressed in various ways, including orthodox, liberal and reformed traditions.

Christianity

Christianity (2 billion)[3] developed from within the Hebrew tradition and, at least until the Jewish–Roman war of *c.* 70 CE, was initially understood

---

2   The true figure for Taoism is actually very difficult to estimate, partly because it is more a philosophy than an institution, and partly because it overlaps with traditional Chinese religion. The actual worldwide adherence is therefore probably nearer 20 to 50 million.

3   More space is devoted here to Christianity, and later to Islam, than to other faith traditions based on the number of worldwide adherents. Approximately a third of the world's population today identify themselves as Christian and approximately one-fifth as Muslim.

as a sect within Judaism rather than as a separate religion. Central to the Christian tradition are four accounts (known as Gospels) of the life of Jesus of Nazareth, a prophet who lived in Palestine and who was executed by the Romans around 30–33 CE. The Gospels record the teachings of Jesus, miraculous healings, his birth, death and, crucially, his resurrection by God. They present a picture of a man popular with ordinary people, known for the wisdom and compassion of his teaching and unpopular with religious authorities, who felt threatened by the following that he attracted. This appears to have led to his being handed over to the Roman executioners for death by crucifixion. This historical event was subsequently taken up by the Gospel writers and others as being central to Christian faith. In it was found a basis for meaning in human suffering, forgiveness for moral evil (or 'sin'), and relationship between God and human beings.

The belief that God raised Jesus from the dead was defining of early Christianity, based on accounts of an empty tomb and of a series of personal encounters with the risen Jesus by anything from one to several hundred individuals. In this belief was found hope of resurrection from the dead and eternal life for all Christians. After several centuries of theological debate, the Church Councils asserted that Jesus was God 'incarnate' – that is, in Jesus God had come to earth in human form. It was claimed not only that Jesus was fully God, but also that he was fully human – thus asserting two apparently irreconcilable opposites. From this there developed a similarly paradoxical belief that God, being indivisibly one, is also three persons in the form of the Trinity of Father, Son and Holy Spirit. In addition to the Gospels, Christian scriptures (*The New Testament*) include an account of early Church history (*The Acts of the Apostles*), various letters written by apostles (leaders of the early Church) and a prophetic book (*The Revelation to John*). A division into Eastern (Orthodox) and Western (Catholic) branches of the Christian Church took place at the great schism of 1054 CE. Contemporary Western Christianity recognises two further divisions, into Protestant and Catholic, which developed in the course of the 16th-century European Reformation.

Christianity today is expressed in diverse ways. Creedal orthodoxy proclaims the historical events of the birth, life, death and resurrection of Jesus, the doctrine of the Trinity, and the forgiveness of sins. But, in practice, differences are most often found in variations of expression of the relationship between God and human beings. For Catholics, Christ becomes present in a real and special way in the bread and wine consumed at the Eucharist (or mass: a service deriving from the last meal of Jesus with his disciples). For most Protestants the bread and wine are received more as symbols and encounter with God is seen more as taking place through the words of scripture and preaching. For Pentecostal Christians, and so-called 'charismatics' in other denominations, the emphasis is on encounter with God the Holy Spirit, mediated by experiences such as glossolalia ('speaking in tongues'), prophecy and the ministries of both healing and deliverance from the forces of evil.

Islam

Islam (1.2 billion) derives from the Semitic word for peace (*shalom*), meaning submission to God, or peace through surrender to God. Islam shares the Abrahamic traditions of Judaism and Christianity but affirms the pre-eminence of the ministry of the Prophet Muhammad (*c.* 570–632 CE). The Islamic tradition recognises a series of revelations made known to the Prophet Muhammad by the archangel Gabriel during 610–632 CE, which were subsequently written down and collected together as the Holy Qur'an. The Qur'an is understood as having been dictated by God and is the pre-eminent source of legislative authority within Islam. It is interpreted in part by the Hadith – a collection of the teachings of the Prophet Muhammad. The five 'pillars' of Islam are profession of faith ('I testify that there is no God but Allah, and I testify that Muhammad is his prophet'), prayer (five times each day), alms-giving, fasting (which is obligatory at the time of Ramadan), and hajj (or pilgrimage, to Mecca).

The two major divisions of Islam today, Shia and Sunni, date back to early divisions over leadership after the death of Muhammad. Shia Muslims believe that leadership should have passed directly to Muhammad's cousin/son-in-law, Ali. The word *shia* in Arabic means a group or supportive party of people, shortened here to stand for 'shia-t-Ali' or 'the party of Ali'. Sunni Muslims do not hold this belief. The word *sunni* in Arabic comes from a word meaning 'one who follows the traditions of the Prophet'. Sunni Muslims make up the majority (85%) of Muslims all over the world. Significant populations of Shia Muslims can be found in Iran and Iraq, with large minority communities in Yemen, Bahrain, Syria, and Lebanon.

An aspect of Islam that has been of particular interest to many Westerners is Sufism, a mystical tradition within Islam which seeks an intimate and personal experience of God. As in the mystical traditions of other religions, this experience is not to be sought for its own sake, but rather out of devotion to God.

Islam teaches that on the Judgement day every individual will be held accountable for his or her deeds. They will either be granted admission to Paradise, where they will enjoy spiritual and physical pleasures forever, or condemned to Hell to suffer spiritual and physical torment for eternity. According to the Qur'an, human beings cannot in reality either perceive or imagine the pleasures and tranquillity of Paradise.

Bahaism

The Baha'i faith (7.1 million) was founded by Bahaullah (1817–1892) in Iran (then Persia) in the 1860s and is also sometimes considered to be an Abrahamic religion. Claiming to represent a 'single religion of God', its cornerstone has been the spiritual unity of humankind across diversity of race, creed and culture.

The Baha'i faith soon began to attract converts in the Western world as well as, more recently, in the developing world (although not generally

239

in Muslim countries). It is a monotheistic faith which emphasises the unknowability and transcendence of God but which also teaches a series of 'manifestations of God' in particular persons, among whom are said to be: Abraham, Moses, Zoroaster, Gautama, Jesus and Muhammad, as well as Bahaullah. Although relatively small in number, the Baha'i faith nevertheless holds a strong, contemporary appeal for those who believe that all religions serve one and the same ultimate spiritual truth.

The Eastern traditions

Hinduism

Hinduism (811 million) traces its origins to the Stone Age in India and is thus one of the most ancient of the world's faith traditions, as well as having the third largest number of adherents worldwide. The collection of scriptures, or Vedas, is variously defined, but is acknowledged by virtually all Hindus to include the *Bhagavad-Gita* (the most sacred scripture of Hinduism, an account of the conversation between Krishna and Arjuna). Hinduism teaches the existence of a human self or soul (*atman*) that persists through a repeated process of birth, death and rebirth known as reincarnation. Through the moral law of karma (of cause and effect), each successive rebirth may be in a better or worse condition, with the possibility of eventual release from this cycle (*moksha* or liberation) and experience of nirvana (or *samadhi*), in which the soul merges with Brahman, the supreme soul (God). Hinduism may appear (at least to outsiders) as polytheistic, since aspects of Brahman manifest as a variety of gods, such as Vishnu and Shiva, but many Hindus would consider themselves to be monotheistic. In fact, terms such as monotheism and polytheism tend to oversimplify the complexity and diversity of Hindu belief. The three paths to moksha within Hinduism are described as the way of good works (karma yoga), the way of knowledge (jnana yoga) and the way of devotion to God (bhakti yoga). Yoga, meaning union (with God), has now become a discipline in its own right. Hinduism has no personal founder, and it does not have a central authority or structured organisation. The beliefs and practices of individual Hindus tend to be highly diverse because Hinduism has assimilated much from other faith traditions.

Buddhism

Buddhism (360 million) has its historical origins in the life and teachings of Siddhartha Gautama in the 6th to 5th century BCE in India. It is believed that Gautama was a prince who, aged 29, gave up all his worldly possessions to become a mendicant and seek enlightenment. This is said to have taken place while he was seated under the Bhodi Tree, and so he was thereafter known as the Buddha or 'awakened one'. Drawing upon Hindu cosmology, Buddhism broadly shares the Hindu understanding of reincarnation. However, the Buddha also introduced fundamentally new ideas. According to Buddhism, all things are transient and suffering arises as a result of inappropriate attachment to these things, whether to material objects or the inner world (thoughts). Because all things are impermanent, there is no individual, everlasting soul and there is no unchanging, eternal Deity. Buddhists seek to live by the 'Four Noble Truths' of Buddhism:

1   The universal nature of impermanence and suffering.
2   The origins of suffering in attachment to things that are impermanent.
3   The cessation of suffering where desire for impermanent things is eradicated.
4   The teaching of the 'Eightfold Path' as a means to achieving that goal.

There are two major strands of Buddhism today: Theravada and Mahayana, each further subdivided. There are many Buddhist scriptures, including the written teachings of the Buddha, but less emphasis is given to these than to oral transmission of his teachings.

Sikhism

Sikhism (23.3 million) was founded in Northern India on the teachings of Guru Nanak (born 1469 CE). Althoguh a guru can be any religious teacher, the term is applied in Sikhism especially to God, then specifically to ten historical Indian gurus, from Guru Nanak through to Guru Gobind Singh (died 1708), and finally also to the Sikh scriptures (Guru Granth Sahib). Sikh means 'learner' or 'disciple' and Sikhism advocates the pursuit of salvation through the study of Sikh scriptures, the teachings of the Guru and disciplined, personal meditation on the nature of God. Sikhism is monotheistic and is characterised by religious tolerance, holding that all religious paths lead eventually to God. According to Sikhism, the way to escape from the cycle of reincarnation is to move one's disordered human inclinations into alignment with the will of God.

Jainism

Jainism (4.2 million), mainly based in India, is also an ancient religious tradition, dating back to prehistoric India. Jainism does not recognise a creator God of the kind usually understood by other theistic traditions, but believes every human to have an eternal soul subject to the law of karma. The aim is to free the soul from karma through a radical programme of self-discipline based on five vows:

1   non-violence
2   to speak the truth
3   not to steal
4   chastity
5   non-attachment to material things.

Absolute reverence for all living things, including insect and plant life, is a fundamental precept.

Folk religion, syncretism and the subjectivity of faith

The major faith traditions have been described here in outline in their 'official' or orthodox forms, but in practice popularly held beliefs and practices often differ. So-called 'folk religion' tends to be eclectic, consisting of beliefs, superstitions and rituals transmitted from generation to generation of a specific culture and often blended with the major religions, i.e. 'folk Christianity,' 'folk Islam' and so on.

Folk religion serves to help handle everyday problems, provides the need for reassurance in times of trouble and is enlisted in attempting to avert misfortune or to seek healing. When elements of various religions have become combined so as to completely blur the boundaries between them, this is referred to as syncretism. Syncretism is now widespread and in its extreme form offers a complete transcendence of all historical faith traditions in the belief that there is truth in all of them. The Baha'i faith is thus, to a large extent, syncretistic.

Many individuals in Western society show a tendency towards folk religion and/or syncretism, but these are not uniquely Western phenomena. For example, Chinese traditional religion (around 385 million followers) includes varying mixtures of Taoism, Confucianism and Buddhism. African traditional religions spread through slavery to the Caribbean where they merged with Catholicism to give rise to Santeria, Voodoo and Spiritism, the last now having a worldwide diaspora of 12 million.

The complex mix of religious beliefs in contemporary society highlights the need in clinical practice to avoid assumptions about the beliefs of any particular patient. At the individual level, belief is a personal and subjective matter and does not necessarily conform to traditional orthodoxy, culture or other social norms.

Religious experience

Religious experience may be defined as 'the structured way in which a believer enters into a relationship with, or gains an awareness of, the sacred within the context of a particular religious tradition. It is the whole range of spiritual feelings, cognitions and perceptions that are experienced by many people in various religious settings, including worship' (Habel *et al*, 1993: p. 107).

Religious experiences have been classified into the immediate and the mediated types. In the mediated experience, the believer discovers the sacred through mediators such as prayer, fasting, rhythm and chanting. On the other hand, the immediate experience comes to the believer without any intervening agency or mediator. Another classification is based on the content of the experience; experiences can be sensory (visual, auditory, touch and smell), cognitive and affective (including sense of presence), precognitive, or happen through supposed extra-sensory perception (telepathy, clairvoyance and psychokinesis). Religious experiences in general are particularly associated with times of stress and turmoil (Maxwell & Tschudin, 1990).

Sir Alister Hardy built up an impressive body of knowledge of religious experiences by collecting individual first-hand accounts, resulting in an archive of more than 5000 cases. He began analysing the data with his research team in 1925 and continued for over 20 years. The Alister Hardy Research Centre was officially founded in 1969, first in Oxford and then, from 2000, moving to Lampeter. Much was learnt about how religious experiences were 'sensed' or otherwise perceived; when, where, in what circumstances; both the contents and feelings that accompanied these experiences, some profound and wonderful, others anguished and fearful (Hardy, 1979).

Of Hardy's research team, two members have made further notable contributions: David Hay and Michael Jackson. Hay's hypothesis has been that religious or spiritual awareness is biologically natural to the human species and that it has a survival value. It implies that all people, including those who have no religious belief, have a spiritual life (Hay, 2001; 2006; Hay & Socha, 2005). Hay's research has included a number of national and in-depth surveys of reports of religious or spiritual experience in the UK. During the 1990s he directed a 3-year study of the spirituality of young children (Hay et al, 1996). It has been shown that for most children, childhood is a time of great spiritual openness (Hay & Nye, 2006). Hay's research has also revealed that in the UK significantly more people reported religious experiences than expected and that they were more likely to be women (Hay, 1990).

Jackson's research has looked at the relationship between 'healthy' religious experiences and psychotic states. Drawing on the database of 5000 case records, he identified people who had experiences that would have been diagnosed as delusional or hallucinatory had they been referred to the psychiatric services and compared them with an index group that had been formally diagnosed and treated. The diagnosed group had significantly more negative experiences, including the way in which people had reacted to them, and they also reported greater early life trauma than the un-diagnosed group. Yet both groups expressed how valuable their religious experience had been, and how it had contributed to their sense of meaning and purpose in life. All were involved in altruistic work or activities (Jackson & Fulford, 1997).

It is of note that recent research indicates that early life trauma and abuse is over-represented among people with major psychotic illnesses (Read et al, 2004). Jackson (1997; Jackson & Fulford, 2002) has explored the presentation of schizotypy in two papers which provide fascinating case studies of individuals both undiagnosed and diagnosed, and having very similar experiences.

Common elements of profound religious experiences

Maxwell & Tschudin (1990) have identified common features that can be found in profound religious experiences:

- ineffability: religious experiences are of an order that we know very little about and so it is not surprising that we have not enough, or not adequate, language to describe what is happening;
- affect: most people welcome such an experience, accompanied by a variety of fascinating and desirable positive moods; however, the affect can become frightening and occasionally terrifying;
- secrecy: the experience is very personal. Some people consider it so private that talking about it may take away that 'specialness';
- loneliness: most experiences take place when the person is alone, which seems to enhance the element of mystery and of being given something personal and unique;
- transience: many religious experiences last for only a short while in chronological time, yet they may be perceived as having no beginning or end, enfolding everything and therefore timeless;
- passivity: although some people strive and pray for such an experience, its actual occurrence cannot be made to happen – it can only be 'given';
- noetic: a profound sense of understanding of a different order; 'Praise be to God, Who will soon show you His Signs, so that ye shall *recognize* them [emphasis mine]' (The Qur'an, sūrah 27:93; Ali, 2000).

Attuning to the need

When working both individually with patients and to create an integrated therapeutic environment, a generic approach towards people's religious beliefs is likely to help most. Openness to and interest in the religious experiences of patients themselves will make all the difference. The focus is less on what people believe and more on how they believe and how their faith works for (or indeed against) their well-being.

As mental health professionals, we do not have to understand all the details of a person's beliefs. If we listen, patients will tell us about their faith and its importance to their mental health. They may think their illness is caused by their faithlessness or that they are being punished for some failure in living up to their religion's expectations. Equally, they can tell us about what in their religion has helped and supported them in the past and might comfort and help them now.

The following model, developed by Gleeson (1990), has been found to be a useful resource in fostering the clinician's ability to listen and to explore the religious beliefs of patients, irrespective of the therapist's own orientation. Gleeson has adapted the work of James Fowler (1981) (see also chapter 5, pp. 84–86) and Paul Tillich (1957) in a simple and practical way for clergy working in the health services. We think his model is useful for psychiatrists and other mental health workers in helping us understand and value rather than try to influence another person's faith.

Gleeson (1990) categorises people's faith based broadly on four different world views:

1   World View 'A' persons are natural or unconscious literalists. They have no doubts about their faith and whatever life does to them will fit naturally into their belief system. They can appear naive and others may think that they deny the worst in their experience and need to be helped over such denial. However, this is pointless and unnecessary; their faith is sufficient and requires respect and affirmation.

> God has become my everything. I know that without my faith I would not have survived the child sexual abuse; the abusive relationships; the loneliness and abandonment of my parents and the church; the poverty; the depression; the bereavements; the stigma … I could go on and on … However I do thank 'God' for my faith. It allows me to try and forgive, forget and move on [Nicholls, 2002: p. 14].

2   World View 'B' persons are conscious literalists. They appear to believe as strongly as the A person, but harbour doubts about themselves or their faith and are much more affected by their beliefs being questioned or criticised by others. They are likely to hold fundamentalist views and will want to convince others of the rightness of their faith. They are natural evangelists. Sometimes the mental health services are experienced as inhabiting a world view B on account of their medical reductionism.

> I have had a very bad experience with psychiatrists. They will tell me it's all in the mind … it's anxiety or depression, and they don't understand what is going on in me [Nicholls, 2002: p. 25].

Gleeson suggests the best response to world view B persons is to encourage them in the doing and the practice of their faith and if possible to do this with them, reading their sacred texts and fulfilling their religious practices. We have found it helpful to keep in contact with their faith communities, even if they are suspicious of and hostile to psychiatry.

3   World View 'C' persons are much less literalist. They will search for meanings that are symbolic and metaphorical rather than simple facts of truth and falsity. They will want to discern the meaning in their suffering and distress, both in terms of the science of psychiatry and personally in the significance the illness has for their lives.

> My boundaries became much wider, much broader … I suppose I found a lot inside myself that I didn't know existed … I can stop trying to achieve perfection, it's impossible, I'm a human being [Nicholls, 2002: p. 18].

World view C people need time, space and attention in order to follow their instincts and find the meaning that is theirs. Many have valued psychotherapy as an aid to this search but others have appreciated the mere presence of their families, friends, fellow patients and professional carers who have accompanied them on their journeys.

4   Gleeson says that we will be lucky to meet many World View 'D' people for they are the exceptions to the rule, the mystics and saints who, like those in group A, are seemingly unaffected by the ups and downs of life. Though lifelong members of a religion, they will sit lightly with its traditions and continually look beyond them, but not with the same struggles as those in group A. Crises may affect them, but they will look to find ways to incorporate the worst of their trials into their contemplation of the infinite meaning of all things.

This schema provides the busy professional with ways of understanding how peoples' beliefs can affect their well-being, how to help them make the most of their religious resources and how to concentrate care upon those concerns most important to the individual at any one time. Inevitably, however, there are limitations due to over-generalisation and some patients will not fit into any one category, or may well change category over time.

Implementing the therapeutic focus

A number of strategies for counselling and psychotherapy with religious content have been reviewed (Richards & Bergin, 1997); many psychotherapists now use an eclectic, integrative approach to match the needs of each patient. A generic approach to religious belief can then be supplemented by a more specific focus upon the individual's own faith tradition or denomination with the help of the appropriate religious guides from that tradition. The aim is to use the patient's religious support system, helping him or her to draw on his or her own religious resources, whether based on individual, group or social interventions.

Individual guidance

The religious guide is a long-established figure in most faith traditions. Currently, guidance can be offered through a spiritual advisor such as the hospital chaplain, or through pastoral care within the patients' own religious community. The aim is to enable patients to incorporate their personal religious beliefs and practices into their daily life. Cox has argued the case for chaplains to be members of the multidisciplinary team (Cox, 1996).

Religious support groups

Both of us have had experience of providing religious and spiritual support groups in which the aim has been to help identify patients' religious needs and foster their resources by incorporating a religious component into the dynamics of the group and using supportive, behavioural, cognitive and existential techniques.

One of us (MS) was responsible for planning and establishing a religious and spiritual support group at the Medway Maritime Hospital in Gillingham, Kent. First, a planning group was organised and met regularly for 8 months to define the aims of the group and to address its practicalities. The planning group included a consultant psychiatrist, the two hospital chaplains and two psychiatric nurses. Then, an open support group was set up, to run on a weekly basis for a 45-minute session, facilitated by a psychiatric nurse and a chaplain and supervised by the consultant psychiatrist. Patients with acute psychotic symptoms were excluded. The subjects discussed were designed to be relevant to a multi-faith membership and focused on: meaning of life, from despair to hope, worth and self-esteem, guilt and forgiveness, and religious experiences. Many of these themes were suggested by the participants themselves.

At heart, these groups touched people in their humanity rather than in their illness. Self-worth was affirmed and encouraged as participants shared their experience and insights and as they recognised and supported the worth of each other.

The strength of individual religious guidance is in its being able to tune in to each individual's own world view and the need, as required, specifically to focus on religious beliefs, values and practices. On the other hand, the strength of group work is that it generates its own momentum, allowing individuals to find things they have in common and to be less isolated with their fears and their uncertainties. World view C people are most likely to flourish in groups that question and explore the inner world, while world view A and B people are more inclined to benefit from participating in a group of their own faith tradition, finding reinforcement of their own beliefs and to join with fellow worshippers in religious practices.

The social and communal focus

Much of what we have already written reflects the predominant practice of psychiatry in focusing on the individual patient and the individual member of staff. Looking beyond that focus takes us first to the patient's immediate family and friends, and possibly those involved in their occupation, education or housing. However, religions also place great emphasis upon the faith community. Mental health services have done little to recognise this, let alone exploit its considerable resources.

The hard-pressed mental health professional does not have to be an expert in religion to support this aspect of care. If he or she cares to look, they will find they are in the midst of a plethora of religious communities. When mental health services and faith groups overcome their suspicion of one another, the potential for care in the community is enormous. An example of this vision was expressed by a leading psychiatrist in the national press.

> Emotional access can be a big barrier ... Our research with Punjabi women in Southall [west London] showed they wanted help to overcome depression,

247

but the stigma of the illness made it difficult for them to seek support. It would be far easier if we took our services to temples and mosques [*The Guardian*, 2006].

Taking services from the hospital and the GP practice to the church, the mosque, the temple and the synagogue sounds a revolutionary move. The service that has done most to provide a foundation for this kind of revolution is in the London borough of Newham. In two groundbreaking accounts, Copsey (1997; 2001) sets out the way in which this service developed with the cooperation of many religious groups and how it has transformed spiritual care provided by the East London and City Mental Health NHS Trust.

A research grant from the Sainsbury Centre first enabled Nigel Copsey, an Anglican priest and healthcare chaplain, to engage with the religious communities of Newham. In the end, he identified over 200 different groups in a borough where over half of the inhabitants were from Black and minority ethnic groups. There were some 30 000 Muslims, 21 000 Hindus and 5000 Sikhs among the large African, African–Caribbean and Asian communities, together with flourishing traditional Christian churches. When Copsey explored with them their greatest mental health needs and ideas on how the NHS service could better respond to them, he met with a surprising response.

> I imagined there would be deep suspicion of my turning up at many religious centres. However, across the faith communities I was welcomed according to the custom of that particular community. Indeed, many were so pleased that someone wanted to come and listen to them in their own setting [Copsey, 1997: p. 13].

Copsey was struck by how closely culture and religion were intertwined among those he met. People were unused to separating out these fundamental aspects of their life and well-being. He had expected faith groups to be multicultural but he quickly discovered 'that many reflected strong cultural identities (including White cockney) in order to preserve a sense of belonging' (ibid., p. 8). In the face of extreme feelings of isolation, 'religious faith was an integral part of maintaining identity' (ibid.). Copsey understood the importance of religious buildings to these faith groups in providing a focus for their belonging and a major resource for social needs, including those with mental health problems. None were at ease coming out of their communities to get help from strangers. In conversation he heard how important their faith was to their mental distress, but at the same time,

> There was a fear regarding talking about those beliefs because it was thought that if they did so, they would either be sectioned, placed on medication, or seen as exhibiting psychotic symptoms [Copsey, 1997: p. 11].

It became clear that religion was something professionals avoided discussing by using terms like 'cultural or ethnic diversity' instead.

Many mental health workers with whom I spoke saw the whole complexity of religious beliefs as being far too complicated to engage with, and many saw religious belief as contributing to mental health problems [Copsey, 1997: p. 12].

Copsey's research confirmed the findings of the King's Fund's study of London's mental health (1997) in identifying the following priorities: effective, acceptable and appropriate care for members of ethnic minorities; improving the care provided by statutory services to this end; changing professional attitudes and practice to achieve this; widespread dialogue with service users about the provision of access to spiritual and religious places of worship and closer liaison with religious advisers; integration with non-medical and social models of care giving; and training in culturally sensitive practice for professionals.

Consequently, the East London and City Mental Health NHS Trust set up a new department of spiritual, religious and cultural care to meet these diverse needs. The team eventually included coordinators for different faith groups – European, Asian, African–Caribbean and African – translators of the many languages within the community. Two other workers were seconded to the team to work with Muslim groups. Initially, the team worked with the acute in-patient units where users are most likely to be separated from their familiar religious and cultural symbols and practices. Time was spent with unit staff to explain the role of the department. Since then, the team has moved out to work with the community services. A major feature of the department's work has been on building up and training a resource group of volunteers to take the dialogue to more religious communities.

We have been excited to see how a mixture of men and women drawn from very different faith and cultural backgrounds can form a team and listen to and understand each other, whilst at the same time remaining true to their own individual traditions. Our hope is that the resource team will eventually reflect all the faith traditions of Newham [Copsey, 2001: p. 21].

The team have focused explicitly on the views of service users and discovered the following priorities:
- specific times of worship on units to accommodate different groups and traditions
- visits to churches and temples
- appropriate diets
- different ways of praying
- celebrating major religious festivals
- freedom to talk about issues of faith
- requests for prayers for people of all religions (Lau & Bryan, 2002).

Copsey points out both the simplicity of the requests and their complexity when it comes to their organisation within Western-dominated institutions. Much patience and persistence is needed.

A basic premise is that it is not possible for one person to hold all the diverse knowledge. Thus, we have discovered that there was a continuing journey of teaching each other. We have also sought to find a common language devoid of all jargon whereby we are free to ask lots of questions of each other [Copsey, 2001: p. 31].

The team aims to empower catalysts within every religious community to help them out of their isolation and into greater responsiveness to those with mental health problems.

> We are seeking to equip a group of people representing the faith communities of Newham, with the necessary skills to get alongside patients both on wards and also when discharged back home. By establishing this network across the community, it will be possible to prevent further relapses due to isolation and at the same time, to reduce stigma by engaging with the faith communities themselves [Copsey, 2001: p. 23].

The further aims of the spiritual care service are:
- to provide holistic care to all service users of whatever faith;
- to arrange an initial spiritual assessment for all new patients and to continue contact with those who wish it thereafter;
- to liaise with the mental health teams;
- to offer a range of choices of different support and spiritual care;
- to provide ongoing training to the team and develop dialogue with both mental health professionals and religious communities (Copsey, 2001).

Similar projects have developed in a number of other centres of very mixed cultural and religious communities. In 1994, the South London and Maudsley NHS Trust appointed the first (and only) Fellow in Religion and Mental Health in the UK. Julia Head, who holds the Bishop John Robinson Fellowship in Pastoral Theology and Mental Health, has developed a wide network of useful resources and projects, which are shared through a regular newsletter (Head, 2007). Service users have played a major part in these developments; Muslims use the hospital chapel for their regular times of prayer, and meditation groups, both Buddhist and Christian, meet weekly on two hospital sites.

Conclusion

Clearly, religion and religious experiences deserve greater recognition and attention from all mental health professionals. Religious experience is associated with the quality and purpose of life as a whole and with the ultimate destiny of the person. Certain special times and events in the course of life are occasions that direct human thought to the divine and the sacred with peculiar forcefulness. These occasions, often life crises, are potentially dangerous because they are transitional from one stage of life to another and open to view the relation of life as a whole to its sacred ground. These events can progress to serious consequences of distress and mental illness in vulnerable persons, if their experience is not understood and their needs are not properly addressed.

Religion provides rich resources that can help people cope better with mental health crises. This is confirmed by the results of most research in the field of spirituality and mental health, especially as the majority of it is drawn from religious sources (Shams & Jackson, 1993). Therefore, cultural and religious factors must be considered when working with patients in the community as well as in hospital. All agencies involved in the mental healthcare of patients should have an integrated view of the person as a whole – as body, mind and spirit – and we would urge that mental health professionals are made fully aware of the constructive role that religion can play in promoting mental well-being and in the alleviation of mental distress.

References

Ali, A. Y. (ed.) (2000) *The Holy Qur'an: Translation and Commentary*. IPCI: Islamic Vision.

Barrett, D. B., Kwian, G. T. & Johnson, T. M. (2001) *World Christian Encyclopedia*. Oxford University Press.

Batson, C. D., Schoenrade, P. A. & Ventis, W. L. (1993) *Religion and the Individual: A Social–Psychological Perspective*. Oxford University Press.

Copsey, N. (1997) *Keeping Faith*. Sainsbury Centre for Mental Health.

Copsey, N. (2001) *Forward in Faith*. Sainsbury Centre for Mental Health.

Cornah, D. (2006) *The Impact of Spirituality on Mental Health: A Review of the Literature*. Mental Health Foundation.

Cox, J. L. (1996) Psychiatry and religion: a general psychiatrist's perspective. In *Psychiatry and Religion* (ed. D. Bhugra). Routledge.

Foskett, J., Marriott, J. & Wilson-Rudd, F. (2004) Mental health, religion and spirituality: attitudes, experience and expertise among mental health professionals and religious leaders in Somerset. *Mental Health, Religion and Culture*, **7**, 5–22.

Fowler, J. (1981) *Stages of Faith: The Psychology of Human Development and the Quest for Meaning*. Harper & Row.

Gleeson, J. (1990) Spiritual assessment and pastoral response: a schema revisited and updated. *Journal of Pastoral Care*, **XLIV**, 66–73.

Habel, N., O'Donoghue, M. & Maddox, M. (1993) Religious experience. In *Myth, Ritual and the Sacred. Introducing the Phenomena of Religion*. Underdale.

Hassan, R. (1983) *A Way of Dying: Suicide in Singapore*. Oxford University Press.

Hardy, A. (1979) *The Spiritual Nature of Man*. Religious Experience Research Centre, Westminster College.

Hay, D. (1990) *Religious Experience Today: Studying the Facts*. Cassell.

Hay, D. (2001) The biological basis of spiritual awareness. In *Spirituality and Society in the New Millennium* (ed. U. King), pp. 124–135. Sussex Academic Press.

Hay, D. (2006) *Something There: The Biology of the Human Spirit*. Darton, Longman & Todd.

Hay, D. & Nye, R. (2006) *The Spirit of the Child* (revised). Jessica Kingsley.

Hay, D. & Socha, P. (2005) Spirituality as a natural phenomenon: bringing biological and psychological perspectives together. *Journal of Religion and Science*, **49**, 589–612.

Hay, D., Nye, R. & Murphy, R. (1996) Thinking about childhood spirituality: review of research and current directions. In *Research in Religious Education* (eds L. Francis, W. K. Kay & W. S. Campbell), pp. 47–71. Gracewing Press.

Head, J. (2007) *The Bishop John Robinson Newsletter*. South London and Maudsley NHS Trust.

Hunt, R. A. & King, M. B. (1972) The intrinsic–extrinsic concept: a review and evaluation. *Journal for the Scientific Study of Religion*, **10**, 339–356.

251

Jackson, M. (1997) Benign schizotypy? In *Schizotypy: Implications for Illness and Health* (ed. G. Claridge), pp. 227–250. Oxford University Press.

Jackson, M. & Fulford, W. (1997) Spiritual experience and psychopathology. *Philosophy, Psychiatry and Psychology*, **4**, 41–65.

Jackson, M. & Fulford, W. (2002) Psychosis good and bad: values-based practice and the distinction between pathological and non-pathological forms of psychotic experience. *Philosophy, Psychiatry and Psychology*, **9**, 387–394.

Khavari., K. A. & Harmon, T. M. (1982) The relationship between degree of professed religious belief and use of drugs. *International Journal of Addictions*, **17**, 847–857.

King's Fund (1997) *London's Mental Health*. King's Fund.

Koenig, H. G., Cohen, H. J., Bazer, D. G., *et al* (1992) Religious coping and depression in elderly hospitalized medically ill men. *American Journal of Psychiatry*, **149**, 1693–1700.

Koenig, H. G., Ford, S. M., George, L. K., *et al* (1993) Religion and anxiety disorder: an examination and comparison of associations in young, middle-aged and elderly adults. *Journal of Anxiety Disorders*, **7**, 321–340.

Koenig, H. G., George, L. K., Meador, K. G., *et al* (1994) Religious practices and alcoholism in a southern adult population. *Hospital and Community Psychiatry*, **45**, 225–231.

Koenig, H. G. (1997) *Is Religion Good for Your Health?* Haworth Press.

Lau, S. & Bryan, J. (2002) Building bridges with faith communities. *Mental Health Today*, January, 22–23.

Lawrence, R. (2003) The integration of spirituality in psychiatric teaching: the lesson to be learnt from our patients. *Newsletter of the Royal College of Psychiatrists Special Interest Group*, **13**, 18–22.

Levin, J. (1994) Investigating the epidemiological effects of religious experience: findings, explanations and barriers. In *Religion in Aging and Health* (ed J. Levin), pp. 3–17. Sage.

Loewenthal, K. (1995) *Mental Health and Religion*. Chapman and Hall.

Macmin, L. & Foskett, J. (2004) 'Don't be afraid to tell: the spiritual experience of mental health service users in Somerset. *Mental Health, Religion and Culture*, **7**, 23–40.

Mahy, G. (1993) Suicide behaviour in the Caribbean. *International Review of Psychiatry*, **5**, 261–269.

Maxwell, M. & Tschudin, V. (1990) *Seeing the Invisible: Modern Religious and Other Transcendent Experiences*. Arkana.

Neeleman, J. & King, M. (1993) Psychiatrists' religious attitudes in relation to clinical practice. *Acta Psychiatrica Scandinavica*, **88**, 420–424.

Neeleman, J & Persaud, R. (1994) Why do psychiatrists neglect religion? *British Journal of Medical Psychology*, **68**, 169–178.

Nicholls, V. (2002) *Taken Seriously: the Somerset Spirituality Project*. Mental Health Foundation.

Paloutzian, R. F., Richardson, J. T. & Rambo, L. R. (1999) Religious conversion and personality change. *Journal of Personality*, **67**, 1047–1079.

Pargament, K. I. (1997) *The Psychology of Religion and Coping*. Guilford.

Read, J., Mosher, L. & Bentall, R. (2004) *Models of Madness*. Routledge.

Richards, P. S. & Bergin, A. E. (1997) *A Spiritual Strategy for Counseling and Psychotherapy*. American Psychological Association.

Salem, M. O. (2006) Religion, Spirituality and Psychiatry. *Royal College of Psychiatrists Spirituality and Psychiatry Special Interest Group Newsletter*, **21**, 1–15.

Shams, M. & Jackson, P. R. (1993) Religiosity as predictor of well-being and moderator of the psychological impact of unemployment. *British Journal of Medical Psychology*, **66**, 341–352.

Sims, A. C. P. (1994) 'Psyche' – spirit as well as mind? *British Journal of Psychiatry*, **165**, 441–446.

Stack, S. (1983) The effect of religiosity on suicide. *Journal for the Scientific Study of Religion*, **22**, 239–252.

The Guardian (2006) *The struggle for 'cultural competence'*. 12 April (http://www.guardian.co.uk/money/2006/apr/12/publicfinances.politics6).

Tillich, P. (1957) *Dynamics of Faith*. Harper.

Trivedi, P. (1992) *Survivors Poetry: From Dark to Light* (ed. P. Campbell). Survivors Press.

Trivedi, P. (2007) Aum shanti, shanti. In *Spirituality, Values and Mental Health: Jewels for the Journey* (eds M. Coyte, P. Gilbert & V. Nicholls). Jessica Kingsley.

CHAPTER 13

Pathological spirituality

Nicki Crowley and Gillie Jenkinson

> It is possible to fall into the heights, as well as the depths.
>
> Holderlein, in Lind (2000)

'Pathological spirituality' is, on one level, a misnomer and a contradiction in terms. The quality of spirituality, for the purposes of this book (see p. 4), is by definition the opposite of pathological dysfunction and disease, though it does embrace an approach to suffering.

The Jonestown massacre in the jungle of Guyana in 1978, the deadly Sarin nerve gas attacks in the Tokyo underground by Aum Shinrikyo in 1995, the suicide bombers of 9/11 in the USA in 2001 and the 7 July bombings in the UK in 2005 all illustrate how pathological and harmful spiritual values can be when doctrines take precedence over human health and well-being.

Two questions can be asked about the concept of pathological spirituality:

1   When do spiritual beliefs, practices and experiences become pathological?
2   Can apparently psychopathological mental states ever be understood as spiritual?

The second question has been explored in the context of a transpersonal understanding of the psyche in chapter 11, see 'spiritual emergency' (pp. 227–230).

Path or pathology?

The past hundred years has witnessed immensely destabilising changes within our society. Traditionally cohesive social structures, such as the church and the family unit, are losing their status (Murray, 2004). Different influences are exerting their effects far more powerfully than before via the media and the internet. We use, and are influenced by, technology beyond our understanding and are bombarded by information beyond our absorptive capacity. 'Information disease' (Conway & Siegelman, 2005) is a new category of disorders describing the lasting changes of mind and personality that may be brought on by, among other things, reckless or excessive use of popular spiritual and personal growth practices. Our cultural background and education has often not prepared us to navigate safely this new territory.

Seeking a clearly guided path that promises relief from suffering, answers important existential questions and offers some form of self-improvement or self-transformation feels necessary to many. The advent of psychoanalysis in the 20th century, with its own controversial dismissal of religious or mystical experience as merely regressive, the subsequent evolution of numerous different schools of psychology and psychotherapy, together with the New Age movement and popular psychology self-help books, each provide a different perspective on what it is to be human. But when does adherence to a spiritual, religious or therapeutic path lead to pathologically de-humanising or even life-threatening consequences?

Healthy v. pathological spirituality

A distinction needs to be made between those spiritual practices and beliefs that foster the healthy development of a person within his or her community and those that have been incorporated into a person's lifestyle and subsequently cause them or others harm.

The issue of harm is complex. Kendall (2006) notes that some groups (including religious and spiritual groups) may be positive in certain respects, display sect-like (or cult-like) characteristics in other respects and be innocuous in others.

Rather than attempting to classify groups into 'good or bad', 'harmful and not harmful', and their beliefs into 'true' and 'false', it can be helpful to consider a continuum with a critical point after which a group can progress to become harmful, if it takes its beliefs and/or practices to the extreme (Chambers et al, 1994; Kendall, 2006).

Battista (1996) describes pathological spirituality by exploring both spiritual defences and offensive spirituality.

Spiritual defences

Spiritual defences are spiritual beliefs that prevent people from expressing their actual, embodied, emotional self, for example:

- submission to 'the other', or to authority, rationalised as the spiritual quality of humility;
- inability to develop intimacy in relationships, rationalised as God being the primary and only necessary relationship in life;
- failure to deal with interpersonal or sexual needs, rationalised as ascetic practice;
- failure to deal with the practical materialistic aspect of life rationalised as 'God will provide'.

Spiritual defences enable a 'spiritual bypass', a premature transcendence of personal pain and suffering and denial of the real substance of a grounded life that, if not ignored, can instead be viewed as the 'ore' that shapes our development and yields valuable qualities (Hillman, 2004).

Offensive spirituality

This refers to the assertion of one's self as spiritually developed as a means of constraining another person. It is the narcissistic use of a spiritual persona or spiritual identification (Battista, 1996). The narcissistic misuse of both spiritual and psychoanalytic principles has been addressed by cultural critics (Lasch, 1979; Frank & Frank, 1993; Masson, 1994; Raubolt, 2006). Lack of recognition of this quality can be a serious pitfall for those on the path of psycho-spiritual exploration.

False spiritual teacher or guru

Storr (1996) defines a guru as a teacher who 'claims special knowledge of the meaning of life, and therefore feels entitled to tell others how life should be lived' (p. xi). He differentiates between 'morally superior individuals [who] exist [with] integrity, virtue and goodness … beyond the reach of most of us' (p. xii), and self-appointed experts who promise their followers new ways of self-development and new paths to salvation. The latter tend to demonstrate narcissistic personality traits. Storr observes that guru-types tend to have experienced isolated childhoods. They possess a limited capacity to form friendships, tend to be elitist, anti-democratic and are often intolerant of criticism. They hold their belief systems with unshakeable conviction and this certainty, together with their persuasiveness, adds to their charisma. Barker (1989) states that: 'Almost by definition, charismatic leaders are unpredictable, for they are bound neither by traditions or rules; they are not answerable to other human beings' (p. 13).

Unshakeable convictions may follow a period of chaotic suffering in the guru's life, thus giving meaning to it. They may have experienced a period of mental illness, involving paranoia or grandiosity. Regardless of whether their experience fulfils psychiatric diagnostic criteria, the essential question remains: is their behaviour harmful to others or not? Deikman (1983) asserts that a teacher who is guilty of financial or sexual exploitation represents a drastic failure of responsibility that disqualifies them from any special consideration. Various cult disasters illustrate how grandiose and paranoid cult leaders occasionally self-destruct, taking their group with them.

Harmful groups

The beneficial aspects of belonging to a group, be it religious or otherwise, are well-recognised in psychological and sociological literature. It is a matter of moral, ethical, religious, political and sometimes clinical opinion whether the influences of being part of a particular group have, or have not, been good for the individual and, hence, society.

Definitions of groups that may be harmful derive from different epistemologies and can be ambiguous, pejorative and controversial (Barrett, 2001; Langone, 2007). Attempts at defining and understanding lead to polarisation of views (Lalich, 2004). Although there are a good number of attempts at defining harmful spiritual groups, the following categories, from the cultic studies field will be considered:

- cults
- sects
- new religious movements
- charismatic groups.

Cults

There are numerous definitions of cults: dictionary, theological, psychological (which describe the effects of cult involvement on individuals' and their families' psychosocial well-being) and sociological (which tend to view behaviour as it occurs in social interactions with a group or a movement). Langone (1993) defines a cult from a psychological perspective thus:

> A cult is a group or movement that, to a significant degree, (a) exhibits great or excessive devotion or dedication to some person, idea, or thing, (b) uses a thought-reform program to persuade, control, and socialise members (i.e. to integrate them into the group's unique pattern of relationships, beliefs, values, and practices), (c) systematically induces states of psychological dependency in members, (d) exploits members to advance the leadership's goals, and (e) causes psychological harm to members, their families and the community [p. 5].

At the extreme, the term 'destructive cult', sometimes called 'doomsday cult' (Singer, 2003), can be used to refer to quasi-religious groups that have intentionally killed people.

There are many religious groups, new and old, that are not cults as defined here. A group should not be assumed to be a cult simply because it exhibits one or two of the above features.

Sects

A sect is generally viewed as 'a separate, exclusive entity, with abstract ideas, existing within another, larger religious organisation' (Reber & Reber, 2001: p. 656).

New religious movements

The term 'new religious movement' (Barker, 1989) was adopted by sociologists of religion in the 1970s to refer to a religious faith or an ethical, spiritual or philosophical movement of recent origin that is not part of an established faith tradition. Some modern religious groups have been called thus by writers attentive to the potential of cult-style groups for finding a place in society.

Charismatic groups

The model of the charismatic group has been developed by Galanter (1989), who uses this term to describe modern cults and zealous self-help movements. He proposes that members of charismatic groups are characterised by the following psychological elements:

- a shared belief system
- a high level of social cohesiveness
- strongly influenced by the group's behavioural norms
- impute charismatic (or sometimes divine) power to the group or its leadership (ibid.: p. 5).

Galanter asserts that charismatic groups, including some therapy groups, can relieve certain aspects of psychopathology, as well as precipitate psychiatric symptoms.

Harmful v. healthy groups

Religious, spiritual and therapy groups can be positive and life-affirming or inherently authoritarian and manipulative. Some key differences are drawn out in Table 13.1.

Group dynamics are powerful and can exert considerable influence on their members' psychiatric status (Galanter, 1990). Certain therapy

Table 13.1 Healthy and potentially harmful spiritual groups, comparison (adapted from Haworth, 2001)

Healthy religious/spiritual group	Potentially harmful, cult-style group
Conversion or 'worldview shift' (Lalich, 2004)	Coercion or 'coercive persuasion conversion' (Lalich, 2004)
commitment freely chosen	commitment via psychological force
between individual and God	between individual and group
empowers members	dis-empowers members
increases discernment	decreases discernment
unconditional love for members	conditional love for members
recognises and values the family	alienates members from the family
growth and maturing of members	regression and stunting of members
individual uniqueness	cloned personalities
happiness and fulfilment	artificial 'high'
unity	uniformity
truth leads to experience	experience becomes 'truth'
accountability of leadership	no accountability of leadership
questioning encouraged	questioning discouraged
honesty prevails	the end justifies the means
does not hide behind fronts	hides behind fronts

groups have been described as applying orthodox methods of psychological treatment in an unorthodox and ill-directed manner (Singer, 2003). Both professionals and non-professionals alike have been involved in such groups (Temerlin & Temerlin, 1982; Temerlin & Temerlin, 1986). Some psychoanalysts have commented on the cult-style aspects of psychoanalytic training and institutes (Arlow, 1972; Kernberg, 1986; Masson, 1994; Raubolt, 2006).

Frank & Frank (1993) take the view that all psychotherapies are a vehicle for influence and persuasion. Indeed they define psychotherapy as a form of influence, characterised by: a healing agent, 'typically a person trained in a socially sanctioned method of healing believed to be effective by the sufferer'; 'a sufferer who seeks relief from the healer'; and 'a healing relationship' in which the healer 'tries to bring about relief of symptoms' (p. 2). Their definition of psychotherapy therefore encompasses Western psychotherapy, the placebo effect in medicine, religio-magical healing including religious revivalism, the activity of cults, thought reform and brainwashing. They refer to the power imbalance in the therapeutic encounter and comment that 'in long term therapy, the patient and therapist progressively shape each others' behavior, with the patient increasingly fulfilling the therapist's expectations' (p. 176).

The reality is usually less polarised, but there is a warning here for the psychiatric and psychotherapeutic professions to be aware of the inherent power imbalance and to avoid causing harm (Table 13.2).

To empirically measure the abusiveness of groups while acknowledging the continuum of healthy to harmful, and to address academic disputes as

Table 13.2   Key differences between healthy and potentially harmful therapeutic groups (adapted from Haworth, 2001)

Healthy therapeutic group	Potentially harmful, cult-style therapy group
rehabilitates	debilitates
objectives: goals agreed by client	objectives: therapist or leader's goals
promotes healthy relationships with others	fosters alienation from others
aim: independence of client	aim: dependence of member
psychologically enables the client	psychologically disables the member
questioning encouraged	questioning discouraged
decision making ability enhanced	decision making ability impaired
therapist accountable	cult leader not accountable
qualifications recognised by outside body	self-appointed
fees agreed in advance	fees often inflated once member fully involved
for benefit of client	for benefit of leader
does not hide behind fronts	hides behind fronts

to whether or not 'thought reform' or 'brainwashing' exists, Chambers and colleagues (1994) developed the Group Psychological Abuse Scale (GPA). The 28-item GPA was originally built from a 20-page questionnaire with 112 descriptive items. The items fall into three domains of interest:

- the purpose of the group
- the relationships within the group
- the relationships with others outside the group.

This was developed in the USA from a factor analysis of 308 former cult members' descriptions of the characteristics of their groups; 101 groups were represented (Chambers *et al*, 1994).

Some descriptions of cult dynamics

Terms such as 'conversion', 'brainwashing', 'coercive persuasion', 'mind control techniques' and 'snapping' are all attempts to describe psychological methods employed by cult-style groups to recruit and maintain new members.

Conversion

It is widely recognised that conversion to a religious faith is, for many, deeply significant, life-enhancing and can bring with it a huge sense of relief (Storr, 1996).

The term is used here in a broader sense. Lalich (2004) notes that conversion is typically thought of as a process of religious change but that it also takes place in social contexts. She notes that conversion is a process by which a person develops a new perspective on life; that external pressure may or may not be present; and it may be sudden or gradual. Again, it occurs on a continuum. Conversion may, in some cases, be genuine in spite of external pressure or coercion.

Lalich (2004: p. 15) adopts the term 'worldview shift' to describe the internal change that takes place as a person adopts this new perspective (the term is not restricted to religious settings). If the worldview shift has taken place within a coercive environment (a 'coercive persuasion conversion'), the initial sense of relief at 'having found the answer', which is associated with a kind of personal freedom, may also result in a loss of sense of self and the development of the cult pseudo-personality (Lalich, 2004; Jenkinson, 2008).

Brainwashing and thought reform

'Brainwashing' is a popular term coined in 1951 by journalist Edward Hunter and is a loose translation of the Chinese *hsi nao*, 'wash brain'. It describes the process by which individuals captured in the Korean War and in Communist China could quickly reverse their allegiance and confess to fictional war crimes (Lifton, 1989; Hassan, 2000).

Robert Jay Lifton (1989), who studied this process, noted that the term 'brainwashing' quickly 'developed a life of its own', sometimes causing fear at one end of the continuum or ridicule at the other. He noted that the term is 'far from precise with a questionable usefulness'. To describe the process of conversion from one ideology to another, Lifton preferred to use the term 'thought reform'. He describes eight psychological components that are used to create the 'totalist' environment in which this takes place:

1   milieu control – the control of information and communication;
2   mystical manipulation – the manipulation of experiences that appear spontaneous but in fact were planned and orchestrated;
3   demand for purity – the world is viewed as black and white and the members are constantly exhorted to conform to the ideology of the group and strive for perfection;
4   confession – sins, as defined by the group, are to be confessed either to a personal monitor or publicly to the group;
5   sacred science – the group's doctrine or ideology is considered to be the ultimate truth, beyond all questioning or dispute;
6   loading the language – the group interprets or uses words and phrases in new ways which restrict critical thinking and that the outside world does not understand;
7   doctrine over person – the member's personal experience is subordinated to the sacred science and any contrary experiences must be denied or reinterpreted to fit the ideology of the group;
8   dispensing of existence – the group has the prerogative to decide who has the right to exist and who does not.

Lifton (1999) later came to believe that thought reform could be accomplished without physical coercion (as used with Korean and Chinese prisoners of war) and acknowledged that it is used in some cults. There is some evidence of this type of psychosocial conditioning in the training of terrorists and suicide bombers (Stahelski, 2004; Lalich & Tobias, 2006).

Coercive persuasion

Coercive persuasion is a term coined by Edgar Schein (1961), following his study of the Chinese prisoners' of war indoctrination. Schein asserted that the essence of coercive persuasion is to produce ideological and behavioural changes in a fully conscious, mentally intact individual. Psychologist Margaret Singer has adapted these theories and applied the term 'co-ordinated programs of coercive influence and behavioural control' (Ofshe & Singer, 1986) to the practices of certain religious, spiritual or other types of groups.

Mind control techniques

Mind control techniques are strategies to manipulate another person's thoughts, feelings and behaviour, within a given context over a period of time, resulting in a relatively greater gain for the manipulator than for those being manipulated (Zimbardo, 1993). Examples include: hypnosis, sleep deprivation and control of diet, peer group pressure, rejection of old values, financial commitment, forbidding questioning, fear and replacement of relationships (Haworth, 2001).

Snapping

Conway & Siegelman (2005) applied the term snapping to describe the phenomenon of 'sudden, drastic alteration of personality in all its many forms' (p. 6), precipitated specifically by intentional manipulation by others. Their research concluded that this phenomenon was more than a superficial alteration of behaviour or belief, and that it could bring about deeper, 'organic' changes in awareness and personality structure.

Who joins or is recruited?

There is no particular type of person who joins or is recruited into a cult (Lalich & Tobias, 2006). Individual vulnerability factors, such as being friendly, obedient, altruistic and malleable, are a more accurate predictor than personality type. The individual may be vulnerable to cult recruitment simply because they are at a transition point in their lives, bereaved, slightly depressed, lonely (Singer, 2003) or simply in the wrong place at the wrong time (Langone, 2007). Most individuals go into a religious or spiritual practice or group in the hope that it will be life-enhancing. Some groups mask their true intention using deceitful recruitment techniques (Martin, 1993).

The researches increasingly refer to those joining cults as adults as 'first generation' and those spending all or part of their childhood in a cult as 'second generation' (Kendall, 2006).

Psychiatric intervention

Occasionally, a psychiatrist or psychotherapist will be asked to help someone who has recently left a cult, or be told that the patient under their care has been under the influence of such a group. The patient may present with symptoms of anxiety, depression, a dissociative state, perhaps with psychotic symptoms, or be described by their friends or relatives as having completely changed in their personality. It may also be the case that a person with a strong psychosis talks about being damaged or chased by a cult. Some cults continue to threaten their former members after leaving and so this information may need to be verified (Singer, 2003).

The following case studies (13.1–13.3) are compositions based on real clinical situations. All names and identifying details have been changed.

Case study 13.1

Taylor: born and raised in a cult, recovering from and re-engaging with spiritual practice

Taylor is a 44-year-old married woman, of Anglo-Native American (Cherokee) descent, originally from the southern states of America. She was born into a religious-group that was later exposed as a cult in the 1970s. This group held a mixture of

---

Case study 13.1 *(contd)*

fundamentalist, charismatic, Christian teaching and pseudo-Christian views, along with ideas from other sources. It included teaching on the need to 'crucify the shadow'; that there would be 'a second coming of Jesus'; predicted 'the tribulation' (a 7-year interval where a world religious–political leader called the Anti-Christ takes power); 'Armageddon' (a terrible war provoked by the Anti-Christ in which most people on earth will die); and 'The Rapture' (a miraculous event when Christ will descend from the heavens and save 144 000 believers).

Taylor's mother was a member of the group but her father lived away from it. He was a highly intelligent man, 'a genius' in mathematics, a recluse who lacked some social skills, but who she describes as gentle in nature. Taylor describes her mother as a beautiful, strong, impassioned woman, who had spiritual gifts such as prophetic dreaming and the ability to speak in tongues, but who also had a dark, violent side to her nature.

Ritualistic abuse occurred on a regular basis. At the age of 5, Taylor took part in a staged 'live judgement day'. The right hand side of the room was cast as heaven with cult members, including her mother, dressed in white, singing to beautiful angelic music. The other side was cast as hell with people dressed as Satan moving to loud demonic music. Her aunt was painted white, lying as if dead in a coffin, waiting for resurrection. Her uncle was cast as God, directing cult members to one side or another. Taylor and her little brother were cast over to the devil's side. She remembers her little brother screaming hysterically, wanting to be with his mother. The children were indoctrinated with the fact that they were part of the devil from then on.

Sunday school lessons consisted of learning from a book called *Lucifer*. There were hundreds of demonic names associated with each of the negative emotions that needed to be rote learnt and chanted. Anger was not thought to come from the self, it was thought to be given in spirit from the devil.

Rebuke circles were common events, where the person thought to be full of demons would be surrounded by cult members dancing, speaking in tongues, singing in rapture, and touching them to force out the devil. Taylor was defiant, she disagreed that she was the devil. She was beaten, so severely that her whole face and body would be covered in welts, and remembers looking at herself in the mirror shouting to the adults 'now I am like Jesus.'

She was also sexually abused in the cult by one of its elders and two of her brothers. Her source of refuge was her father's home outside of the cult. Sexual abuse was a regular occurrence here also, from both her father and grandfather, but the environment and experience of it was much gentler, so she would prefer it to the cult environment.

By the time she was 12, she was so full of anger and murderous rage that she declared that if any man ever touched her again she would kill them. She was believed, and the abuse stopped. Following this she started to experience nightmares full of terrifying, violent, dark and erotic material. Severe panic attacks started lasting up to 30 minutes at a time, at least three times a day, that lasted for years.

She left the cult aged 14, the age when parents were no longer deemed responsible for the souls of their children. She survived in the outside world. Soon after, the group was exposed as a cult in a local newspaper.

Case study 13.1 *(contd)*

Part of Taylor's recovery has been to work on connecting with her spirituality without dissociating from her body. The practice of martial arts has been useful in this regard. In her recovery, she has also needed to recognise felt emotions such as joy or anger and to disentangle these from the alternative demonic or spiritual names attached to them in her psyche. She has had to learn to recognise emotions as coming from herself. This also meant that later in her recovery she had to accept that the dark negative energies which she naturally experiences are also from within her. This was especially hard, as her early survival from the cult had been to defy her elders' projections that she was a demon. As a mature woman she has been able to work on integrating both sides of herself at a deep level.

For the vast majority of the time she spent in the cult, both she and the other cult members were in various altered states of consciousness, 'as if we were all hypnotised.' Traumatic memories from that time were stored at that altered level of consciousness, and were barely accessible in everyday normal waking consciousness. Straight-talking therapy, therefore, provided vital containment and support, but it was not able to touch and hence adequately process the unconscious, damaging material in her psyche, driving her agoraphobic symptoms and 'emotional seizures'.

Taylor has since engaged in well-run shamanic and breath-work practices. These processes have allowed her to access this material in a safe setting with the guidance of a qualified practitioner and in doing so her symptoms have completely abated. She currently has a strong psychotherapeutic and spiritual focus in her life. She works as a mental health professional within the psychiatric system, drawing upon her experience working with indigenous cultures, as well as her own training in shamanic and breath-work techniques.

Case study 13.2

Steve: anxiety, quasi-psychotic thoughts and dissociation

At the age of 15, Steve became involved in a pseudo-Buddhist group which promoted the idea of enlightenment. He had been seduced into the group by an older woman whom he recalled had stared at him in a strange and powerful way, exerting a hypnotic effect on him; he had fallen in love with her. He later discovered that the founding leader of the group was homosexual and was himself persuaded over time that he was in fact homosexual, although he had never previously had sexual inclinations towards men. He was traumatised by the cult leader who had homosexual sex with him when he was just over the age of consent. This act, apparently necessary for 'enlightenment,' was essentially non-consensual, but Steve complied due to subtle threats that non-compliance would lead to expulsion from the group and therefore loss of enlightenment.

Part of the group practice would involve long periods of time meditating, chanting and rocking back and forth. At irregular intervals someone would stand at a microphone giving out very loud injunctions to 'surrender to the Buddha', via the cult leader.

Case study 13.2 (contd)

Steve left the group when he was in his mid-twenties and had considerable problems adjusting back into mainstream life. He sought specialist help for his panic attacks and episodes of feeling 'spaced out.' Because Steve had spent long periods of time effectively in a dissociated state, he was now struggling to focus his mind and critical faculties.

During the therapeutic intervention it was noted that some of his ideas sounded rather paranoid; for example, he was convinced that the group were out to kill him and remembered someone mentioning making him into a suicide bomber. He remembered veiled threats about what would happen to him if he left the group. He also expressed some bizarre ideas, that people are really reptiles, which his group had believed along with more classic Buddhist beliefs. He believed he had a reptile living in him and said he could see the reptile eyes blinking inside others.

Steve was calmly helped to recall what he could in a non-judgemental atmosphere. His fears relating to threats to his safety and that of others, from this apparently peace-loving Buddhist group, were taken seriously. He was encouraged to challenge the more bizarre ideas by using cognitive techniques including critical thinking and reasoning.

His levels of dissociation and the bizarre ideas indoctrinated into him began to lessen as he adjusted to the 'real' world. He had a supportive family and was slowly able to normalise back into a functional day-to-day routine.

Case study 13.3

Gina/Martha: cult pseudo-identity

By her mid-twenties, Gina had become disillusioned with being a teacher and was disenchanted with her local church. She heard about a new radical Christian community that had started up a few miles away and although she heard it was a bit 'wacky', and knew little about it, she felt there would be no harm in going along and seeing what they were up to.

She quickly became involved with the community, drawn in by their apparent genuineness, caring and desire to see her join. The leader was attractive, charismatic and seemed to think she was special.

Gina visited increasingly often, not fully listening to her gut feeling that perhaps it was too good to be true, yet not seeing anything that she felt should put her off. She spent a good deal of time in groups reading the Bible and being taught new ways of interpreting it. This included a teaching that you must leave your family and friends to show commitment to 'God'. She decided to leave her flat and job and to give her full time to the community. Her family and friends were very concerned about this but she didn't care as her new friends were pushing her to 'lay down her life for Christ' and to 'surrender' herself for the work of the community. She was excited at being accepted into this special group of people. They suggested she change her name to Martha to show her commitment to God and to them. She felt more connected to them than ever.

Case study 13.3 *(contd)*

After being a member for some months she was asked to cook the evening meal but politely declined as she was busy. The demeanour of her new 'friend' suddenly changed. She became cold, hard and chastised her. Gina/Martha was shocked by this sudden change. She could barely comprehend it and became confused. Initially, she felt a spark of anger, but quickly turned this anger against herself for questioning in the first place. This incident was followed by a period of silence from members of the group. Gina/Martha soon learnt that if she complied, she would feel accepted, and if she did not, she would receive similar rebukes and silences.

One Sunday Gina/Martha went for a walk and came back 'full of the joys of spring'. The leader told her to make some breakfast and she immediately felt resentful and let him know by a small huff that she did not want to. He insisted and so she complied. When the community met for their worship meeting later that day, Gina/Martha was received with a chillingly cold atmosphere, was told God was angry with her for her 'bad attitude' and that they wanted to talk to her privately. She was filled with dread. Later, they told her God would reject her if she did not change her attitude – Gina/Martha was deeply shocked by this and was shaking and frightened. From that time Gina became Martha in actuality. She became quiet, serious and religious, complying fully with the beliefs and practices of her new group of people, her new 'family'. She dressed differently, wore her hair differently and had no contact with her own family.

Not long after, she was told that God wanted new members to join the community and although at one time Gina would have questioned 'going out and dragging people in', and would have absolutely refused, on some level Martha remembered the anger and shock of being rebuked, which had happened unpredictably many more times, and she complied. She was told that any tactics were sanctioned in order to bring people in. She was assigned to bring men into the group. Martha understood the implications and Gina was truly buried deep within. Martha believed that sleeping with men in order to 'convert them' and obeying without question was the work of God.

Gina's personality was profoundly altered by this experience. She had grown up in a middle class, well-adjusted family, done well at school and as a young woman enjoyed partying, travelling and fun. She had had a few boyfriends and had slept with one but since then had felt she wanted to wait until she was in a long-term, stable relationship before sleeping with anyone again.

After she left the group, Gina said: 'Martha was "born" in order to become the person they expected me to be: hating my parents, rejecting all outside the community, and doing things I would never have done before – I was a stranger to myself. Martha is still present in me, and her voice is different to mine.'

Gina's therapist understood that she had developed a 'cult pseudo-personality' which was compliant with the cult, and informed her that this is usual following an abusive cult experience. Her therapist held in mind the fear that Gina had been under and took a gentle, non-challenging, empowering stance with her. Gina was helped to recall what she was like before her time in the community and she began a process of remembering and reconnecting with her pre-cult personality.

Her therapist encouraged her to get in touch with her family and old friends again, to think carefully about what she wanted to wear, how she wanted her hair and what she wanted to eat, in order to assist this process. She was encouraged to

> **Case study 13.3** *(contd)*
>
> use critical thinking and challenge the way the Bible and her belief in God had been used to control her, including finding other ways of interpreting the Bible. Gina's family were supportive and learnt as much as they could about harmful and abusive cults. They supported Gina financially for some months as she had no savings – the cult had taken all her money and she struggled with dependency issues. In time, she began to reconnect with her pre-cult self, although her therapist could see her 'floating' between the two personas.
>
> She talked about how ashamed she felt having had sex with men to bring them into the group. Her therapist explained to her that within the coercive belief system of the community it made sense (Lalich, 2004). This helped normalise her feelings and to disarm her shame. She suffered traumatic reactions, such as nightmares and flashbacks and these were worked with, again, in the context of helping Gina understand the cult control and helping her to ground herself in the reality that she had been abused. (Adapted from Jenkinson, 2008.)

Post-cult psychopathology

Leaving a cult-style group is often a traumatic experience. The way individuals leave may have an impact on their recovery process. They may walk away, be expelled (Singer, 2003), leave by means of an intervention by an ethical 'cult exit-counsellor' (Giambalvo, 1995) or leave when their parents leave the cult (Kendall, 2006).

Post-cult psychological problems include increased social dependency and decreased autonomy (Walsh & Bor, 1996), high degrees of dissociation (Martin *et al*, 1992) and significant adjustment difficulties (McKibben, *et al*, 2000). On top of these specific findings, there is generally a wide degree of agreement between a number of authors and researchers concerning general post-cult characteristics and symptoms, including: persistent emotional states such as shame, guilt, fear and cognitive deficiencies, dependence, conformity, difficulty in decision-making, cult-induced phobias, anxiety and panic attacks, depression, dissociation, derealisation, depersonalisation, complex post-traumatic stress disorder including persistent nightmares, and psychotic symptoms (Langone, 1993; Martin, 1993; Hassan, 2000; McKibben *et al*, 2000; Singer, 2003; Conway & Siegelman, 2005; Lalich & Tobias, 2006). Individuals have also attempted suicide, manifested eating disorders and been rendered mute following traumatic cult experiences (Tylden, 1995).

The term 'cult pseudo-identity' describes the phenomenon where a person's identity has been distorted or altered, and as a result a different persona emerged. It is well acknowledged that certain types of childhood trauma can be psychodynamically understood as contributing to a resulting clinical picture of dissociative identity disorder or other conditions along the same spectrum, such as fugue, amnesia or somnambulism. Not so well studied, however, is how particular forms of environmental stress in

267

adults can disrupt the normally integrative function of identity. A pseudo-identity can be generated by particular types of external stress in a person who may have previously been quite free of any signs or symptoms of personality malfunction (West & Martin, 1996; Jenkinson, 2008). There can be an abrupt switching back and forth between behaviours characteristic of the two identities, with the new personality primarily reflecting the new situational forces and requirements. Lalich (2004) suggests that the pre-cult personality fades into the background, whereas the cult persona emerges and becomes stronger:

> This is not schizophrenia, not the eruption of a split personality, as might be described in the psychology literature. Rather, the cult member undergoes the development of a personality that stands for, and with, the newly adopted world view and its practices. Total and unquestioning commitment requires a new self [Lalich, 2004: p. 19].

Kendall (2006) looked at whether the indications of harm and/or benefits were different for those becoming part of a cult as adults (first generation), as compared with those who spent all or part of their childhood in a cult (second generation). She compared their scores on psychological distress scales in adulthood as well as childhood experiences and concluded that the second generation had higher scores in adulthood for psychological distress than the samples of either first-generation former members or those who had spent no time in a sect.

Diagnosis

Perlado (2003) reviews some diagnostic proposals on the clinical complexity of those affected by cult-like organisations. He concludes that criteria unification as well as more work on specific diagnostic outlines could help in the research of this problem. He suggests that diagnosis should increase understanding of the complex psychopathology involved and warns against it adding to 'a sense of omnipotence and control over the problem'.

Martin et al have stated that 'the collective profiles for these [ex-cult member] populations appear to be sufficiently dissimilar to established clinical profiles as to warrant labelling as a distinct syndrome' (Martin et al, 1992: p. 239). Sirkin (1990) raises the difficulty of discerning whether the psychopathology is a function of cult involvement or whether it was pre-existing. He notes this question may never be resolved but suggests DSM–IV diagnosis on Axes I and II should be the rule rather than the exception. Rapid resolution of symptoms that are cult-related should usually be achieved on exiting the cult, and if so, this fits in with Axis I spectrum disorders. More long-standing personality problems that may have rendered the person vulnerable to the cult initially would be in line with Axis II.

Hassan (2000) recommends further research into the cult phenomenon and predicts that a study of in-patients in mental hospitals in the USA will reveal that a significant percentage have been recipients of destructive cult-style behaviour. Haworth (2001) notes there are well over 500 different cults operating in the UK and Hassan's prediction may therefore also be true for the UK.

Treatment

Psychiatric and psychotherapeutic help is unlikely to be of benefit to former members unless the full history and context of their cult involvement is known and understood (Martin, 1993; Singer, 2003). Psychiatric care will be dictated by the nature of the illness, the pre-morbid personality and the patient's remaining available strengths.

Specialist counselling with first-generation cult members needs to focus on:

- discerning between cult-induced psychopathology and inherent mental illness; attention to what the individual has been taught in the group will be necessary;
- education aimed at empowering the ex-cult member to understand their cult experience and undo indoctrinated teachings, beliefs and practices that compromise their autonomy;
- addressing cult-related issues before any childhood or family of origin issues;
- disarming shame (cults often use shame as a control mechanism (Lalich & Tobias, 2006) and ex-members can feel a sense of shame at having been involved);
- attending to post-traumatic stress and post-traumatic stress disorder;
- reconnecting with the pre-cult personality and moving away from the cult pseudo-identity (which may include changing appearance, reconnecting with creativity and learning to trust family, friends and new people) (Jenkinson, 2008);
- integrating the experience and moving on (see Langone, 1993; Martin, 1993; Hassan, 2000; Singer, 2003; Lalich & Tobias, 2006).

John Clarke, from Harvard Medical School, in 1979 testified before a special committee of the Vermont State Senate investigating 'the effects of some religious cults on the health and welfare of their converts'. In his statement he cited the known health hazards, both physical and psychological, and concluded:

> The fact of a personality shift in my opinion is established. That this is a phenomenon basically unfamiliar to the mental health profession I am certain of. The fact that our ordinary methods of treatment don't work is also clear, as are the frightening hazards to the process of personal growth and mental health [Conway & Siegelman, 2005: p. 78].

Specialist counselling for second-generation cult survivors needs to acknowledge their different and unusual needs. They will have no, or very little, pre-cult experience and may need a wide range of practical as well as psychological support in order to integrate into the very different and alien world outside the cult.

Conclusion

The modern world is characterised by a search for meaning in the midst of the breakdown of traditional structures and beliefs. Many people are exploring new ideas and are being attracted to a wide range of spiritual approaches. Amid this chaos a significant number will fall victim to false gurus and pathological spirituality.

Mind-altering techniques exert their influence along a continuum, but when used in an environment where there is an imbalance of power, they may cause harm. Groups that use techniques such as 'brainwashing', 'persuasive coercion', 'thought reform' and 'mind control' may be damaging to individuals, their communities and society at large. When such techniques are used, spiritual beliefs, practices and experiences may become pathological.

Psychiatry must be prepared to understand the potent effects of 'pathological spirituality' not only on the mindset of individuals but also, from the cultic studies' perspective, on the dynamics within groups. Only then can psychiatrists hope to recognise the signs and help those involved in the most effective way.

Acknowledgements

Thanks go to Lois Kendall, PhD, for reviewing the information on cults.

We also thank Ian Haworth of the Cult Information Centre UK for his kind permission to reproduce the tables.

This chapter is dedicated to Dr Elizabeth (Betty) Tylden who worked as a Consultant Psychiatrist in the NHS until her retirement in 1985. She has generously given of her time and expertise and helped innumerable ex-cult members and their families both in exiting cults and also in recovering from the after-effects. She often saw people on a charitable basis and her work was marked by her intelligence, compassion and generosity. Dr Tylden continued to work in treating individuals and their families and as an expert court witness up until 2005. She died on 3 February 2009.

References

Arlow, J. (1972) Some dilemmas in psychoanalytic education. *Journal of the American Psychoanalytic Association*, **20**, 556–566.

Barker, E. (1989) *New Religious Movements*. HMSO.

Barrett, D. V. (2001) *The New Believers: Sects, 'Cults' and Alternative Religions*. Cassell.

Battista, J. R. (1996) Offensive spirituality and spiritual defences. In *Textbook of Transpersonal Psychiatry and Psychology* (eds B. W. Scotton, A. B. Chinnen & J. R. Battista), pp. 250–260. Basic Books.

Chambers, W. V., Langone, M. D., Dole, A. A., *et al* (1994) The group psychological abuse scale: a measure of the varieties of cultic abuse. *Cultic Studies Journal*, **11**, 88–117.

Conway, F. & Siegelman J. (2005) *Snapping, America's Epidemic of Sudden Personality Change*. Stillpoint Press.

Deikman, A. J. (1983) The evaluation of spiritual and utopian groups. *Journal of Humanistic Psychology*, **23**, 8–19.

Frank, J. D. & Frank, J. B. (1993) *Persuasion and Healing: A Comparative Study of Psychotherapy*. The Johns Hopkins University Press.

Galanter, M. D. (1989) *Cults: Faith, Healing and Coercion*. Oxford University Press.

Galanter, M. D. (1990) Cults and zealous self-help movements: a psychiatric perspective. *American Journal of Psychiatry*, **147**, 543–551.

Giambalvo, C. (1995) *Exit Counselling: a Family Intervention*. American Family Foundation.

Hassan, S. (2000) *Releasing the Bonds, Empowering People to Think for Themselves*. Freedom of Mind Press.

Haworth, I. (2001) *Cults, a Practical Guide*. Cult Information Centre.

Hillman, J. (2004) *A Terrible Love of War*. Penguin.

Jenkinson, G. M. (2008) An investigation into cult pseudo-personality – what is it and how does it form? *Cultic Studies Review*, **7**, 199–224.

Kendall, L. (2006) *A Psychological Exploration into the effects of Former Membership of 'Extremist Authoritarian Sects'* (PhD Thesis). Department of Psychology, Buckinghamshire Chilterns University College.

Kernberg, O. (1986) Institutional problems of psychoanalytic education. *Journal of the American Psychoanalytic Association*, **34**, 799–834.

Lalich, J. (2004) *Bounded Choice*. University of California Press.

Lalich, J. & Tobias, M. (2006) *Take Back Your Life: Recovering from Cults and Abusive Relationships*. Baytree Publishing.

Langone, M. D. (ed.) (1993) *Recovery from Cults, Help for Victims of Psychological and Spiritual Abuse*. WW Norton.

Langone, M. D. (2007) Responding to Jihadishm: a cultic studies perspective. *Cultic Studies Review*, **5**, 268–306.

Lasch, C. (1979) *The Culture of Narcissism*. WW Norton.

Lifton, R. J. (1989) Ideological totalism. In *Thought Reform and the Psychology of Totalism: A Study of Brainwashing in China*. pp. 419–437. WW Norton.

Lifton, R. J. (1999) *Destroying the World to Save It: Aum Shinryko, Apocalyptic Violence, and the New Global Terrorism*. Metropolitan Books.

Lind, R. E. (2000) *The Seeking Self: The Quest for Self Improvement and the Creation of Personal Suffering*. Phanes Press.

Martin, P. R. (1993) *Cult-Proofing Your Kids*. Zondervan Publishing House

Martin, P. R., Langone, M. D., Dole, A. A., et al (1992) Post-cult symptoms as measured by the MCMI before and after residential treatment. *Cultic Studies Journal*, **9**, 219–240.

Masson, J. M. (1994) *Against Therapy*. Common Courage Press.

McKibben, J. A., Lynn, S. J. & Malinoski, P. (2000) Are cultic environments psychologically harmful? *Clinical Psychology Review*, **20**, 91–111.

Murray, S. (2004) *Post-Christendom: Church and Mission in a Strange New World*. Paternoster.

Ofshe, R. & Singer, M. R. (1986) Attacks on peripheral verses central elements of self and the impact of thought-reforming techniques. *Cultic Studies Journal*, **3**, 3–24.

Perlado, M. (2003) Clinical and diagnostic issues of cultism: group dependence disorder. *Cultic Studies Review*, **2** (2). [internet edn]

Raubolt, R. (2006) *Power Games: Influence, Persuasion and Indoctrination in Psychotherapy Training*. Other Press.

Reber, A. S. & Reber, E. (2001) *The Penguin Dictionary of Psychology* (3rd edn). Penguin.

Schein, E. H. (1961) *Coercive Persuasion: A Socio-Psychological Analysis of 'Brainwashing' of American Civilian Prisoners by the Chinese Communists*. WW Norton.

Singer, M. (2003) *Cults in Our Midst* (revised). Jossey-Bass.

Sirkin, M. I. (1990) Cult involvement: a systems approach to assessment and treatment. *Psychotherapy*, **27**, 116–123.

Stahelski, A. (2004) Terrorists are made, not born: creating terrorists using social psychological conditioning. *Journal of Homeland Security* (www.homelanddefense.org/journal/Articles/stahelski.html).

Storr, A. (1996) *Feet of Clay: A Study of Gurus*. Free Press.

Temerlin, J. W. & Temerlin, M. K. (1986) Some hazards of the therapeutic relationship. *Cultic Studies Journal*, **3**, 234–242.

Temerlin, M. K. & Temerlin, J. W. (1982) Psychotherapy cults: an iatrogenic perversion. *Psychotherapy: Theory, Research and Practice*, **19**, 131–141.

Tylden, E. (1995) *The Church, Medicine and the New Age* (ed. J. Watt). Churches' Council for Health and Healing.

Walsh, Y. & Bor, R. (1996) Psychological consequences of involvement in a new religious movement or cult. *Counselling Psychology Quarterly*, **9**, 47–60.

West L. J. & Martin P. R. (1996) Pseudo-identity and the treatment of identity change in captives and cults. *Cultic Studies Journal*, **13**, 125–152.

Zimbardo, P. (1993) Understanding mind control: exotic and mundane mental manipulations. In *Recovery from Cults, Help for Victims of Psychological and Spiritual Abuse* (ed. M. Langone). WW Norton.

CHAPTER 14

Ageing

Robert M. Lawrence and Julia H. Head

> For the suffering individual ... what he makes of his suffering – whether it becomes a triumph or a tragedy of the human spirit, whether hope gains, or despair – matters, not just to himself, but to the creation itself ... Whatever anyone may think then, the response of the suffering individual matters: he is not powerless. But his power is not apparent: its true measure is relative not to the achievement of others, but to the suffering individual's own condition [Boyd, 2000: p. 88].

Old age psychiatry is a discipline of particular 'confluence', where medical and psychological sciences meet in more integrated and interrelated presentations than at any other time in a patient's life. Pathology increases and psychopathology becomes more frequent, the latter being brought about by the substantial occurrence of dementia or functional illness, or both. The social profile of an older person can be marked by the accumulation of progressive losses in social meaning and networks. For example, their relationship with family members and friends may undergo significant changes as a result of relocation to supported accommodation or residential and nursing facilities. The challenge of a personal journey into degrees of fragility and isolation creates fertile ground for increased vulnerability and the generation of specific needs, related to mental, emotional, spiritual and physical well-being. The relevance of a multidimensional and holistic approach therefore becomes paramount in the teaching and training of old age psychiatrists.

It appears that in the assessment of the older person insufficient attention has been paid to core aspects of the personality, which can convey important information on coping skills and how they influence responses to treatment, and thus overall outcome. Deep among these lie the root constructs of a person's vision of life and personal meanings, and the presence of a spiritual core. This may or may not be accompanied by formal religious adherence and integration into a faith community.

The scope of this chapter is to review the ageing process and the emerging psychopathologies of old age psychiatry, the role of spirituality in ageing and the diverse ways in which individuals approach the transition to later life. In addition, we consider an approach that goes beyond standard medical practice.

Psychopathologies commonly emerging in old age psychiatry

Physical pathologies

Levels of physical ageing vary between individuals. Mechanisms at play are both genetic and related to 'wear and tear' of body systems and organs. The expectation is that gradually eyesight, hearing, skin, reproductive, neurological, metabolic and endocrinological functions, bone structure and mobility will become less efficient, rendering individuals more prone to the development of disease (Bittles, 2002; Stuart-Hamilton, 2006).

Outward signs of ageing include graying of hair, wrinkling of skin, changes in posture, slowness and hesitancy in gait and coordination. Hearing and eyesight can also be affected. The reduction of bone density increases the risk of osteoporosis and the urogenital system becomes less effective. There is an increased incidence of heart disease, hypertension and gastrointestinal pathologies. Respiratory function is reduced and atherosclerotic changes appear, bringing a risk of peripheral and cerebrovascular damage.

Psychological pathologies

In the older individual, cognitive functions slow down, together with the ability to learn new information (Persson *et al*, 2006; Townsend *et al*, 2006). This translates into diminished ability to accustom to new situations and the acquisition of more rigid personality traits. This may also be understood as part of a reactive strategy to stave off the disintegration of function in the face of reduced skills.

There is no unitary personality theory that may be applied to ageing. However, it has been observed that introversion increases and neuroticism decreases with age, in principle promoting a quieter and more contented outlook (Eysenck & Eysenck, 1969). Erikson's theory of stages of development throughout one's lifespan depends on the accomplishment or failure, partial or total, of successive life transitions. In this 'nested', multi-staged life history, chronological age is not as relevant as the outcome of transition from stage to stage (Erikson, 1963, 1982). Erickson posits a final stage from around age 65 as 'integration *v*. despair', which can be viewed as a basic conflict affecting many people that are seen in old age psychiatry services.

Social pathologies

Social milestones in the transition to old age include retirement from employment, reduction in income and the ever-increasing likelihood of bereavement. Previous relationships and supportive networks shrink and may disappear altogether. Health problems are likely to add to the burden of advancing years, contributing to the decision to move away from one's house and a familiar neighbourhood to the new environment of sheltered housing or care homes.

Within Western society, ageing may be stereotyped both by the young and the old as a phase of decline, social and financial redundancy, and as the target of humour ranging from benevolence to outright disrespect. This phenomenon speaks of a 'financial, power-driven' morality present in modern society which may intrinsically disenfranchise the old. This 'morality' does not promote caring attributes and intergenerational responsibility. Fortunately, a current of opinion is slowly emerging today that is attempting to reinstitute respect and dignity to the role of older adults. However, it is far from overcoming the predominant trend, which is well-rooted in our modern history (Department of Health 2001; Age Concern & Mental Health Foundation, 2006; Department of Health & Care Services Improvement Partnership, 2006; Royal College of Psychiatrists, 2006).

The physical decline that does not spare higher cortical functions erodes social networks and challenges the psychological transitions of old age and may also attack the core of a person's long-term inner constructs. This can affect the ability to hold on to a sense of personal integrity. Personal resources may waver under the strain and even collapse altogether when facing the magnitude of the task at hand. However, this challenge can serve as a process enabling the individual to reaffirm identity and self-esteem.

Depression and dementia

Depression is very common in the dementias; it has been described as both a predisposing factor and integral to clinical presentation, as well as reactive to patients' degree of awareness concerning their diagnosis and its implications (Amore et al, 2007; Chinello et al, 2007; Pfennig et al, 2007). Up to 15% of older people experience symptoms of depression and 3% have a depressive episode (Baldwin, 2002), but in association with physical illness and cognitive dysfunction prevalence increases to about 20%, affecting about a third of those in residential and nursing homes.

Depression in old age has been linked to physical factors such as heightened vulnerability to cerebrovascular changes and primary neurodegenerations (Allen & Burns, 1995; Banerjee et al, 1996; Robert et al, 1997; Baldwin, 2007), as well as the overall increased frequency of health problems and disability. Psychological and social factors also play a part by adding loss of role, low self-esteem, expectations of a bleak future and progressive marginalisation.

Depression is directly related to suicide and the elderly are very vulnerable here, particularly older men (Pearson et al, 1997; Pritchard & Baldwin, 2000). For men, the act of suicide is 'often planned and rational', indicating 'not an unwillingness to live or inability to live but a willingness to die' (Hassan, quoted in MacKinlay, 2001: p. 73).

In practice, the old age psychiatrist deals with only the most severe cases of depression and/or cognitive and/or behavioural problems, especially where the cognitive deficit has reached the stage of causing substantial concern in patient and/or carer. The diagnostic process is complex and leads to different strands of action for diverse needs to be met. Old age psychiatrists are trained to recognise physical contributors to psychopathology. For this reason, the initial assessment includes detailed investigations and identification of acquired sensory deficits and of issues around poor mobility. Such assessments are carried out 'at home', where the absence of support networks, vulnerability and risk factors are more promptly identified. At the completion of investigations, medication may be prescribed, support care packages are put in place and skills in activities of daily living maximised, if possible. All this effort is directed at improving mental well-being as well as quality of life. The formal and informal burden of care can be considerable.

The elderly person is dealing with getting older and frailer. They may be depressed or concerned about forgetfulness. Depression strips an individual of positive feelings about him- or herself and the world, and in the older person it may find perverse validation in stereotypical self-degradation and lack of social support. An individual in this state feels lonely, anxious, frightened, hopeless, abandoned and, at best, ambivalent about his or her future. He or she may begin to think that death or euthanasia are preferable since there is nothing left in life to do or enjoy. There may be thoughts of 'altruistic suicide', where an individual, feeling a burden to others, may contemplate taking his or her life for their benefit. Medication attempts to repair the biochemical imbalance, 'activities of daily living' training addresses rehabilitation and psychology seeks to explain maintaining and precipitating factors. The care programme, however, steps into true human focus only when the person can be reached at more intimate emotional levels, commencing with true acknowledgement and respect for his or her singular and unique humanity. This acknowledgement is based on a non-verbal disposition that allows respectful contact at a deep level and in principle does not exclude those individuals where the gift of spoken language is irreparably lost or was never there.

Through a person-centred approach, the care of the older person requires a holistic stance that goes beyond the generic medical model. It stands to reason, therefore, that the old age psychiatrist should be encouraged to develop skills in recognising and assessing a broader range of factors that are relevant to individual care patterns. These may include spiritual reawakening and validation, religious coping and resurgence of faith, reactions to loss, and death anxieties and their psychopathological manifestations.

All these factors highlight the interface of religion/spirituality and physical and mental well-being. They are also important in helping practitioners understand how older people's perspectives on the meaning of life and suffering may influence the nature of therapeutic relationships and health outcome.

We shall first discuss aspects of this interface, before addressing the quest for meaning and integration in later life.

The role of spirituality in ageing

Resurgence in spiritual interest in older people

Older people often resume aspects of behaviour relating to internal and formal religiousness (Idler *et al*, 2001, Wink & Dillon, 2002, 2003; Dalby, 2006). This suggests an internal shift towards seeking security and control when they become less accessible to the individual. Factors that appear to correlate with return to spirituality in older adults are religious upbringing, life events and introspective and insightful personality traits. The personal meaning is the affirmation of one's continuity despite changing appearance and decline in physical strength and health (Ross, 1995; Isaia *et al*, 1999). The social meaning, especially in the context of religious networks and activities, also serves to counteract the feeling of isolation experienced through separation and bereavement (Folkman & Lazarus, 1984; Koenig *et al*, 1988a; Guignon, 2000).

Older people recognise the value of religion, the pursuit of specific interests, healthy lifestyles, will power and socialisation as coping mechanisms. They are also aware of the possible benefits of spiritual approaches in providing a framework of meaning to one's experience (Pieper, 1981). It seems that spirituality has an existential purpose, mediating a process of reconnection with oneself at the end of life (Sabat & Harre, 1992; Slater, 1995). In fact, spiritual conduct may be more relevant to outcome in terms of well-being than either social support or financial status (Koenig *et al*, 1988b; Fry, 2000; Koenig, 2006).

General health outcomes and spirituality/religion in older people

Current evidence suggests that religion and spirituality have an important role in the health of the elderly. Spirituality has been linked with more positive perceptions of one's general health, whereas older people spontaneously refer to religious coping in health surveys (Bosworth *et al*, 2003) and to coping better with the pain and disability of a range of conditions, such as rheumatoid arthritis, cardiac surgery, hypertension (Koenig *et al*, 1997, 1999; Bartlett, 2003).

Religiousness appears also to be linked with better health through participation in more wholesome patterns of behaviour, such as not smoking, drinking moderately, more physical activity and socialisation. In groups where social support networks are dedicated to mutual care, individuals become aware of problems in other members of the group; identification of problems may be easier and earlier and compliance with treatment more likely than for those who are socially isolated (Koenig *et al*, 1999). A higher degree of self-esteem may also indirectly reflect upon the resilience of the immune system (Lutgendorf *et al*, 2004).

Religious practice and health outcomes

Religious practice has been found to effect a degree of protection against the more serious symptoms of depressive disorder, although less has been reported about the actual correlation between depression and individual spiritual make-up. However, the prevalence of depressive symptoms varies in populations drawn from different faith groups (Kennedy *et al*, 1996; Braam *et al*, 1997; Koenig *et al*, 1997; Butler & Orrell, 1998; Dein, 2006). Studies of older people suggest that rates of depressive illness are lower among some faith groups such as Roman Catholics, and higher in other groups such as Pentecostals. This may reflect the extent of support of a faith community (Meador *et al*, 1992; Braam *et al*, 2001).

Religious practice has been described as protecting against depression when individuals are also physically ill (Wink *et al*, 2005), in hospital (Koenig, 2004) or a nursing home (Milstein *et al*, 2003), and in lessening anxiety symptoms linked to specific situations, such as fear of falling (Reyes-Ortiz *et al*, 2006). Studies have also highlighted the complexity of interaction between depression and the dimensions of organised, non-organised and intrinsic religiosity (Parker *et al*, 2003); here, those with less severe depression score higher on all three dimensions than those with more severe depression. Conversely, depression and poor quality of life have been linked to lack of belief in external and/or divine means and a negative attitude towards faith communities and organised religion (Koenig *et al*, 1988*b*).

The importance of faith and formal religious practice in older people has been the subject of much psychosocial exploration in recent years. The evidence points to a positive correlation with mental health, and in coping with disease (Koenig *et al*, 1988*a*; Koenig, 1994; Pargament, 1997; Krause *et al*, 1999; Fry, 2000; Post *et al*, 2000).

In a project looking at 2676 individuals aged between 17 and 65 at baseline in 1965 and who were alive in 1994, those who worshipped regularly were found to be generally healthier, particularly women. Results suggested about 23% lesser risk of dying during the study period for those individuals who worshipped regularly (Strawbridge *et al*, 1997; 2001).

The Swiss longitudinal study of individuals older than 80 years of age suggests that religious practice correlates with longevity (Spini *et al*, 2001), and a 6-year longitudinal study in North Carolina of individuals older than 64 years of age (Koenig *et al*, 1999) confirmed generally healthier lifestyles and a survival rate as much as 46% higher among church attendees than non-attendees.

The relationship between better survival and private religious activity was described by Helm *et al* (2000) in older people who had participated in religious worship before developing impairment in activities of daily living. Longer survival of older people has also been observed in religious *v.* secular kibbutzim in Israel (Kark *et al*, 1996), unrelated to diverse sociological cohort profiles. Religious beliefs have further been associated with health and well-being in elderly men, more so than religious practice (Kroll & Sheehan, 1989; Pressman *et al*, 1990), a positive correlation that extends to an association between religion and lesser risks of both mortality and depression (Post, 1995; Post *et al*, 2000).

Looked at the other way round, in a study of elderly physically ill men, after controlling for baseline physical and mental health and demographics, higher mortality during a 2-year follow-up was found to be associated with feelings of loss of faith, of being abandoned by God or of being the victim of evil forces (Pargament *et al*, 2001).

Spirituality, meaning and health outcomes

Spirituality has been linked with higher self-esteem (Krause *et al*, 1999), more positive mood states and improved psychiatric treatment outcome (Bosworth *et al*, 2003). Individuals with dementia may still clearly be concerned with spiritual themes. The qualitative analysis of interviews carried out on 23 individuals with early dementia (Katsuno, 2003) identified a primary separate category of 'faith in God', with six subcategories. These were: belief, support from God, sense of meaning/purpose in life, private religious practice, public religious practice and changes due to dementia.

Spiritual themes may also discretely nest in psychopathology. In a study of 'musical' hallucinations, older individuals with a diagnosis of dementia commonly described hearing religious tunes (Warner & Aziz, 2005). This phenomenon may relate to the uncovering of culture-bound unconscious mechanisms. An individual's spiritual life may facilitate a sense of not feeling alone in the experience of pain, being part of a 'grand design' and attributing a meaning to the experience of pain as atonement, purification, transition, maturation, spiritual progress and salvation, which may apply to older people in a poignant way.

Nomothetic research method does not reveal this unique, more complex process taking place at an individual level. There are diverse degrees of appreciation, definition and expression of the individual's experience and personal views of health and sickness. Individuals will have their own sense of why they are unwell, alongside what they are told by doctors, religious people or even their own faith tradition.

Why then should 'religion' and spirituality help with better outcomes? What is the nature of the relationship between these factors? Apart from rational and more superficial accounts of any individual's experience of illness, distress, pain and suffering, there is a deeper, symbolic level of meaning to the event. We would suggest that this is what (consciously or unconsciously) influences a relationship with health outcomes, requiring the assuaging intervention of healing and coping methods. This is the level at which it is possible to discern and understand how spiritual and religious factors are embedded in health states; helping to make these more explicit is part of the caring and healing process. Illich (1990) illustrates this point well:

> When I suffer pain, I am aware that a question is being raised... Pain is the sign for something not answered; it refers to something open, something that goes on the next moment to demand, 'What is wrong?' 'How much longer?' Observers who are blind to this referential aspect of pain are left with nothing but conditioned reflexes. They are studying a guinea pig, not a human being. A physician, were he able to erase this value-loaded question shining through a patient's complaints, might recognise pain as the symptom of a specific bodily disorder, but he would not come close to the suffering that drove the patient to seek help [p. 149].

The symbolic level of meaning provides a strong argument for de-objectifying the experience of illness and distress in favour of a more anthropocentric and holistic approach. Creative use of pain and suffering by all individuals involved in the process means engaging more with the movement towards healing, recognising the 'mystery' of pain and suffering as part of the human condition, being creative with that experience and willing to explore the 'mystery.' An individual's ability to do that does not diminish with mental and emotional crises – it is often heightened – but doing so from a place of pain and distress can be a difficult and courageous journey to make (Head, 2004).

Individuals will have their own resources and will also seek them out in order to counteract the loneliness, isolation and unsupported sense of self that so often accompanies the experience of disease and pain. For many, this will include their religious and spiritual resources as well as looking to their immediate carers as a major part of their resources. The studies relating to older adults with mental health needs reveal very powerfully the subjective nature of the experience that they are going through on physical, psychological, social, emotional and spiritual levels. Psychological states involved in the process of ageing as it interfaces with mental disturbance and organic dysfunction include (Head 2006):

loss	depression	grief	anxiety
despair	forgetfulness	terror	emptiness
isolation	alienation	deterioration	suspicion
paranoia	devaluation	unpredictability	denial
confusion	avoidance	fear	aggression
frustration	restlessness	diminishment	sadness
anger	blaming		

The practitioner who cannot hear questions associated with 'Why is this happening to me?' may miss a vital opportunity for enhanced outcome and patient well-being. Not paying attention to these questions may also have the effect of causing/increasing spiritual distress.

Prayer and old age

Prayer is both personal and congregational. Fundamentally based on terms of relationship and hope, it can become an emotional bridge to 'optimism'. In the older individual, personal prayer reflects striving towards integrity of the mature self in the face of age-inherent weakness, in relation to a transcendent entity believed to be watching, listening, understanding and holding in empathy and love. It is not possible to properly describe personal prayer as content, but rather as a function of individual 'connection'. In this special relationship with the Transcendent, the self-worth of the older individual is affirmed (Krause, 2004).

In its congregational aspects, prayer acquires the symbolism of rituals that are performed as a group. This group engagement enables adaptation and cohesion (Searle, 1992). Emotional validation and companionship are therefore also promoted through a set of basic spiritual meanings represented in the performing together of specific acts derived from religious tradition and culture.

Prayer is said to have healing attributes in both physical illness and mental disturbance (Mackenzie *et al*, 2000; Ai *et al*, 2002). For example, prayer as therapy is a source of spirituality for the elderly with dementia (Abramowitz, 1993; Higgins, 2003; Shamy, 2003; Higgins *et al*, 2004). In an unpublished recent pilot project, individuals in moderate and severe stages of dementia, both believers and non-believers, freely took part in a prayer ritual especially adapted to their needs with the help of an experienced spiritual advisor. A qualitative analysis of the feedback from fourteen consecutive participants identified eight categories of feelings that arose as a result:

- feeling good
- human dignity
- feeling accepted
- being together/sharing
- company *v.* isolation
- coping
- caring for others
- faith/religion are relevant.

In the group, participants generally felt at ease and expressed their wishes for themselves and others. This helped them feel valued, accepted and supported (Higgins 2005, personal communication).

Loss and bereavement

Loss on many different levels affects older adults in mental healthcare and their caregivers to a disturbing degree (Head 2006). Speaking of the many losses and threats of loss that most human beings have to negotiate, Cheston & Bender (2000) report that:

psychiatric disturbance increases in proportion to the severity of multiple losses. It is not just that the loss and its subsequent handicap creates emotional disturbance as part of its process, but also that the burden of a handicap depletes the individual's resources, leaving him or her prey to what is internally unresolved and disturbed [p. 157].

For an older person, the death of one's partner or finding that one is increasingly the lone survivor of a long list of departed friends and relatives can easily tip over the balance from coping with an already large number of adverse personal events into despair. However, in addition to the demise of nearest and dearest, bereavement and loss take many different forms. The older person has left behind his or her youth, physical strength, looks, ambitions and a number of unfulfilled dreams, employment, a more active role in society, the public acknowledgement of his or her usefulness and so often a family home. Transition into old age strips the individual of material references and a sense of external security, never to be replaced. At this difficult time, spiritual constructs, for example a belief in an afterlife or the contentment of having usefully achieved the completion of one's life cycle, sustain emotional and psychological endurance (Fry, 2001).

Tragically, however, when mental disturbance strikes, the loss can reach into the very meaning of one's existence, and compromise the journey to integrity by destroying the basis of self-esteem on which it started. Worse still, it can erase the functional memory of the journey, producing a devastating vacuum of fear. The spiritual encounter is dedicated to healing through patiently journeying with the individual who has depression and sifting through themes that can still bring comfort. This can include searching for traces of past conflict, guilt or lack of forgiveness for oneself or others, still nested in spiritual anguish and needing resolution. In dementia, one may need to go 'beyond words'. When the use of language is no longer accessible to the individual, touch, lights, colours and sounds from the past may still give a sense of connection and comfort (Lawrence, 2003; 2007).

Patients, caregivers and spirituality

Myriads of devoted informal carers walk alongside older individuals who experience physical and/or mental distress. Caring for someone who is close to us is difficult enough at any age; yet additional problems arise in the care of older people. Diseases are more likely to be chronic and complex, accompanied by physical and emotional pain. The carers of the seriously and chronically ill are also vulnerable to stress and illness, even more so because those who care for an older person are likely to be their spouse and themselves elderly, or else their children. The old age psychiatrist is called to place them too in a framework of holistic care and support and to understand their needs.

Reviews of available studies are inconclusive as to the real impact of spirituality or formal religious practice on caregivers' well-being, but there are more than anecdotal indications of some positive effects, both on themselves and on those they care for. In terminal cancer, for example, the spiritual caregiver is described as being more willing to engage in carrying the burden of care and deriving more satisfaction in the process (Hebert *et al*, 2006; Pearce *et al*, 2006). For those who lose a loved one to a terminal illness, the process of grief and vulnerability to depressive breakdown may be lessened through a foundation of faith in an afterlife and the support of a spiritual network (Walsh *et al*, 2002; Fenix *et al*, 2006). Carers of people with a mental illness may find support in spiritual means of coping – personal religiousness has been found to be more effective in this case than congregational activities (Murray-Swank *et al*, 2006). Indeed, the caregiver does not need to belong to a faith tradition or to a religious community to derive a personal spiritual meaning from the experience of caring (Stuckey, 2003).

There is evidence that caregivers of people with dementia not only pray frequently but also cope better with their role, if they perceive it to be within a spiritual and/or religious context (Dudley & Kosinski, 1990; Guberman *et al*, 1992; Stolley *et al*, 1999). Spouses of individuals with dementia face a long journey during which their known marital relationship will erode from its original form and move to a completely different level. Here intimacy is lost, communication is no longer at the same level and responsibility is no longer shared. They can become depressed and also physically ill (Meller, 2001). However, the more stable the history of the relationship with the caregiver before dementia developed and the more spiritual its foundation, the more successful the emotional itinerary of the caregiver appears to be (Dudley & Kosinski, 1990; Guberman *et al*, 1992; LoboPrabhu *et al*, 2005). The experience of caring for someone with dementia may therefore also produce a 'positive outcome' by providing the context for spiritual growth, which may in part counteract the stress of the burden of care (Acton & Miller, 2003; Sanders, 2005). As the latter increases, so recourse to spiritual matters may grow (Skaff, 1995; Picot *et al*, 1997; Vernooij-Dassen *et al*, 1997; Chang *et al*, 1998). In some cases, church communities can contribute to caregiver support by providing key emotional and practical help (Ragno, 1995).

End-of-life issues

End-of-life issues have both sociocultural and personal existential implications. From society's viewpoint, old age is linked to the expectation that the individual will make a final will and testament and also provide advance directives for one's continued care and quality of life with, where appropriate, lasting powers of attorney. This has cultural and intercultural ramifications.

End-of-life decisions reflect cultural and ethnic backgrounds. Qualitative analysis of a community of Chinese elders in Canada revealed that decisions concerning approaching death were intrinsically linked to concepts of hope and ending one's life cycle according to Buddhist, Taoist and Confucian religious perspectives (Bowman & Singer, 2001).

Management of terminal illness is also interpreted within the framework of the individual's culture and beliefs. Jewish, Catholic and Protestant residents from thirteen nursing homes in the USA participated in a survey examining their last given instructions on life-sustaining measures, half having given 'advanced directives'. Those of higher education and with less hope appeared to desire more intervention at the end of their lives. In this study, the Jewish participants expressed a stronger wish to receive life-sustaining interventions (Ejaz, 2000).

At an existential level, the ageing process is likely to mean facing the fear of one's own death and annihilation of existence. The negotiation of this process is supported not only by faith constructs in an afterlife but also by a sense of personal esteem fed by the successful completion of one's life cycle, as well as one's existence having contributed to future generations (Cicirelli, 2002).

The quest for meaning

What does it all mean? People have their own answers to existential questions. Some view suffering as just part of getting older, others as a punishment from God and yet others as confirmation that there is no God or higher power. Resentment or regret over one's life may develop, the whole experience becoming passive in the face of what could also be seen as life's final challenge. However, getting older can also be a period in which the individual brings into focus real priorities and achieves the contentment of having discovered the meaning of his or her life after all, not least the resignation and freedom to accept one's final fate. In an older person this private quest for meaning can be hijacked by levels of emotional disturbance and thrown into chaos by the experience of dementia.

Negotiating life's final challenge

In being alongside individuals as they face life's final challenge, the question remains how clinicians can find encouragement to work with the full spectrum of Erikson's final stage of 'integration v. despair' mentioned earlier. This is not so much about prescribed modes of 'doing to' the patient but more about modes of 'being with' those who are negotiating end of life issues as they interface with their mental and emotional health. A starting point is for clinicians themselves to be able to reflect on the meaning of suffering and the existential questions it raises – for the world of one's patients is never very far removed from that of one's own.

A fundamental aspect concerning the nature of suffering is that it changes one's sense of self, testing the way a person approaches life and its exigencies (Head, 2006). Pain and suffering may impart a sense of meaninglessness but it is more often about the way it disturbs connections to others, as we struggle to remain connected to the world we have known, which of course will never quite be the same again. Yet as practitioners, we can uphold the possibility that human beings continue to be actors in events that threaten their personhood, especially in relation to a person's inner world, when the effects may not be so visible to the outside world. Perhaps it is important also for practitioners to acknowledge that it is virtually impossible to know when this movement towards personal development and spiritual integrity has ceased.

Our concern must be to find the dignity that belongs to personhood within the midst of suffering, pain and decline. The Royal College of Psychiatrists' 'Changing Minds' booklet on Alzheimer's disease and dementia seems to suggest that we can do that, and that the question 'If your mind goes, do you go with it?' can be answered firmly in the negative. For example:

> The change comes slowly. Who is to say that this is the moment at which you stop seeing him as himself? He loses his dignity when you stop treating him with dignity.
>
> When a person can't remember or do the things he used to do, he is like a different person. If he also acts differently, you might say he is not the man he was. But that depends on what makes him the man he is.
>
> Just because he cannot speak, it does not mean he cannot understand.
>
> The person gradually loses his intelligence, his memory and his personality. Some go quietly, others rebel. This is distressing for people close to them. But for the man himself? Perhaps it is better than being invisible [Royal College of Psychiatrists, 2004].

With people who are ageing, can we embrace the possibility that they may continue to be on their progressive journey towards 'spiritual maturity', even though there may be 'ways forward and ways backward ... directions which enhance our humanity, and ... directions which diminish and endanger it' (Macquarrie, 1982: p. 228). Can we think that it is possible for us to journey with people in terms of their experiences being transforming and transcending, even when journeying together appears to come to nothing? When our own perspectives on the nature of suffering and pain do not allow for this, we might otherwise conclude that little can be done in terms of communication and interaction, and we are just waiting for death.

> Pain, sickness and suffering ... are part of what it means to be human. But not necessarily for everyone, at least as far as physical pain and suffering are concerned ... Nor does everyone respond to these experiences in the same way. For some, they are the making of character; for others its destruction. Some reach for aspirin, others turn to prayer. Pain, sickness and suffering thus raise questions both about how we should understand them and about how we should respond to them [Boyd, 2000: p. 81].

Perhaps all of this is about being able to entertain the idea that in later years we still have the capacity to transform old parts of ourselves and not get rid of them, or that we can hear and relate to the pain and suffering that is an inevitable part of life from a different place, that is, to change our relationship with it.

MacKinlay (2001) suggests that 'spiritual development and growth as a process towards achieving spiritual integrity has been identified as a developmental task of ageing' (p. 220). Much of her language in discussing the interface of spirituality and ageing includes the notion of people transforming and transcending their difficulties. From her research, she identifies characteristics associated with growth and development that include:

> An openness to change and learning; an attitude of searching for the ultimate meaning in their lives; relationship with a confidante and/or membership of a long-term small group. It also included transcendence of disabilities and losses encountered in ageing; acceptance of their past life and a readiness to face the future, including the ability to live with uncertainty, and, finally, a sense of freedom and a move to a greater degree of interiority [MacKinlay, 2001: p. 220].

The spiritual tasks of ageing include transcending disabilities and loss, finding final meaning and hope, intimacy with God and/or others – all of which centre on responding to the ultimate meaning in life. Again, we have this notion of interiority, of the individual's inner world, evoking the idea of a realm of thinking, feeling, desiring and imagining not always available to objective scrutiny but holding vital energy in terms of the person's spiritual/ transpersonal journey.

In our engagement with older adults, it may be difficult for us to discern, particularly where communication through words is minimal, quite what is going on in their spiritual and religious life. It may be that we have to be more creative in offering an empathic response that looks beyond what is most immediately obvious. Killick's reflections on the experience of dementia remaining a fundamental mystery – but a mystery that is part of the broader mystery of life itself – provide us with an example of this creative thinking:

> Looking at this woman before me I am led to speculate on her life – what events have shaped her, has she experienced the highs and lows of existence, or has she maintained an equilibrium, living largely uneventfully and untroubled? Has her frame been stirred with passion, and the only just supportable knowledge of its being returned? Or have her days been informed by a steady and constant affection, to lull her into the illusion of permanence? Does this love still sustain her in her present removed state? [Killick, 2002: p. 23]

Pain and suffering occur, and call for healing, on all levels – physical, psychological, social and spiritual. We are not dealing with suffering in old age as a static category but with individuals from different contexts and cultures, with varying responses to life events all the way through their lives. We often deal with individuals who find it difficult to exercise autonomy over personal growth, who may desire to dwell in the past and who may be fearful of opening up to the future. On the other hand, we also encounter people who have been journeying with life's meanings and mysteries for many years.

Perhaps another vital element of spiritual accompaniment is to recognise that in many cases we are not talking about major and one-off moments of transformation. Neither are we talking about linear progression of one's spiritual life such that it reaches its pinnacle with old age – although some kind of progression and maturity in the same might be expected. We are talking very often about 'moments' of transformation/transcendence and of the forgetting of such moments, and about starting right from the beginning when working with some people, although we cannot always be so sure about this either.

Spiritual care

Spiritual care is aimed at maintaining personhood and upholding the dignity and respect of individuals, which is particularly relevant for those whose mental powers are failing (Kitwood, 1997). Practitioners play a potentially important role in the spiritual care process. However, this depends on developing the ability to use skills of empathic listening and validating presence – concepts that should not be alien to practitioners.

Most people find themselves caught in the realities of life, which include pain and suffering. Sometimes the pain we face incapacitates our very response to it. However, staying with the tension of the distress caused by suffering and not aiming for quick 'resolution' is the art of anyone who considers that there can be movements towards health even in the midst of pain and distress. This indicates the importance for practitioners of revisiting their own philosophies on health and sickness, because spiritual care depends first on being in a 'right relationship' with ourselves before we can be in an authentic relationship with others. This is a factor that is often overlooked in the mental health context.

> Right relationships begin with ourselves. This exploration will inevitably transcend the very limited scientific view of what we are as human beings, and cause us to re-examine and incorporate spiritual values into our caring work. When this occurs, the healing potential expands ... New relationships can come into existence which recognise the value of being with people as much as doing to them. Carers can let go of the intense effort required to give compassion, and relax into *being* compassionate, *being* healing, in short, *becoming* the sacred space in which healing occurs [Wright & Sayer-Adams, 2000: p. 41].

People who have struggled with their own meaning can recognise that same spiritual endeavour in others. A person who is distressed needs another person who may be able to open up to them the experience of being genuinely understood. Those who are mentally distressed are very keenly aware of the chaos involved with the loss of self. It is only when individuals can accept this within themselves, which they will do at many different levels, that the growth towards 'personhood' advances. What is important is that practitioners can commit themselves to 'be with' the person in distress. Sometimes giving a 'space' wherein the person may experience presence, but not necessarily have to act in it, is the only thing one can share with the other. The silence of encounter is more expressive and indicative of authentic solidarity with another than words could ever be.

To sit with someone who is not communicating is the real test of empathy in encounter – to listen to what the person might be trying to communicate in ways other than through language, and to think oneself into the experience of what life is like for them. This is the same for all forms of disturbance and age, but the difference may show itself in how we attempt to enable a person's resources for communicating what they most need.

> Is any life worth the selfless devotion that would be necessary to sustain this commitment? And yet, if relationship is to mean anything, then surely this is just the circumstance which provides the testing-ground – the greatest need existing where no need is manifest? [Killick, 2002: p. 23]

All of the elements of authentic relationship, presence, encounter, empathy and listening, will honour an individual's spiritual quest at any time of life – enabling the discernment and respecting of spiritual need and nurturing the dignity of personhood.

Conclusion

Many contemporary writers describe the notion of an innate movement of human beings towards health and the maintaining of personhood. This often expresses itself precisely in the struggle of coping with adversity and decline – a struggle that can lead to oscillation, an either/or position relating to Erikson's stage of integrity *v.* despair. However, given the right support, a different reality can emerge, that of adopting a more synthesised position of working with the 'given' (Head, 2006). The theologian, John Macquarrie (1982) speaks of two possible reactions to pain and suffering, in terms of rebellion and resignation/passive acceptance. However, he effectively promotes a third way – a synthesis of these two positions which represents a more spiritual, transpersonal movement and journey.

> There is the possibility of realistically accepting that suffering is inevitable in the human condition, but at the same time of seeking to transform it and integrate it into human life in such a way that we come to see that life would be poorer without it. It may not be possible to integrate it without remainder. Perhaps there remains a surd, an irremovable question mark. But at least we must see how far along this road we can go [p. 224].

If we can hold to a notion that life imposes its own wounding, sometimes to the extent that we can lose sight of our selves/our souls, we might be able to view life also as a journey to 'health', to reconnect to our selves/souls, a process that does not cease in later years. Reflecting this stance,

James Hillman, in his book *The Force of Character and the Lasting Life* (1999: pp. xiii–xv), advances a fascinating perspective that is in tune with much contemporary thinking concerning the meaning of this period of life. He suggests that 'ageing is no accident. It is necessary to the human condition, intended by the soul', and that old age is a '*structure* with its own essential nature'. Whereas one may think of ageing as being a process leading to dying, Hillman desires to elevate thinking on this issue to include the notion that 'the last years confirm and fulfil character'. In questioning whether the soul has to be 'aged' properly before it leaves, he suggests we might then be able to 'imagine aging as a transformation in beauty as much as in biology'. He enquires:

> Can a person become an epiphany? Can we entertain the idea that all along our earthly life has been phenomenal, a showing, a presentation? Can we imagine that at the essence of human being is an insistence upon being witnessed – by others, by gods, by the cosmos itself – and that the inner force of character cannot be concealed from this display. The image will out, and the last years put a final finish to that [Hillman, 1999: p. 201].

Thomas Moore (2004), a contemporary spiritual writer, describes growing old as a 'matter of growing deep', growing into the earthiness of identity, becoming less interested in the 'surface glitter of culture' and living more from the soul than the self. This is to understand oneself as being a part of nature and to conceive of the soul, which is the source of identity, as a piece of the world's soul. He suggests that our 'roots reach downward, not into the brain, but into the soil' (p. 294) and that all people can prepare through life for this opportunity of 'growing deep', although not all people take this up so readily as others. He tells us we do not have to understand this deep level of our existence, but we do have to trust it.

> There can be no doubt that as you grow old, you must come to terms with the arc of your life, its rising and setting. You have to see its elephant ears as things of beauty and signals of a divine design. You have to move gracefully with that downturn and dimming so that you will benefit from its special powers. Then all your dark nights will begin to make sense and fold themselves into the ultimate passing of the light. You will enter the darkness knowing something about the territory. You will understand that it has its own luminosity and beauty [Moore, 2004: p. 300].

Inevitably, the process of ageing draws the older person towards reappraising the meaning of life. Transition into old age involves the involution of physical strength and the need to readdress the continuum of one's own psychological identity. Here the human psyche bids for integrity in the light of less empirical yet increasingly transpersonal relationships. Within a body that is externally weakening, the intimate core of one's constructs and personality comes to relatively outshine material parameters, now progressively obsolete for loss of beauty and physical strength. The intimate core is one's whole unqualified 'I am', containing the zest of core experiences of childhood, the formative years of young adulthood, indeed all the hard and pleasant lessons learnt along life's path. The feelings of hurt and joy posited in one's emotional memory, together with acquired and deeply held convictions and beliefs now come to cushion the impact of the pain of growing older. If these feelings and beliefs are strong enough, they provide a most powerful coping mechanism and emotional survival tool (Lawrence, 2003; 2007).

References

Abramowitz, L. (1993) Prayer as therapy among the frail Jewish elderly. *Journal of Gerontological Social Work*, **19**, 69–75.

Acton, G. J. & Miller, E. W. (2003) Spirituality in caregivers of family members with dementia. *Journal of Holistic Nursing*, **21**, 117–130.

Age Concern & Mental Health Foundation (2006) *Promoting Health and Well-Being in Later Life: A First Report from the UK Inquiry*. Age Concern & Mental Health Foundation.

Ai, A. L., Peterson, C., Bolling, S. F., *et al* (2002) Private prayer and optimism in middle aged and older patients awaiting cardiac surgery. *Gerontologist*, **42**, 70–81.

Allen, N. H. P. & Burns, A. (1995) The non-cognitive features of dementia. *Reviews in Clinical Gerontology*, **5**, 57–75.

Amore, M., Tagariello, P., Laterza, C., *et al* (2007) Subtypes of depression in dementia. *Archives of Gerontology and Geriatrics*, **44**, 23–33.

Baldwin, R. (2002) Depressive disorders. In *Psychiatry in the Elderly* (eds R. Jacoby & C. Oppenheimer), pp. 627–676. Oxford University Press.

Baldwin, R. (2007) Recent understandings in geriatric affective disorder. *Current Opinion in Psychiatry*, **20**, 539–543.

Banerjee, S., Shamash, K., Macdonald, A., *et al* (1996) Randomised controlled trial of effect of intervention by psychogeriatric team on depression in frail elderly people at home. *BMJ*, **313**, 1058–1061.

Bartlett, S. J. (2003) Well-being and quality of life in people with rheumatoid arthritis. *Arthritis Care & Research*, **49**, 778–783.

Bittles, A. H. (2002) Biological aspects of human ageing. In *Psychiatry in the Elderly* (eds R. Jacoby & C. Oppenheimer), pp. 3–24. Oxford University Press.

Bosworth, H. B., Park, K.-S., McQuoid, D. R., *et al* (2003) The impact of religious practice and religious coping on geriatric depression. *International Journal of Geriatric Psychiatry*, **18**, 905–914.

Bowman, K. W. & Singer, P. A. (2001) Chinese seniors' perspectives on end-of-life decisions. *Social Science and Medicine*, **53**, 455–464.

Boyd, K. (2000) Pain, sickness and suffering. In *Spiritual Dimensions of Pastoral Care: Practical Theology in a Multidisciplinary Context* (eds D. Willows & J. Swinton). Jessica Kingsley.

Braam, A. W., Beekman, A. T., van Tilburg, T. G., *et al* (1997) Religious involvement and depression in older Dutch citizens. *Social Psychiatry and Psychiatric Epidemiology*, **32**, 284–291.

Braam, A. W., Van Den Eeden, P., Prince, M. J., *et al* (2001) Religion as a cross-cultural determinant of depression in elderly Europeans: results from the EURODEP collaboration. *Psychological Medicine*, **31**, 803–814.

Butler, R. & Orrell M (1998) Late-life depression. *Current Opinion in Psychiatry*, **11**, 435–439.

Chang, B., Noonan, A. E. & Tennstedt, S. L. (1998) The role of religion/spirituality in coping with caregiving for disabled elders. *Gerontologist*, **38**, 463–470.

Cheston, R. & Bender, M. (2000) *Understanding Dementia: the Man with the Worried Eyes*. Jessica Kingsley.

Chinello, A., Grumelli, B., Perrone, C., *et al* (2007) Prevalence of major depressive disorder and dementia in psychogeriatric outpatients. *Archives of Gerontology and Geriatrics*, **44**, 101–104.

Cicirelli, V. G. (2002) Fear of death in older adults: predictions from terror management theory. *Journals of Gerontology*, **57B**, 358–366.

Dalby, P. (2006) Is there a process of spiritual change or development associated with aging? A critical review of research. *Aging and Mental Health*, **10**, 4–12.

Dein, S. (2006) Religion, spirituality and depression: implications for research and treatment. *Primary Care and Community Psychiatry*, **11**, 67–72.

Department of Health (2001) *National Service Framework for Older People*. Department of Health.

Department of Health & Care Services Improvement Partnership (2006) *Everybody's Business: Integrated Mental Health Services for Older Adults. A Service Development Guide*. Department of Health & Care Services Improvement Partnership.

Dudley, M. G. & Kosinski, F. A. (1990) Religiosity and marital satisfaction: a research note. *Religious Research*, **32**, 78–86.

Ejaz, F. K. (2000) The influence of religious and personal values on nursing home residents' attitudes toward life-sustaining treatments. *Social Work in Healthcare*, **32**, 23–39.

Erikson, E. H. (1963) *Childhood and Society*. Norton.

Erikson, E. H. (1982) *The Life Cycle Completed: a Review*. Norton.

Eysenck, S. B. & Eysenck, H. J. (1969) Scores on three personality variables as a function of age, sex and social class. *British Journal of Social and Clinical Psychology*, **8**, 69–76.

Fenix, J. B., Cherlin, E. J., Prigerson, H. G., *et al* (2006) Religiousness and major depression among bereaved family caregivers: a 13-month follow-up study. *Journal of Palliative Care*, **22**, 286–292.

Folkman, S. & Lazarus, R. S. (1984) *Stress, Appraisal and Coping*. Springer.

Fry, P. S. (2000) Religious involvement, spirituality and personal meaning for life: existential predictors of psychological wellbeing in community-residing and institutional care elders. *Aging and Mental Health*, **4**, 375–387.

Fry, P. S. (2001) The unique contribution of key existential factors to the prediction of psychological well-being of older adults following spousal loss. *Gerontologist*, **41**, 69–81.

Guberman, N., Maheu, P. & Mailee, C. (1992) Women as family caregivers: why do they care? *Gerontologist*, **32**, 607–617.

Guignon, C. (2000) Authenticity and integrity: a Heideggerian perspective. In *The Psychology of Mature Spirituality: Integrity, Wisdom, Transcendence* (eds P. Young-Eisendrath & M. E. Miller), pp. 62–67. Routledge.

Head, J. (2004) 'Please pray for me': the significance of prayer for mental and emotional well-being. *Spirituality and Psychiatry Special Interest Group Newsletter*, **14** (April).

Head, J. (2006) A rich tapestry: emergent themes in spirituality in the care of older adults with mental health needs. *Spirituality and Psychiatry Special Interest Group Newsletter*, **21** (June).

Hebert, R. S., Weinstein, E., Martire, L. M., *et al* (2006) Religion, spirituality and the well being of informal caregivers: a review, critique and research prospectus. *Aging and Mental Health*, **10**, 497–520.

Helm, H. M., Hays, J. C., Flint, E. P., *et al* (2000) Does private religious activity prolong survival? A six-year follow-up study of 3,851 older adults. *Journals of Gerontology Series A: Biological Sciences and Medical Sciences*, **55**, 400–405.

Higgins, P. (2003) Holding a religious service for people with dementia. *Journal of Dementia Care*, **11**, 10–11.

Higgins, P., Allen, R., Karamat, S., *et al* (2004) Candlelight Group: a pilot project for people with dementia. *Spirituality and Psychiatry Special Interest Group Newsletter*, **14** (April).

Hillman, J. (1999) *The Force of Character and the Lasting Life*. Random House.

Idler, E. L., Kasl, S. V. & Hays, J. C. (2001) Patterns of religious practice and belief in the last year of life. *Journals of Gerontology Series B: Psychological Sciences and Social Sciences*, **56**, S326–S334.

Illich, I. (1990) *Limits to Medicine: Medical Nemesis – The Expropriation of Health*. Penguin.

Isaia, D., Parker, V. & Murrow, E. (1999) Spiritual well-being among older adults. *Journal of Gerontological Nursing*, **25**, 15–21.

Kark, J. D., Carmel, S., Sinnreich, R., *et al* (1996) Psychosocial factors among members of religious and secular kibbutzim. *Israel Journal of Medical Sciences*, **32**, 185–194.

Katsuno, T. (2003) Personal spirituality of persons with early-stage dementia. *Dementia*, **2**, 315–335.

Kennedy, G. J., Kelman, H. R., Thomas, C., *et al* (1996) The relation of religious preference and practice to depressive symptoms among 1,855 older adults. *Journal of Gerontology Series B: Psychological Sciences and Social Sciences*, **51**, 301–308.

Killick, J. (2002) Approaching the mystery. *Journal of Dementia Care*, March/April, 23–4.

Kitwood, T. (1997) *Dementia Reconsidered: The Person Comes First*. Open University Press.

Koenig, H. G. (1994) *Aging and God: Spiritual Pathways to Mental Health in Midlife and Later Years*. Haworth Pastoral Press.

Koenig, H. G. (2004) Religion, spirituality, and medicine: research findings and implications for clinical practice. *Southern Medical Journal*, **97**, 524–529.

Koenig, H. G. (2006) Religion, spirituality and aging. *Aging and Mental Health*, **10**, 1–3.

Koenig, H. G., George, L. K. & Seigler, I. C. (1988*a*) The use of religion and other emotion-regulating coping strategies among older adults. *Gerontologist*, **28**, 303–310.

Koenig, H. G., Kvale, J. N. & Ferrel, C. (1988*b*) Religion and well-being in later life. *Gerontologist*, **28**, 18–28.

Koenig, H. G., Hays, J. C. & Larson, D. B. (1999) Does religious attendance prolong survival? A six-year follow-up study of 3,968 older adults. *Journals of Gerontology. Series A: Biological Sciences and Medical Sciences*, **54**, M370–M377.

Koenig, H. G., Hays, J. C., George, L. K., *et al* (1997) Modeling the cross-sectional relationship between religion, physical health, social support, and depressive symptoms. *American Journal of Geriatric Psychiatry*, **5**, 131–144.

Krause, N. (2004) Assessing the relationships among prayer expectancies, race, and self-esteem in late life. *Journal for the Scientific Study of Religion*, **43**, 395–408.

Krause, N., Ingersoll-Dayton, B., Ellison, C. G., *et al* (1999) Aging, religious doubt and psychological well-being. *Gerontologist*, **39**, 525–533.

Kroll, J. & Sheehan, W. (1989) Religious beliefs and practices among 52 psychiatric inpatients in Minnesota. *American Journal of Psychiatry*, **146**, 67–72.

Lawrence, R. M. (2003) Aspects of spirituality in dementia care: when clinicians tune into silence. *Dementia: the International Journal of Social Research and Practice*, **2**, 393–402.

Lawrence, R. M. (2007) Dementia: a personal legacy beyond words. *Mental Health, Religion and Culture*, **10**, 553–562.

LobhoPrabhu, S., Molinari, V., Arlinghaus, K., *et al* (2005) Spouses of patients with dementia: how do they stay together 'till death do us part'? *Journal of Gerontological Social Work*, **44**, 161–174.

Lutgendorf, S. K., Ullrich, P., Wallace, R., *et al* (2004) Religious participation, interleukin-6, and mortality in older adults. *Health Psychology*, **23**, 465–475.

Mackenzie, E. R., Rajagopal, D. E., Meibohm, M., *et al* (2000) Spiritual support and psychological well-being: older adults' perceptions of the religion and health connection. *Alternative Therapies in Health and Medicine*, **6**, 37–45.

MacKinlay, E. (2001) *The Spiritual Dimension of Ageing*. Jessica Kingsley.

Macquarrie, J. (1982) *In Search of Humanity: A Theological and Philosophical Approach*. SCM Press.

Meador, K. G., Koenig, H. G., Highes, D. C., *et al* (1992) Religious affiliation and major depression. *Hospital and Community Psychiatry*, **43**, 1204–1208.

Meller, S. (2001) A comparison of the well-being of family caregivers of elderly patients hospitalized with physical impairments versus the caregivers of patients hospitalized with dementia. *Journal of the American Medical Directors Association*, **2**, 60–65.

Milstein, G., Bruce, M. L., Gargon, N., *et al* (2003) Religious practice and depression among geriatric home care patients. *International Journal of Psychiatry in Medicine*, **33**, 71–83.

Moore, T. (2004) *Dark Nights of the Soul: A Guide to Finding Your Way through Life's Ordeals*. Gotham Books.

Murray-Swank, A. N., Lucksted, A., Medoff, D. R., *et al* (2006) Religiosity, psychosocial adjustment, and subjective burden of persons who care for those with mental illness. *Psychiatric Services*, **57**, 361–365.

Pargament, K. I. (1997) *The Psychology of Religion and Coping: Theory, Research and Practice*. Guilford Press.

Pargament, K. I., Koenig, H. G., Tarakeshwar, N., *et al* (2001) Religious struggle as a predictor of mortality among medically ill elderly patients: a 2-year longitudinal study. *Archives of Internal Medicine*, **161**, 1881–1885.

Parker, M., Roff, L. L., Klemmack, D. L., *et al* (2003) Religiosity and mental health in southern, community-dwelling older adults. *Aging and Mental Health*, **7**, 390–397.

Pearce, M. J., Singer, J. L. & Prigerson, H. G. (2006) Religious coping among caregivers of terminally ill cancer patients: main effects and psychosocial mediators. *Journal of Health Psychology*, **11**, 743–759.

Pearson, J. L., Conwell, Y., Lindesay, J., *et al* (1997) Elderly suicide: a multinational view. *Aging Mental Health*, **1**, 107–111.

Persson, J., Nyberg, L., Lind, J., *et al* (2006) Structure–function correlates of cognitive decline in aging. *Cerebral Cortex*, **16**, 907.

Pfennig, A., Littmann, E. & Bauer, M. (2007) Neurocognitive impairment and dementia in mood disorders. *Journal of Neuropsychiatry and Clinical Neurosciences*, **19**, 373–382.

Picot, S. J., Debanne, S. M., Namazi, K. H., *et al* (1997) Religiosity and perceived rewards of Black and White caregivers. *Gerontologist*, **37**, 89–101.

Pieper, H. (1981) Church membership and participation in church activities among the elderly. *Activities, Adaptation and Aging*, **1**, 23–29.

Post, S. G. (1995) Medicine and religion. In *The HarperCollins Dictionary of Religion* (eds J. Z. Smith & W. S. Green), pp. 690–691. HarperCollins.

Post, S. G., Puchalski, C. M. & Larson, D. B. (2000) Physicians and patient spirituality: professional boundaries, competency and ethics. *Annals of Internal Medicine*, **132**, 578–583.

Pressman, P., Lyons, J. S., Larson, D. B., *et al* (1990) Religious belief, depression and ambulation status in elderly women with broken hips. *American Journal of Psychiatry*, 147, 758–760.

Pritchard, C. & Baldwin, D. (2000) Effects of age and gender on elderly suicide rates in Catholic and Orthodox countries: an inadvertent neglect? *International Journal of Geriatric Psychiatry*, **15**, 904–910.

Ragno, J. G. (1995) Volunteers of the spirit: quality of life programming with religious volunteers. *Activities, Adaptation and Aging*, **20**, 35–39.

Reyes-Ortiz, C. A., Ayele, H., Mulligan, T., *et al* (2006) Higher church attendance predicts lower fear of falling in older Mexican-Americans. *Aging and Mental Health*, **10**, 13–18.

Robert, R., Kaplan, G. A., Shema, S. J., *et al* (1997) Does growing old increase the risk for depression? *American Journal of Psychiatry*, **154**, 1384–1390.

Ross, L. (1995) The spiritual dimension: its importance to patients' health, well-being and quality of life and its implications for nursing practice. *International Journal of Nursing Studies*, **32**, 457–468.

Royal College of Psychiatrists (2004) *Alzheimer's Disease and Other Dementias*. Royal College of Psychiatrists.

Royal College of Psychiatrists (2006) *Raising the Standard: Specialist Services for Older People with Mental Illness. Report of the Faculty of Old Age Psychiatry*. Royal College of Psychiatrists.

Sabat, S. & Harre, R. (1992) The construction and deconstruction of self in Alzheimer's disease. *Ageing and Society*, **12**, 443–461.

Sanders, S. (2005) Is the glass half empty or half full? Reflections on strain and gain in caregivers of individuals with Alzheimer's disease. *Social Work in Healthcare*, **40**, 57–73.

Searle, M. (1992) Ritual. In *The Study of Liturgy* (eds C. Jones, G. Wainwright, E. Yarnold, *et al*). Society for Promoting Christian Knowledge.

Shamy, E. (2003) *Worship for People with Alzheimer's Disease and Related Dementias: A Guide to the Spiritual Dimension of Care for People with Alzheimer's Disease and Related Dementias.* Jessica Kingsley.

Skaff, M. M. (1995) *Religion in the Stress Process: Coping with Caregiving.* Paper presented at the Annual Scientific Meeting of the Gerontological Society of America, Los Angeles.

Slater, R. (1995) *The Psychology of Growing Old.* Open University Press.

Spini, D., d'Epinay, L. & Pin, S. (2001) Religious practice and survival in old age. *Médecine et Hygiène*, **59**, 2258–2262.

Stolley, J. M., Buckwalter, K. C. & Koenig, H. G. (1999) Prayer and religious coping for caregivers of persons with Alzheimer's disease and related disorders. *American Journal of Alzheimer's Disease*, **14**, 181–191.

Strawbridge, W. J., Cohen, R. D., Shema, S. J., *et al* (1997) Frequent attendance at religious services and mortality over 28 years. *American Journal of Public Health*, **87**, 957–961.

Strawbridge, W. J., Shema, S. J., Cohen, R. D., *et al* (2001) Religious attendance increases survival by improving and maintaining good health behaviors, mental health and social relationships. *Annals of Behavioral Medicine*, **23**, 68–74.

Stuart-Hamilton, I. (2006) *The Psychology of Ageing.* Jessica Kingsley.

Stuckey, J. C. (2003) Faith, aging, and dementia: experiences of Christian, Jewish, and non-religious spousal caregivers and older adults. *Dementia*, **2**, 337–352.

Townsend, J., Adamo, M. & Haist, F. (2006) Changing channels: an fMRI study of aging and cross-modal attention shifts. *Neuroimage*, **31**, 1682–1692.

Vernooij-Dassen, M., Felling, A. & Persoon, J. (1997) Predictors of change and continuity in home care for dementia patients. *International Journal of Geriatric Psychiatry*, **12**, 671–677.

Walsh, K., King, M., Jones, L., *et al* (2002) Spiritual beliefs may affect outcome of bereavement: prospective study. *BMJ*, **324**, 1551–1554.

Warner, N. & Aziz, V. (2005) Hymns and arias: musical hallucinations in older people in Wales. *International Journal of Geriatric Psychiatry*, **20**, 658–660.

Wink, P. & Dillon, M. (2002) Spiritual development across the adult life course: findings from a longitudinal study. *Journal of Adult Development*, **9**, 79–94.

Wink, P. & Dillon, M. (2003) Religiousness, spirituality and psychosocial functioning in late adulthood: findings from a longitudinal study. *Psychology and Aging*, **18**, 916–924.

Wink, P., Dillon, M. & Larsen, B. (2005) Religion as moderator of the depression–health connection: findings from a longitudinal study. *Research on Aging*, **27**, 197–220.

Wright, S. & Sayer-Adams, J. (2000) *Sacred Space: Right Relationship and Spirituality in Healthcare.* Churchill Livingstone.

Index

Compiled by Linda English